HUMAN DISEASES AND CONDITIONS

Supplement 1:
Behavioral Health

HUMAN DISEASES AND CONDITIONS

Supplement 1: Behavioral Health

Neil Izenberg, M.D. • Steven A. Dowshen, M.D.
Editors in Chief

David Sheslow, Ph.D. • Richard S. Kingsley, M.D. • D'Arcy Lyness, Ph.D.
Volume Editors

Published in Association with the
Center for Children's Health Media,
The Nemours Foundation

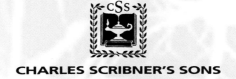

CHARLES SCRIBNER'S SONS

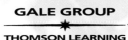

GALE GROUP

THOMSON LEARNING

New York • Detroit • San Diego • San Francisco
Boston • New Haven, Conn. • Waterville, Maine
London • Munich

The information in *Human Diseases and Conditions Supplement 1: Behavioral Health* is not intended to take the place of medical care by physicians and other health care professionals. This book does not contain diagnostic, treatment, or first aid recommendations. Readers should obtain professional advice in making all health care decisions.

Library of Congress Cataloging-in-Publication Data

Human diseases and conditions / Neil Izenberg, editor in chief.
    p. cm.
    "Published in association with the Center for Children's Health Media, the
       Nemours Foundation."
    Contents: V. 1. Abscess-Dysrhythmia.
    Includes bibliographical references and index.
    Summary: present articles dealing with all kinds of diseases and disorders, from acne
      and brain tumor to tobacco-related diseases and yellow fever.
    ISBN 0-684-80543-X (set: alk. paper) —ISBN 0-684-80541-3 (v.1 : alk. paper)
    1. Medicine, Popular—Encyclopedias Juvenile. [1. Diseases—Encyclopedias. 2.
      Health—Encyclopedias.] I. Izenberg, Neil.

RC81.A2 H75 2000
616'.003—dc21

                                     99-051442

  ISBN 0-684-80542-1 (vol. 2)
  ISBN 0-684-80621-5 (vol. 3)
  ISBN 0-684-80643-6 (supp. 1)

1 3 5 7 9 11 13 15 17 19 20 18 16 14 12 10 8 6 4 2

Printed in the United States of America

The paper used in this publication meets the minimum requirements of the American National Standard for Information Services—Permanence of Paper for Printed Library Materials, ANSI Z39.48-1992.

Editorial and Production Staff

Project Editor
Sarah Feehan

Consulting Editor
Faye Zucker

Writers
Linda Wasmer Andrews • Allan Cobb • Kristine Connor • Helen Davidson
Tish Davidson • Joan Huebl • Johnna Laird • Marge Lurie • D'Arcy Lyness
Daphne Northrop • Theodore Zinn • Faye Zucker

Editors, Researchers, Proofreaders
Linda Wasmer Andrews • Mary Flower • Lynn M. L. Lauerman • Marcia Merryman Means

Artist
Frank Forney

Photo Researcher
Martin Levick

Indexer
Julia Marshall, Marshall Indexing Services

Production Manager
Evi Seoud

Compositor
GGS Information Services

Designer
Cindy Baldwin

Cover Design
Michelle DiMercurio

Senior Editor
Stephen Wagley

Associate Publisher
Timothy J. DeWerff

Publisher
Frank Menchaca

Contents

Contents

Preface

Behavioral Health, the first supplement to *Human Diseases and Conditions*, covers almost 100 topics on a wide range of emotional, developmental, and psychological issues. Why did we choose these areas to add to our three-volume base set? Because human health includes not just the mechanics of how the body functions—but also how we learn, how we feel, and how we emotionally develop throughout our life span. What can be more fascinating than how the mind functions and how our body and mind work together—or sometimes have problems working together?

The human mind has intrigued people throughout history, although it was not until relatively recently that we could put aside many age-old prejudices and fears about mental health issues and explore them scientifically, using a growing body of knowledge gained through research. New understandings about brain chemistry, anatomy, and genetics are adding to our appreciation of the complexity and beauty of the human brain—and of human behavior.

Every person—every family—has emotional issues to wrestle with at some time. Just as no one's body is "perfect," the same is true about mental health. People become physically ill from time to time and need a doctor's care or medication, and people with mental health issues also need medical attention. The use of mental health therapy, psychotherapy, or counseling, combined sometimes with medication, can be very helpful for many at some time in their lives.

Just as our bodies grow and change throughout the years, our emotional development changes, too. And just as our bodies may sometimes have problems, humans can have illnesses and conditions affecting their ability to think and learn, the ways they experience the world, their feelings, and their behaviors. Many medical conditions have important effects on mental health. So do life experiences—and many of those important issues, such as divorce or violence, are discussed here.

You'll find that a few of the topics that were discussed in the first three volumes of *Human Diseases and Conditions* are also included here in different and expanded ways. If you're particularly interested in a topic covered in this volume, we encourage you to consult the other volumes for additional information and resources.

For this volume, we have worked with guest editors David Sheslow, Ph.D., Richard Kingsley, M.D., and D'Arcy Lyness, Ph.D. Each combines a long-standing interest and talent in teaching with years of practical experience in providing behavioral health care. We thank them for their dedicated work.

Much of life's journey has to do with learning about yourself and your own emotions. That includes your relationships with others—family, friends, teachers, acquaintances, and strangers. We hope that *Behavioral Health* will help you better understand and appreciate yourself and others. Please drop us an email at info@KidsHealth.org to let us know what you think.

Neil Izenberg, M.D.
Steven A. Dowshen, M.D.
Editors in Chief
Nemours Center for
Children's Health Media
The Nemours Foundation
www.KidsHealth.org

What Is Behavioral Health?

The Human Brain, Emotions, and Behavior

Every moment of our lives, our brains orchestrate a complex symphony of ideas and emotions. Our brains determine how we reason, how we behave, how we feel, and how we understand our everyday experiences. This truly amazing system is what allows us to be fully human—to feel emotion, to reason and make choices, to think and plan, to form memories and relationships, to act wisely at times and foolishly at others. It is no wonder that the human brain and behavior—both normal and abnormal—have been the source of fascination for centuries.

When problems arise within the intricate communications between the mind and body, people may develop conditions that affect how they think and behave. These conditions disrupt their day-to-day lives in ways that can be harmful to themselves or to others. In this volume you will learn how a variety of factors—including genes, environment, relationships, and learned behavior—shape new understandings of certain emotional and behavioral disorders.

What Is Normal?

Every person is different and unique. A person's individual experiences and genetic makeup combine in a way that influences how his or her emotions and behavior develop. While no two people are completely alike, we may say things like "My mom and I have similar personalities." Despite all of our differences, we can recognize reliable personality traits in people, or tendencies to behave certain ways—whether kindly, aggressively, or fearfully, to name a few examples. These traits make up a consistent style of behaving that we call a person's personality. As you read through this book, you will find out that the way psychiatrists and psychologists thought about personality often became the basis for how to help people suffering from mental illness.

But if everyone is different, then how can we decide what is normal? What is considered normal behavior varies widely, depending on the person's age and maturity, expectations within the family and culture, and the context or situation. For example, while in one family it might be normal to be highly emotional, it might be normal in another to be reserved and rarely express strong emotion. Or, behavior that might be seen as normal on the playground may not be considered normal in the classroom. In other words, being "normal" includes a whole spectrum of possible behaviors and different situations.

What is considered normal also changes during a person's development. We would expect a toddler to be afraid of strangers, and a nine-year-old to complete her homework with relatively little help. We would expect teenagers to be thinking about dating and relationships, what they may want to do when they grow up, and even the meaning of being alive. It is normal to wrestle with certain issues at certain stages of development. When events or situations prevent development from progressing smoothly, however, emotional problems may arise.

What Causes Behavioral and Emotional Conditions?

Some conditions develop largely from biological factors. Genetic makeup and brain chemistry can create conditions that result in extreme behaviors, such as autism or schizophrenia. Having a learning disability, chronic illness, or developmental disorder also poses special psychological challenges. With recent medical developments, physicians and psychiatrists are becoming increasingly able to prescribe medicines that help alleviate the difficulties of these disorders.

Many other conditions are understood through the experiences or environments in which they are most likely to occur. Stress is a major factor in many of these conditions, as the ability to cope with stress is closely linked to behavioral and emotional health. Hans Selye, the father of modern stress research, defined stress as the body's response to troublesome demands. Modern stress researchers see stress as any situation that might threaten our sense of well-being to the point where our abilities to cope might be overwhelmed. Almost everyone has experienced the physical and emotional effects of stress at some point in their lives, although not all situations are considered stressful by all people. Phobias, anxiety disorders, and obsessive-compulsive disorder are a few of the topics discussed here that closely relate to how a person copes with, or struggles to cope with, a particular stress.

An important part of how we deal with stress is how well we learn to solve problems, handle frustration, and get help when needed. Some life events can be so painful or traumatic that even the calmest among us can become overwhelmed. For example, it is normal for someone to experience grief or depression following the death of a loved one, a divorce, or another type of loss. Even with good coping skills and supportive friends and family, a person may need a therapist's help to fully recover from a difficult time.

There are other, more general topics that should be included in discussions about mental health. For example, many of the stresses of modern life can lead to the development of behavioral disorders. Homelessness, violence, and discrimination are social conditions that affect us all, whether or not we experience them directly. *Behavioral Health* also includes chapters about how disorders are treated, and takes a look at common treatments, as well as some that are more unusual or even controversial.

Everyone Is a Behavioral Health Expert

No one can disagree with you about how you feel. Therefore, when it comes to understanding yourself, you are your own behavioral health expert. But sometimes even an expert needs to consult with other experts to solve difficult problems. As you will see in this volume, there are many emotional or behavioral conditions that can affect people in ways that cloud their thinking, confuse their emotions, and interfere with day-to-day functioning. Some conditions are the result of being overwhelmed by choices we've made, by events that happen to us, or simply by life's stressors.

You may recognize yourself or someone you know in some of the chapters. If it helps you understand a personal problem that needs to be talked about, find a trustworthy adult and he or she will direct you to a psychiatrist, psychologist, social worker, counselor, or therapist who can help.

We have included almost 100 topics that range from disorders that are common, such as depression and anxiety, to disorders that are rare, such as dissociative identity disorder and fugue. There are also topics about social issues that affect behavioral health, such as peer pressure, families, divorce, love and intimacy, violence, abuse, and homelessness. Other chapters describe how biology affects behavior—you will find chapters on the brain and nervous system, memory, intelligence, sexual development, and genetics. You may identify with the problems discussed, or you may just be intrigued by a particular topic. To encourage further research, there are resources at the end of the chapters to help you learn more. We hope you will enjoy reading about behavioral health and conditions, and that this volume may spark your interest to explore how relationships between the brain, behavior, and emotions help determine who we are.

David Sheslow, Ph.D.
Richard Kingsley, M.D.
D'Arcy Lyness, Ph.D.
Volume Editors
Nemours Center for
Children's Health Media

HUMAN DISEASES AND CONDITIONS

Supplement 1:
Behavioral Health

The Brain and Nervous System

The nervous system is the complex body system that most directly determines and organizes a person's reactions to the world in which he or she lives. It includes the central nervous system, which is made up of the brain and spinal cord, and the peripheral (per-IF-fer-ul) nervous system, which includes all of the nerves and other nervous structures in the rest of the body.

KEYWORDS
*for searching the Internet
and other reference sources*

Central nervous system

Neurology

Neurotransmitters

Peripheral nervous system

Orchestrating Everyday Life

If life is a symphony of activities—both voluntary activities, such as walking, talking, reading, or going to class, and involuntary activities, such as breathing, digesting food, pumping blood, and perspiring—then the nervous system is the orchestra that makes it all happen. This system controls all of the adjustments people need to make in response to their environment, from basic functions such as sweating on a hot day to more sophisticated tasks such as concentrating attention during a particularly difficult lecture. Without the nervous system and its conductor, the brain, people would not experience joy at seeing an old friend or automatically pull their hand away from a hot stove.

Injuries and diseases that affect the nervous system not only demonstrate how important the system is to everyday life but also show how the brain really determines who a person is as a human being. The actor Christopher Reeve, most famous for his movie role as Superman in the 1970s and 1980s, was thrown from his horse and his spinal cord just below his brain was crushed. Because of his spinal cord injury, he cannot move or breathe on his own, and machines now do some of his bodily functions for him. But because his brain was not injured, Reeve can talk, experience emotions, and plan and make decisions (for example, after the accident he directed a movie). Though being physically active is no longer a part of his identity, Reeve can still enjoy his roles as husband, father, friend, and filmmaker. Since his injury he has participated in acting and directing projects, and has taken on a new role as spokesperson and advocate for spinal cord injury research. A book he wrote about his experiences since his injury is aptly titled *Still Me.*

Injuries and diseases of the brain are often devastating in a different way than are spinal cord injuries. They may affect movement, but they

Positron emission tomography (PET) records electrical activity inside the brain. These PET scans show what happens inside the brain when it is resting and when it is stimulated by words and by music. The red areas indicate concentrations of brain activity. Notice how language and music appear to produce responses in opposite sides of the brain. *Roger Ressmeyer/Corbis* ▶

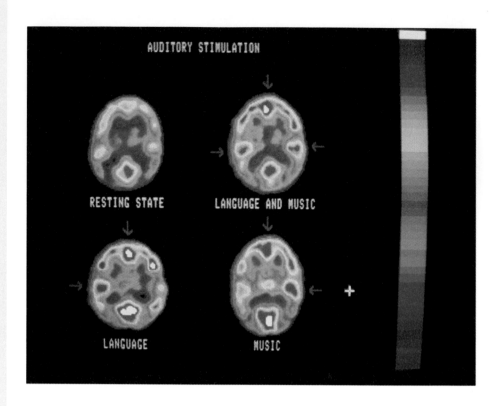

also can literally change a person's personality. Former U.S. President Ronald Reagan is now living with Alzheimer disease, which causes gradual deterioration of the brain. Over time, people with this condition seem less and less like themselves and exhibit drastic mood swings, unpredictable changes in temperament, inability to recognize loved ones, and increasing helplessness. People with Alzheimer disease lose most or all of the traits that once made them the individuals they were.

Because people tend to think of personalities and character traits as fixed, it is strange to realize that injury or disease could really change who a person is. While people can receive a new kidney, lung, or heart to replace a diseased one, they cannot receive a new brain or spinal cord: currently, these structures are irreplaceable.

Many Systems in One

The nervous system is a network of fibers that starts in the brain and spinal cord and branches out to the rest of the body, with each branch getting progressively smaller. The nervous system can be thought of as a pine tree, with the brain and spinal cord forming the trunk and the nerve fibers forming the branches. In the human body, the trunk is called the central nervous system, or CNS, and the branches are known as the peripheral nervous system.

Central nervous system The CNS includes the brain, which is encased in the skull, and the spinal cord, which is a long tube that extends

150 Years Ago: The Famous Case of Phineas Gage

In 1848, a Vermont railway foreman named Phineas Gage was helping to expand the nation's growing network of railway tracks. His job was to make way for new track by blowing up any obstacles in its path, such as rock formations. Gage would use a long rod to push the dynamite down into a hole. One day, the dynamite exploded too soon, and the iron rod was actually driven into the left front side of his skull. After a brief period of unconsciousness, Gage recovered from the injury, and the wound around the rod healed. He could still walk, talk, and move as he did before.

However, the people around Gage began to notice some major changes in his personality. Before the explosion, Gage had been friendly and hardworking, but after the accident he became indecisive, uncaring, and stubborn. Gage was just not the same person he had been. Eventually he left his railway job to take part in what were then called freak shows at fairs.

Gage's experience provided an important clue about how the brain works. Clearly the prefrontal cortex (the front part of the brain where the rod was imbedded) was not important for life functions such as breathing, body temperature control, sensory perception, or movement. Instead, it appeared to be associated with the individual's personality. Later studies have confirmed that the front portion of the cortex really is where a person's character lies. Damage or injury to this area has the potential to change the qualities that people consider so essential to who they are.

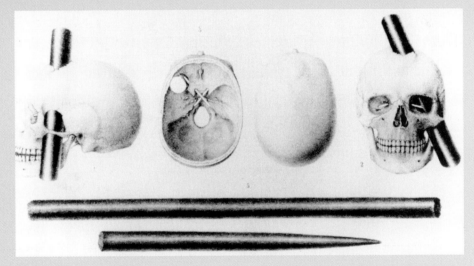

In 1848, a railroad worker named Phineas Gage was injured when an explosion drove a steel rod through his cheek and skull. Gage survived the incident but, according to doctors' reports at that time, he underwent a sudden and complete change of personality. Instead of being the polite, productive, and well-organized worker he had been before the accident, Gage was transformed into a disorganized, impulsive, stubborn slacker who no longer had direction or self-control. When Gage died, an autopsy showed that the accident had destroyed most of his frontal lobe, the part of the brain that controls planning, emotions, and behavior. *National Library of Medicine*

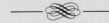

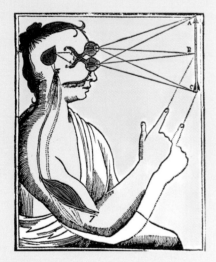

This is an illustration from *De homine,* a book by the French philosopher and mathematician René Descartes (1596-1650). Descartes studied how the mind and the body influence each other in perception and bodily reflexes. *Photo Researchers, Inc.*

out of the brain and down through the spine, or backbone. Higher nervous system functions, including movement, perception, memory, learning, emotion, and consciousness, are carried out within the brain. The spinal cord has other roles. It controls simple reflexes like the knee-jerk that happens when a doctor taps just below the knee (a familiar part of a routine physical examination) and rhythmic movements such as walking or scratching. It also relays sensory information such as touch, temperature, and pressure from the various parts of the body into the brain. A crossover effect occurs after the information is received: information from the right knee goes up the spinal cord on the opposite side from which it was received, eventually reaching the brain on the left side. The spinal cord also carries signals that control movement (motor signals) out of the brain to the rest of the body. The left side of the brain sends signals to the right side of the body, and vice versa.

Peripheral nervous system The nerve cells and other nervous structures in the body outside of the CNS are known as the peripheral nervous system (peripheral means outside). These nerves receive information from body tissues and the outside world and pass it along to the brain and spinal cord. These nerves also carry the signals from the CNS to make body parts move or function. The peripheral system can be divided into three parts:

- The voluntary motor nerves control the muscles of the arms and legs, the head, and other parts of the body. When a person swings a golf club, swats a fly, climbs a flight of steps, or does some other action on purpose, this system comes into play.

- The sensory nerves carry sensory information such as touch, temperature, pressure, and position from the skin and other body parts to the brain.

- The autonomic (aw-to-NOM-ik), or involuntary, system regulates the internal organs, including the heart, digestive tract, lungs, bladder, blood vessels, and glands. These functions happen automatically without a person controlling them. There are two further divisions of the autonomic nervous system: the sympathetic and the parasympathetic systems.

- The sympathetic nervous system, also called the "fight or flight" system, prepares people to deal with frightening or stressful situations, such as a difficult exam, a job interview, or a hostile confrontation. Just about everyone has had the experience of a racing heartbeat and sweaty palms just before a big presentation or a big exam. The sympathetic nervous system primes the body for action by speeding up the heart rate and breathing rate, which sends more oxygen-rich blood to the muscles. The pupils of the eyes dilate to allow more light into the eye, and at the same time, digestive system activity slows down.

■ Parasympathetic nervous system activity, for the most part, causes the body to relax: heart rate and blood pressure drop, the digestive system becomes more active, and the pupils of the eyes constrict. Sometimes called the rest and digest system, it comes into play for most people after finishing Thanksgiving dinner!

Regeneration While the peripheral and central nervous systems work together, they differ in one very important way: the peripheral nerves can regenerate, or grow back, if they are damaged, but damage to the brain or spinal cord is permanent. For example, if someone loses a finger or limb and it is reattached promptly, the severed nerves will usually grow back over time. However, the paralysis that often accompanies spinal cord injuries, as in the case of Christopher Reeve, is permanent. Brain damage is permanent, too, although other parts of the brain sometimes can take over the function of the damaged areas. Doctors have observed this phenomenon in people who are recovering from a stroke, which is usually the result of a blockage in one of the blood vessels that feeds the brain.

The central nervous system (CNS) is made up of the brain and spinal cord. The peripheral nervous system (PNS) is made up of 31 pairs of nerves that travel and branch out through the head, torso, arms, and legs. Together, the CNS and PNS govern thinking, feeling, moving, learning, remembering, and other activities that are conscious and mindful. The autonomic nervous system governs the functioning of the internal organs, and its activities mostly happen outside our awareness. The parasympathetic nerves are most active when the body is calm or sleeping. The sympathetic nerves are most active when the body is responding to stress. ▼

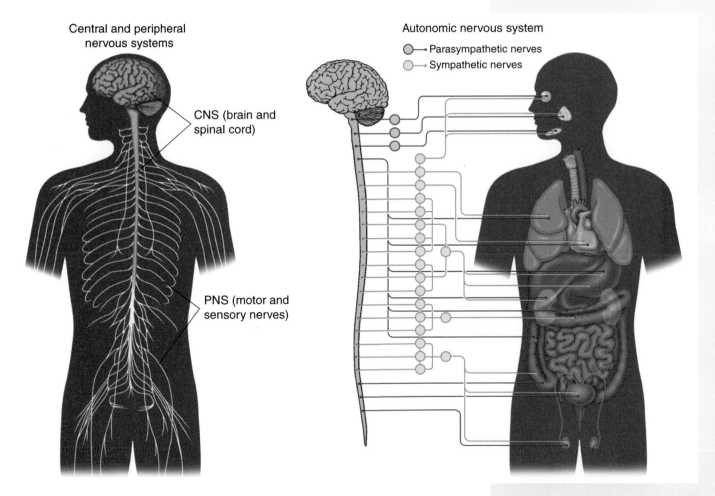

Central and peripheral nervous systems

CNS (brain and spinal cord)

PNS (motor and sensory nerves)

Autonomic nervous system
- Parasympathetic nerves
- Sympathetic nerves

Learning a New Language: The Sooner the Better

A daughter is born to an American father, who speaks only English, and a Spanish mother, who speaks both Spanish and English. If these parents choose to speak both languages to their new daughter, she will likely become fluent in both. While logic might suggest that this would be confusing to the baby, she is actually at the perfect time in her life for learning two languages. If she is raised hearing and speaking only English and waits until high school to take Spanish, learning the new language will be much harder. Why?

As humans get older (and especially after they reach puberty, or sexual maturity), they lose their ability to learn a new language perfectly. Babies and young children are better able to take in and imitate a wide range of sounds. Later in life, if they have grown accustomed to hearing the sounds of just one language, then mastering a second language becomes much harder. Psychologists believe that the synapses and neuronal connections in the brain's language area develop according to the individual's experience. Hearing more than one language from a young age builds the circuits that are needed for each language. In other words, this experience shapes the brain in very specific ways.

In his book *Creating Mind: How the Brain Works*, Harvard professor John Dowling relates the experience of living in Japan for seven months with his five-year-old daughter. Within four months, his daughter was able to speak Japanese fluently, and she did so even better than his wife who had been studying the language for three full years. Dowling saw this as an example of the young brain's plasticity: his daughter's brain had a flexibility that his wife's did not.

The brain tissue that went without oxygen-rich blood is damaged permanently, but other areas sometimes take over its functions (such as movement or speech). Research on spinal cord injuries and other central nervous system disorders continues, and many scientists believe that one day they may find ways to reverse damage that now seems permanent.

What Are the Basic Building Blocks of the Nervous System?

"You're getting on my nerves." "He has some nerve." "I'm all nervous about the test." The word nerve is part of everyday language, but few people think about its literal meaning. The nervous system is made up of nerves, which in turn are made up of smaller units called neurons (NUR-ons), or nerve cells. Despite the important difference between the CNS and the peripheral nervous system in their ability to regenerate, all the parts of the nervous system are made up of these same basic building blocks. Understanding them is the key to understanding how the nervous system as a whole works.

A neuron is a single cell with three main parts: the central cell body, the dendrites, and the axon. Each neuron typically has many dendrites but just one axon. Dendrites look like tree branches that extend from the cell body: they are relatively thick as they emerge from the cell, but they branch out into thinner and thinner structures as they get farther away. These structures receive messages from other neurons and then transmit them into the cell. The axon, on the other hand, transmits messages out of the cell to other organs, such as the muscles and glands, or to other neurons. An axon looks like one long strand that comes out of the cell body, and sometimes its end forks into several branches. Many axons are surrounded by a myelin (MY-uh-lin) sheath, a segmented tube of mostly fatty tissue. The axon-myelin sheath system works in a manner similar to an insulated wire: the insulation (myelin sheath) protects the wire (axon) and allows electrical message pulses to flow smoothly. The disease called multiple sclerosis (skluh-RO-sis) wears away at this protective myelin, which interferes with nerve function and causes symptoms such as weakness, dizziness, and loss of muscle control.

The neuron's cell body is tiny, ranging from about 1/200 to 1/10 of a millimeter. Scientists estimate that the human nervous system has as many as 1,000 billion neurons (which is more neurons than there are stars in the Milky Way!). A neuron can make thousands, even hundreds of thousands, of connections with other neurons. The only part of the neuron that may be relatively large is the axon. Some axons extend all the way from the head to the base of the spinal cord, others from the spinal cord to the fingers and toes. To get a sense of how large such an axon would be in relation to the tiny cell body, imagine a helium balloon with a 14- or 15-mile-long piece of string attached.

There are many different types of neurons that perform different functions within the nervous system. Sensory neurons, for instance, take

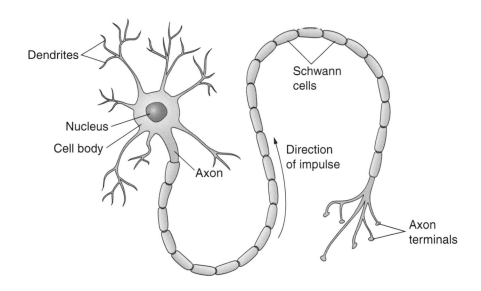

Dendrites

Nucleus

Cell body

Axon

Schwann cells

Direction of impulse

Axon terminals

Neurons are nerve cells. They are designed to transmit electrical signals to body cells, including other neurons. Axons are the transmitting terminals of each neuron, and dendrites are the receivers. Between axons and dendrites are gaps called synapses.

the information received through senses such as vision, hearing, and touch and then transmit it to the rest of the nervous system. Often they are in close contact with receptor cells, which first receive the information from the outside world and turn it into messages that the neuron can understand. Motor neurons make it possible for people to move the muscles in different parts of the body. These neurons' cell bodies are located in the spinal cord or brain and have long axons that transmit messages to muscle cells. Other neurons called interneurons are responsible for sending signals from one neuron to another; in fact, the vast majority of nerve cells are interneurons.

Within the brain and nervous system, neurons cluster together to do their jobs. Ganglia (GANG-lee-uh) are groups of nerves cells that function together, and ganglia are usually found outside the central nervous system. Basically, they are centralized control centers that make sense of messages from different receptor cells and coordinate the activity of different muscle groups. Nuclei (NEW-klee-eye) are groups of nerve cells in the brain and spinal cord that have the same function, such as supporting the sense of hearing or smell.

How Do Neurons Communicate?

The nervous system works only because the neurons are constantly communicating with each other. How does this process happen? Even though it is a complex process to describe, it happens more quickly than the blink of an eye. To simplify things, consider just two neurons: one that is sending a message and the other that is receiving it.

The sending neuron and the receiving neuron are separated by a small space called a synapse (SIN-aps). The end of the sending neuron's axon has small sacs called vesicles (VES-sick-ulz) that store a special chemical messenger called a neurotransmitter (NUR-o-tranz-mit-er). When this chemical is released, it can have one of two effects on the receiving neuron: it can excite it into action or it can inhibit (block or slow down) action. A neuron receiving certain signals produces an electrical impulse and fires off a message to other neurons by releasing its own chemical transmitter. The process can be thought of as an endless chain reaction among billions of neurons.

Scientists have been able to identify a hundred or more different neurotransmitters. One example is acetylcholine (uh-seh-til-KOHL-een),or ACh, which is released at the junction between motor neurons and muscle fibers and makes the fibers contract. Serotonin (sir-uh-TON-in), another chemical messenger in the brain, is involved in the states of sleep and emotional arousal. Decreased levels of serotonin have been linked to depression*. GABA, or gamma-amino butyric (GA-muh uh-MEEN-o byoo-TEER-ik) acid, is a transmitter that inhibits other neurons rather than exciting them into action. (For an illustration of neurotransmission, see "Medications.")

Some drugs that target neurotransmitters can be beneficial in treating certain diseases and conditions. For example, a substance called L-DOPA, which enhances the levels of the transmitter called dopamine* in the brain, has been found to help people with Parkinson's disease by improving symptoms such as tremors and difficulty controlling movements. In people who have this disease, the dopamine-releasing neurons in the brain are not functioning as they should be, and this problem tends to get worse over time. Many people with depression have been helped by medications that increase the availability of neurotransmitters such as norepinephrine* and serotonin in the brain.

Command Central: The Brain

If the nervous system as a whole governs the body's voluntary and involuntary functions, then the brain is the president of that government. This cream-colored, wrinkled organ weighs only about three pounds and has the consistency of gelatin in a mold. The main part of the brain, called the cerebrum (suh-REE-brum), has two hemispheres, or halves, that sit on top of a thick stalk, known as the brain stem, that attaches it to the spinal cord. The very top crinkled layer is called the cerebral cortex (suh-REE-brul KOR-teks): this is where higher mental functions such as thinking, reasoning, and emotion take place. The human cerebral cortex is much more developed that that of other vertebrates (animals with a spinal column), and overall the human brain has more nerve cells than animal brains do. Behind and beneath the cortex is a small, cauliflower-shaped part of the brain called the cerebellum (sir-uh-BELL-um), which literally means little brain. The cerebellum is responsible for coordinating motor activities, from walking to juggling. Some scientists believe that the cerebellum is like a motor computer that controls activities in-

* **depression** (de-PRESH-un) is a mental state characterized by feelings of sadness, despair, and discouragement.

* **dopamine** (DOE-puh-meen) is a neurotransmitter in the brain that is involved in the brain structures that control motor activity (movement).

* **norepinephrine** (nor-eh-pin-EH-frin) is a neurotransmitter that is involved in arousal systems in the brain and in the action of the sympathetic nerves on blood vessels and internal organs.

volving balance and motor skill so that the rest of the brain is free to focus on conscious activities.

Like the other structures of the nervous system, the brain is made up of neurons that receive, process, and transmit information across synapses through chemical means. It is also composed of supporting cells called glia (GLEE-uh), which provide a supporting structure for the neurons.

200 YEARS AGO: MAPPING THE MIND

In the early 1800s, the "science" of phrenology (freh-NOL-uh-jee) was introduced by an Austrian doctor named Franz Gall. Gall theorized that studying the skull surfaces of people who had died would allow him to map their personalities onto the brain. He believed that different areas of the brain were responsible for different traits and that certain bumps or depressions on the skull would correlate with the person's characteristics. Based on these studies, Gall created a map of the mind and started practicing what came to be known as phrenology on living people.

Gall would use a special hat to map a total of 32 qualities, including attachment and friendship, cruelty, cleverness, memory, sense of humor, sense of words, and sense of color. When the hat was placed on the person's head, any bumps on the surface of the skull would push certain pins upward through a piece of paper. The pattern on the paper was viewed as a readout of an individual's character traits.

While this may sound unbelievable to twenty-first century psychologists, phrenology actually became quite popular in the nineteenth century. In addition to paying for phrenology readings, people would buy books and pamphlets on the subject. Some would even get a small personalized model of their head for the tip of their walking canes! In those days, phrenology seemed like a scientific way of understanding how personality is determined. In the twenty-first century, though, it sounds more like a horoscope or palm reading: it may be entertaining, but it has no basis in scientific fact.

Phrenology began to fall out of favor in the mid-1800s, when other discoveries refuted Dr. Gall's theory. In 1861, the French anthropologist Paul Broca examined a man who was unable to speak, except for repeating the word "tan." After the man died, Broca examined his brain and found that the damaged area was completely different from that predicted by phrenology. While phrenology suggested that language was controlled by the lower part of the left eye socket, Broca found that a small region toward the front of the left side of the brain was the true language center.

Nevertheless, Dr. Gall was on the right track in thinking that different regions of the brain are responsible for different functions.

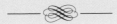

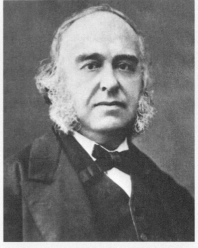

Paul Broca (1824–1880) discovered the area in the frontal lobe of the brain, now known as Broca's area, that controls speech. Patients with damage to this area can understand the speech of others, but are unable to speak themselves. *Hulton-Deutsch Collection/Corbis*

The brain has a left hemisphere and a right hemisphere covered by a layer of nerve tissue called the cerebrum (cerebral cortex). Underneath the cerebrum are other brain structures, including the amygdala, thalamus, corpus callosum, and hippocampus, all of which play important roles in human behavior and emotions. The cerebellum (mammalian brain) and the brain stem (reptilian brain) are believed to be the earliest structures that developed in human and animal evolutionary history. The cerebrum is the larger part of the brain, especially in humans. Each half of the cerebrum has four different lobes. The temporal lobes control speech. The occipital lobes control vision. The parietal lobes control movement. And the frontal lobes control ideas, thinking, planning, and the most complex parts of human emotions and behavior. ▼

Brain cells cannot divide and replace themselves like other cells in the body can. The brain of a human newborn contains as many neurons as it will ever have; in fact, people lose as many as 200,000 brain cells per day as they age. By the time people enter their 60s, 70s, 80s, or 90s, they may have lost anywhere from 5 to 20 percent of their original brain tissue. This helps explain why some older people (though certainly not all!) slow down mentally or have trouble remembering. Just as people need to keep their bodies in shape, they need to keep their brains in shape by taking on new challenges and learning new things. Also, people should wear that bicycle helmet; if brain cells are lost at any age because of injury or disease, they cannot replaced.

The brain has many different regions that are marked by textural or color differences or that are separated by fluid-filled areas. Throughout the twentieth century, researchers made major advances in understanding how different areas of the brain are involved in the control of activities such as movement, hearing, speech, and emotions. Scientists have also learned that these specific areas cannot carry out these functions alone. Instead, it is now known that different areas in the brain have to work together to accomplish all the complex activities that are part of human thought and consciousness. So the brain really does function like an orchestra!

How Does the Brain Develop?

As already noted, the brain's neurons do not divide to make new cells that can replace those that are aging or damaged, as happens with most

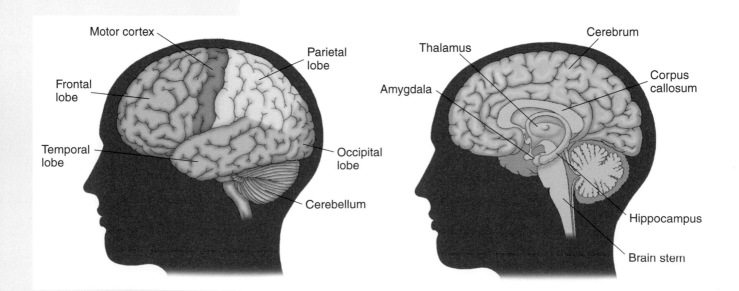

of the cells in the rest of the body. But cell division does happen before a baby is born; in fact, the entire brain and nervous system develop from just a few cells.

The developing human brain looks a lot like the developing brains of other animals, such as rats and rabbits. However, this changes at about seven months of pregnancy when the cerebral cortex of the fetus gets larger and starts to develop the many folds that allow more brain matter to fit inside the skull and gives humans more brain power. Over the next two months, the neurons continue to mature, and their axons and dendrites form increasingly complex branches and interconnections with other nerve cells. By nine months (at or near birth), babies have most of the neurons in their brain that they will ever have.

Although the number of neurons in the brain does not increase after birth, the connections between the neurons continue to develop, especially during the first years of life. Axons keep growing out from

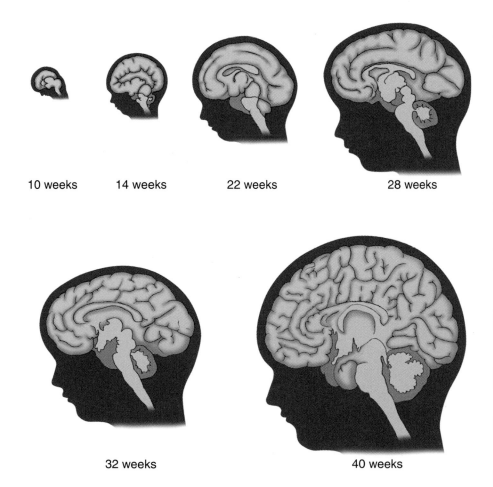

10 weeks   14 weeks   22 weeks   28 weeks

32 weeks   40 weeks

During the 40 weeks (nine months) of pregnancy, the fetal brain increases rapidly in size and complexity. In humans, the cerebrum is the largest part of the brain.

Left Brain/Right Brain: Do People Really Have Two Brains?

It has long been believed that the right hemisphere of the cerebral cortex controls artistic creativity and the use of language and the left side controls analytical thinking and working with numbers. While this is much too simple a division, the right and left hemispheres do appear generally to have different functions. In most left-handed people, the right cortex appears to be dominant, whereas the reverse is true in right-handed people.

Researchers have found that in most people, whether left-handed or right-handed, the areas that control language are located in the left hemisphere. Broca's area, which is located in the frontal lobe (the front of the brain), is concerned mainly with the production of speech. Wernicke's area is located in the temporal lobe (the temporal lobes are located on the two sides of the head) and is concerned with the comprehension of speech and with reading and writing. Both of these areas are named for the scientists who first identified them.

The most compelling evidence that the right and left hemispheres of the human brain function differently has come from split-brain studies, which are studies of people with severe epilepsy (EP-i-lep-see), whose corpus callosum (KOR-pus kuh-LO-sum; the bridge between the two brain halves) was surgically cut to help control seizures. Epilepsy is a condition of the nervous system characterized by recurrent seizures that temporarily affect a person's awareness, movements, or sensations. When these people hold objects in their right hands or look at words or objects flashed at their right eye, they

(continued)

(continued)

can quickly name the object or describe what they are seeing. That is because the information is sent to the left side of the brain where the language areas are (via the brain's crossover effect). However, they cannot say what they are touching or seeing if forced to use their left hand or eye. This information is sent to the right hemisphere, but it has no way to cross the message over to the language areas in the left side. Researchers have also shown that in healthy people, word recognition happens just a bit faster when a word or object is flashed at the right eye, again because it goes right to where the language areas are in the left side. Of course, if the language areas are in the right side, as is true for many left-handed people, the reverse happens.

*mental retardation is a condition in which people have below average intelligence that limits their ability to function normally.

*genetic refers to characteristics that are passed from parent to child by genes.

*metabolism (meh-TAB-o-liz-um) is the process in the body that converts foods into the energy necessary for body functions.

► *See also*

Birth Defects and Brain Development

Brain Chemistry (Neurochemistry)

Brain Injuries

Consciousness

Genetics and Behavior

Mental Retardation

different neurons to connect with others. A baby's brain has many more neuronal connections at age two than it does at birth. This is the basis for urging parents and caregivers to support their child's development by providing a stimulating environment that includes appropriate toys and games, books, music, and conversation.

There are a number of conditions that can result in mental retardation* by interfering with the normal development of the brain before birth, during birth, or even during childhood. For example, genetic* abnormalities can cause disorders that affect a child's development or metabolism*, which in turn can cause problems in the brain. Sometimes, for reasons that are not always understood, the brain is damaged or just does not develop normally before birth, as occurs in the condition called cerebral palsy. If the mother drinks alcohol or does not take in sufficient vitamins or other nutrients in her diet during the pregnancy, brain and spinal cord development can also be affected.

Resources

Books

Brynie, Faith. *101 Questions Your Brain Has Asked About Itself but Couldn't Answer . . . Until Now.* Brookfield, CT: The Millbrook Press, 1998.

Conlan, Roberta, ed. *States of Mind: New Discoveries About How Our Brains Make Us Who We Are.* New York: John Wiley and Sons, 2001.

Ramachandran, V. S., and Sandra Blakeslee. *Phantoms in the Brain: Probing the Mysteries of the Human Mind.* New York: HarperCollins, 1999.

Organization

Neuroscience for Kids is an extensive and entertaining website maintained by Research Associate Professor Eric Chudler at the University of Washington, Seattle. It features easy-to-understand information on a range of topics related to the brain and nervous system. http://faculty.washington.edu/chudler/neurok.html

A

Abuse

Abuse is hurtful mistreatment of other people. It may include physical, sexual, or emotional (ee-MO-shun-al) mistreatment of children or adults.

What Is Abuse?

Abuse is a form of violence in which one person harms another physically or emotionally. The abuser often uses an advantage of size, power, or influence to hurt or mistreat the target of the abuse, who may be smaller, younger, or weaker. Abusers can include:

- a parent, guardian, or teacher who hits a child
- a parent or guardian who neglects a child
- a caregiver who hits or shakes a crying baby
- a caregiver who hits or neglects an elderly or disabled person
- a spouse, a date, or an intimate partner who beats or rapes the other intimate partner
- an adult who asks or forces a child to engage in sexual activity
- anyone who taunts or harms another because of age, race, gender, beliefs, or sexual orientation.

Abuse is a problem for the person who has been abused, for those who witness the abuse, and for society at large. Statistics indicate that abuse may contribute to a cycle of violence whereby abused children can grow up to become abusive adults and parents.

Why Do People Behave in Abusive Ways?

There is no single cause for abusive behavior, but there are many factors that seem to make it likelier that an adult will abuse others. Growing up in an abusive family is one contributing factor. Other factors include:

- alcohol or substance abuse that leads to loss of self-control
- unemployment, lack of education, discrimination, and other factors that cause financial difficulties
- marital problems
- undiagnosed mental illness
- antisocial personality disorder that leads the abuser to disregard the rights of others

KEYWORDS
for searching the Internet and other reference sources

Battering

Child abuse

Child neglect

Child sexual abuse

Family violence

Incest

Interpersonal violence

Intimate partner violence

Shaken baby syndrome

Victimology

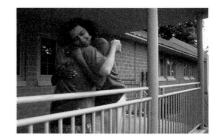

Family violence may lead to "learned helplessness," a form of passivity and hopelessness that people experience when they believe that abuse is an inevitable and inescapable part of their lives. Shelters often offer counseling and therapy to help battered women learn how to overcome learned helplessness and escape from abusive situations.
Stock Boston

Learned Helplessness

"Why doesn't she just leave him?" observers often wonder when they become aware of family violence. The answer most likely is what psychologist and researcher Martin Seligman and his colleagues call "learned helplessness," a form of passivity and hopelessness that people experience when they come to believe that abuse and violence are inevitable and inescapable components of their lives. People who experience violence regularly may give up trying to avoid or escape that violence. They may become passive and unable to create safety for themselves or their families.

In her work on battered wives, psychologist Lenore Walker discovered that these women often remain with battering husbands because of learned helplessness. She found that battered wives who had learned to be helpless and passive needed counseling and therapy before they could learn how to escape from the abusive situation. Even if abused partners want to leave their abusers, leaving may not be an easy option. The abusing partner may increase the level of violence if the abused partner tries to leave the home. The abusing partner also may forbid contact with friends, neighbors, or in-laws; may withhold money or car keys; may stalk the abused partner; or may threaten children or pets.

- lack of coping skills to deal with anger and impulsive behavior
- lack of coping skills to deal with stressful situations, such as the care of a disabled child or a dependent elder.

Abusers often want to deny the seriousness of the problem, evade responsibility for their own abusive behavior, and shift blame to the other person. Abusers may say that the person being abused was "asking for it," but abuse is not the fault of the child or adult who has been abused. No one "deserves" to be abused or neglected.

Emotional Abuse

Abuse does not always cause bruises that one can see. Emotional abuse targets the feelings and spirit of the person being abused, instead of the body. Forms of verbal and emotional abuse may include repeated name calling, hurtful ridicule (RI-di-kyool), harsh criticism, cruel and disrespectful words, bullying, and threats of violence or harm. Emotional abuse can have serious long-term consequences:

- It may damage a developing child's sense of self-esteem.
- It may make it difficult for a child to make friends.
- It may make it difficult for a child to concentrate on schoolwork.
- It may make a child cautious or fearful about his or her safety, even in safe surroundings and situations.
- It may make a child seem too grown-up in behavior.
- It may be contribute to feelings of depression, hopelessness, and anger.

When verbal abuse includes threats of violence, it may indicate that physical abuse and sexual abuse also are occurring.

Physical Abuse

Physical abuse affects the body as well as the head, heart, and spirit. Physical abuse may include a pattern of hitting, kicking, pushing, shoving, shaking, spanking, and harsh physical punishment. It may cause bruising or more serious injury, and even if it is called "tough love," it is in fact a form of violence. Physical abuse, particularly family violence, often is kept secret by the abuser, by the person being abused, and by other family members who fear the consequences of confronting the abuser. Signs that a child may be abused may include:

- unusual injuries that are not the result of normal play activities, for example, black eyes; injuries to cheeks and ears; injuries to stomach, back, thighs, and buttocks; human bite marks; and cigarette burns
- unusual tiredness or trouble sleeping or nightmares
- unusual sadness or crying

- unusual violence toward classmates or siblings or pets
- avoidance of parents or caregivers, such as reluctance to go home after school
- the same behaviors that result from emotional abuse

Family violence Family violence often is referred to as domestic abuse. It includes all forms of intimate partner violence (spouse abuse or wife battering), child abuse and neglect, elder abuse, and child sexual abuse. Intimate partner violence most often involves men who are abusive toward female partners. Female-to-male domestic abuse also occurs, as does male-to-male and female-to-female abuse in same-sex couples.

Research shows that child abuse and spouse abuse often happen in the same families. But even if child abuse does not take place along with spouse abuse, the child who witnesses family violence experiences many problems. Family violence limits the child's ability to feel safe and protected at home, and it may force the child to favor one parent over the other. It also may cause emotional and behavioral (bee-HAY-vyor-al) problems for the child at school or among peers. It may also lead to a broken home or custody dispute if a wife leaves the home for a battered women's shelter or if a child is removed from the home by a government child protection agency.

Child abuse and neglect Child abuse is mistreatment of a child by a parent, older child, or other adult. Physical abuse toward a child may include hitting or kicking, pushing and shoving, or other types of harsh physical punishment. More than half of all cases of child abuse are believed to affect children younger than 8 years old.

Shaken baby syndrome Parents and caregivers who shake a baby to try to make the baby stop crying can cause very serious injuries. Shaking a baby can cause bleeding inside the baby's eyes and brain. This may lead to vomiting, seizures*, brain swelling, blindness, hearing loss, mental retardation, brain damage, coma*, or even death. Shaken babies may or may not have bruises on other parts of their bodies that might signal physical abuse, but researchers estimate that up to 80 percent of serious head injuries in children younger than 2 years are the result of shaking. It is never okay to shake a baby for any reason.

Elder abuse and neglect Elder abuse may occur in families or in institutions such as nursing homes. Abuse may include neglect, hitting, pushing, shaking, giving elders too much medication, and putting elders in restraints that prevent them from leaving a bed or wheelchair. Elders who cannot take care of themselves, who are incontinent*, who need assistance with activities of daily living, or who wander away due to dementia* may be difficult and frustrating to caregivers, but it is never okay to hit or push an elderly person.

---

* **seizures** (SEE-zhurz) are "storms" in the brain that occur when the electrical patterns of the brain are interrupted by powerful, rapid bursts of electrical energy. This may cause a person to fall down, make jerky movements, or stare blankly into space.

* **coma** is an unconscious state, like a very deep sleep. A person in a coma cannot awaken, move, see, or speak.

* **incontinent** means unable to control urination or bowel movements.

* **dementia** (de-MEN-sha) is a term that describes any condition that causes a person to lose the ability to think, remember, and act.

When Children Go to Court

According to tradition and common law, children are the "personal property" of their parents, and parents have the right to decide how to raise their own children. When parents abuse or neglect their children, however, government agencies may step in, because it is the government's responsibility to protect the safety and well-being of all children in the community. Doctors, teachers, school counselors, social workers, or neighbors may report child abuse to the police. Police or local child protection agencies may investigate homes in which possible abuse has been reported. Family courts may remove children from the home and appoint temporary guardians for them. And family courts may order a custody evaluation to decide whether it is safe for a child to be returned to a home in which the child has been abused.

(continued)

Children face many difficulties when they are required to testify in court. Court testimony causes anxiety for all witnesses, but for those who have been abused, the testimony itself can be especially difficult. Being required to remember and discuss past abuses may lead to intensified symptoms of post-traumatic stress disorder. Being challenged by attorneys about the reliability and accuracy of recall of events can be distressing. And being involved in a family court case can carry stigma within a child's peer group. Most important, testifying against a parent or family member whom the child loves may cause the child to feel guilty or disloyal, as if he or she is the abuser who has caused harm rather than the other way around. Doctors, social workers, and foster parents all can create a support network to help children prepare for court testimony and to care for them before and after the court date.

* **pornography** (por-NAH-gra-fee) refers to any material, like magazines or videos, that shows sexual behavior and is meant to cause sexual excitement.

* **genital** refers to the external sexual organs.

* **vagina** (va-JY-na) is the canal in females that leads from the uterus (the organ where a baby develops) to the outside of the body.

* **anus** is the opening at the end of the digestive system, through which waste leaves the body.

Sexual Abuse

Sexual abuse is unwanted, inappropriate, or forced sexual touching, contact, and behavior. Abusers may be male or female, and the person who is sexually abused may be adult or child, male or female, very young or very old, intimate partner or spouse, neighbor, student, or date. Incest is the term for sexual abuse by a member of one's own family. Sexual abusers often believe that the activity is a form of love or intimacy. Abusers may claim that the victim said "no" but that the abuser knew the victim meant "yes." But people who have been abused experience the violation of their personal boundaries and privacy as assault and violence.

Child Sexual Abuse

Child sexual abuse occurs when an adult or an older child pressures or forces a younger child into sexual activity. Sexual activity may involve pornography*, inappropriate touching by the child or the adult, or genital* penetration of the child's vagina*, anus*, or mouth. The abuser may be a family member or someone outside the family, but often it is someone the child knows and trusts. Sometimes sexual abuse happens only once, but in many cases it happens repeatedly with one particular adult.

Consent Children who do not understand sexual behavior cannot give consent for that behavior. An abuser may want to believe that a child is a willing partner in sexual activity, but this is not true. Young children do not understand the complexity or long-term consequences of sexual behavior. They cannot consent to behavior they do not understand.

Secrecy An adult who sexually abuses a child often tells the child to keep the sexual activity secret. Children who have been sexually abused often comply with the request to keep the activity secret because they feel ashamed and confused, because they do not understand the behavior and have difficulty explaining it to responsible adults, and because the behavior makes them uncomfortable and fearful. Children who try to tell their secret to an adult sometimes encounter disbelief, but they need to keep trying to tell the secret, because doctors, teachers, and school counselors can help children improve this difficult situation.

Repressed memories If thinking about the abuse is particularly difficult, children may lock away all knowledge of the abuse in the deepest part of their memories, keeping the abuse secret even from themselves. This form of amnesia (am-NEE-zha), or memory loss, can last for many years according to many experts. Adults who have been abused as children report sometimes discovering a key to the deepest parts of the memory many years after the abuse has stopped. Known as "repressed memory," adult recall of child sexual abuse is considered a controversial topic.

Signs of abuse Even if children deny to themselves or others that sexual abuse has taken place, signs may include:

- redness, swelling, pain, or bleeding of the genitals, anus, or mouth
- questions about sexual activity at a very early age
- sexual acts, words, or drawings at an unusually early age
- avoidance of certain people and places
- unusual fear or jumpiness at the mention of certain people or places
- sudden start of bed-wetting or soiling (losing control of bowel movements)
- sexually transmitted diseases
- urinary tract infections or pregnancy in young girls

Like other forms of abuse, child sexual abuse is never the child's fault. Children who have been sexually abused often benefit from therapy to help heal the emotional hurt caused by abuse.

Discrimination and Hate Crimes

Sometimes people are abused because of race or ethnic background, disabilities, gender, sexual orientation, or religious beliefs. White supremacy, lynching, gay bashing, and ethnic cleansing are a few of the terms associated with these forms of abuse and violence. In many areas of the United States and the world, hate crimes are not yet specifically against the law.

How Do Doctors Treat People Who Have Been Abused?

People who have been abused often try to keep the abuse secret. They may be confused, ashamed, or afraid. They also may be trying to protect the person who has hurt them or trying to protect themselves from further abuse. Remaining silent, however, is not an effective way to end abuse. Confiding in a doctor can lead to protection from further abuse. A doctor who diagnoses abuse can treat injuries and infections that result from abuse and can refer patients to counselors, therapists, social workers, and child protection agencies.

How Do Mental Health Professionals Help People Who Have Been Abused?

Sometimes it is necessary for the person being abused to get immediate protection. Shelters can provide women and children with a temporary safe place to stay. Foster care is a way for children to get immediate protection from abuse in the home. Although this can be a difficult situation for a family, sometimes it is necessary in order to keep abused people safe from severe injury or even death from family violence. Social workers and child protection agencies often provide these kinds of services. After immediate concerns for safety and injury have been attended to, therapists can help people who have been abused with their emotional

Who? Whom? How Often?

While no two abuse cases are *exactly* the same, there are some common patterns.

- Husbands abuse wives more often than wives abuse husbands.
- Male children are beaten more often than female children.
- Child abuse is more likely to occur in families that also experience intimate partner violence.
- Children with disabilities, particularly mental retardation or other cognitive (intellectual) impairment, are at higher risk of sexual abuse than other children.
- Approximately 3 of every 100 men in the United States assault an intimate partner.
- Approximately one of every four girls in the United States experiences sexual abuse.
- Approximately one of every six boys in the United States experiences sexual abuse.
- Approximately 90 percent of cases of child abuse are attributed to parents or other family caregivers. Only 10 percent of cases of child abuse are attributed to strangers.
- Approximately 80 percent of children who are sexually abused know their abusers.

Abuse is an international problem. In 2001, the World Health Organization is scheduled to publish its first World Report on Violence and Health covering child abuse, youth violence, intimate partner violence, sexual violence, elder abuse, and other topics. Find this organization on the Internet at http://www.who.int/violence_injury_prevention.

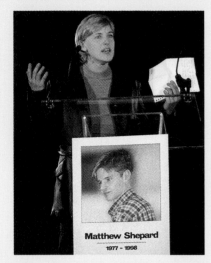

Matthew Shepard
1977 - 1998

▲

Hate crimes are not yet specifically illegal in many areas of the United States and the world. In 1998, actress Ellen DeGeneres spoke out in favor of hate crimes legislation after a college student named Matthew Shepard was killed in a gay-bashing hate crime in Laramie, Wyoming. *Getty Source/Liaison*

▶ *See also*

Antisocial Personality Disorder

Brain Injuries

Bullying

Families

Personality Disorders

Post-Traumatic Stress Disorder

Rape

Therapy

Violence

wounds and post-trauma stress. Family therapists can teach families better coping skills, better parenting skills, and more effective ways to deal with anger, frustration, conflict, and the aftermath of earlier cycles of violence.

Resources

Hotline

National Domestic Violence Hotline. This is a 24-hour hotline. In cases of immediate life-threatening emergency, dial 911.
Telephone 800-799-7233

Books

Lee, Sharice A. *The Survivor's Guide.* Thousand Oaks, CA: Sage Publications, 1995. Written for teens and preteens recovering from child sexual abuse, this guide fits in pocket or backpack.

Pucci, Linda M., and Lynn M. Copen. *Finding Your Way: What Happens When You Tell About Abuse.* Thousand Oaks, CA: Sage Publications, 2000. This easy-to-understand book can help children feel safer in cases when abuse requires legal intervention or a family court appearance.

Organizations

National Center for Injury Prevention and Control, Mailstop K65, 4770 Buford Highway NE, Atlanta, GA 30341-3724. NCIPC is a division of the Centers for Disease Control and Prevention. It posts fact sheets at its website on intimate partner violence, rape, and male batterers.
Telephone 770-488-1506
http://www.cdc.gov/ncipc/factsheets

American Academy of Pediatrics, 141 Northwest Point Boulevard, Elk Grove Village, IL 60007-1098. This organization posts fact sheets at its website on physical and emotional child abuse, child sexual abuse, shaken baby syndrome, and children in court cases.
Telephone 847-434-4000
http://www.aap.org

American Humane Association, 63 Inveerness Drive East, Englewood, CO 80112-5117.

This is an advocacy organization that aims to protect children and animals from abuse, neglect, and cruelty. It posts fact sheets at its website on child abuse and neglect and shaken baby syndrome.
Telephone 800-227-4645
http://www.americanhumane.org

KidsHealth.org is a website sponsored by the Nemours Foundation, created and maintained by the medical experts at the A. I. duPont Hospital for Children, Wilmington, DE. It posts articles and information for kids, teens, and parents about abuse and related topics. http://www.kidshealth.org

Addiction

Addiction (a-DIK-shun) refers to the use of a substance, such as alcohol or another drug, to the point where a person develops a physical or psychological need for it. The term also may be used to describe a harmful habit that is out of control, such as gambling or spending too much time on the Internet.

KEYWORDS
for searching the Internet
and other reference sources
Chemical dependence
Substance abuse
Tobacco addiction

When friends first told Josh that his drinking and drug use were out of control, he ignored them. He liked to party, he said, but he could stop anytime he wanted. He did not stop, though, no matter how much his grades fell and his soccer game suffered. He still did not stop even after he was kicked off the soccer team and lost many of his friends. Eventually, Josh had to admit that his use of alcohol and drugs had gotten out of hand. He had developed an addiction, he now said, and he needed help to fight it.

What Is Drug Addiction?

We often say that people who have an addiction are "hooked" on a substance or behavior. It is an apt choice of words, since addicts often feel as if they are dangling like a trout from a fishing hook and that they cannot break free. Fortunately, this is not true. Treatment can help people with an addiction overcome their bad habits and regain control of their lives.

Physical dependence People with an addiction to alcohol or another drug develop a dependence on it, which is a strong need to use the substance no matter how bad the consequences may be. Sometimes the need is physical. One sign of physical dependence is called tolerance. When someone develops tolerance for a certain substance, it means that over time he or she starts to need more and more of it to get drunk or feel high. If someone keeps using the same amount of the substance, after a while he or she may notice that it does not have the same effect anymore.

Another sign of physical dependence is withdrawal, which means that people who are hooked on a substance can have physical symptoms and feel sick if they stop using it. The symptoms are so unpleasant that people may be driven to start drinking or using drugs again just so they can feel better. This is one effect that keeps people coming back for more of a substance, even after they realize that they have a serious problem.

Without Drugs = Withdrawal

When long-term or heavy drug use suddenly stops, people may soon experience a number of unpleasant symptoms. These symptoms vary, depending on the substance involved. Some common symptoms are:

- **Alcohol and sedatives:** shaking hands, upset stomach, vomiting, anxiety, sweating, rapid heartbeat, restlessness, trouble sleeping, seizures, and hallucinations.

- **Amphetamines and cocaine:** bad mood, tiredness, vivid nightmares, increased appetite, and sleeping too much or too little.

- **Caffeine:** tiredness, sleepiness, depression, anxiety, upset stomach, vomiting, and headache.

- **Heroin and morphine:** bad mood, upset stomach, vomiting, muscle aches, runny nose or eyes, sweating, diarrhea, yawning, fever, and trouble sleeping.

- **Nicotine:** bad mood, depression, trouble sleeping, crankiness, anger, anxiety, short attention span, restlessness, slower heartbeat, increased appetite, and weight gain.

The Tiniest Addicts

What could be sadder than a tiny baby in the throes of drug withdrawal? This tragic scene is played out when babies of drug-abusing mothers are born with an addiction. Babies born addicted to heroin, for example, sneeze, hiccup, twitch, and cry. They also may have such symptoms as restlessness, shakiness, trouble sleeping and eating, a stuffy nose, vomiting, diarrhea, a high-pitched cry, fever, irregular breathing, and seizures*. These symptoms usually start within a few days after birth, and some can last for 3 months or more.

* **seizures** can occur when the electrical patterns of the brain are interrupted by powerful, rapid bursts of electrical energy, which may cause a person to fall down, make jerky movements, or stare blankly into space.

* **heroin** is a narcotic, an addictive painkiller that produces a high, or a euphoric effect. Euphoria (yoo-FOR-ee-a) is an abnormal, exaggerated feeling of well-being.

* **LSD**, short for lysergic acid diethylamide (ly-SER-jik A-sid dy-e-thel-AM-eyed), is a hallucinogen, a drug that distorts a person's view of reality and causes hallucinations.

* **PCP**, short for phencyclidine (fen-SY-kle-deen), is a hallucinogen, a drug that distorts a person's view of reality.

* **cocaine** (ko-KAYN) is a stimulant, a drug that produces a temporary feeling of alertness, energy, and euphoria.

Psychological dependence   Some people feel as if they have lost control of their drinking or drug use, yet they do not show signs of tolerance or withdrawal. While these people may not be physically hooked on a substance, they can still have a strong psychological dependence on it. Like people with a physical dependence, they may feel an intense craving and find themselves drinking or using drugs in larger amounts or more often than they intend.

People who are dependent on alcohol or other drugs, either physically or psychologically, often spend much of their time finding ways of getting the substance, using it, hiding it, and recovering from its ill effects. Friendships, school, work, sports, and other activities all may suffer as a result. As the problems pile up, people may want desperately to give up the substance, yet they find it very hard to do so despite repeated efforts to kick the habit. Often, users will not see the connection between drug use and life problems. They think that the issues in their lives justify their drug and alcohol use and deny that their substance abuse is a real problem.

What Causes Drug Addiction?

Addiction usually begins with a conscious choice to drink or use drugs. People often turn to alcohol or other drugs to avoid things that bother them. For teenagers, this may mean pressure from friends, stress at home, or problems at school. Teenagers also may think that drinking or using drugs will help them fit in, let them overcome their shyness at parties, or make them look older or "cooler." Some just like the feeling of being high. In the long run, though, they end up feeling worse. The more they drink and use drugs, the more problems arise, and the harder it is to stop. By this point, however, people may feel as if they no longer have a choice, because the urge to use alcohol or drugs has become so powerful.

To understand how alcohol and drugs can gain such a strong hold on people, it helps to grasp how these substances act inside the body. Once a substance is taken in through drinking, smoking, injecting, or inhaling, it travels through the bloodstream to the brain, which has its own built-in reward system. When people do things that are important for survival, such as eating, special nerve cells in the brain release chemicals that make people feel pleasure. In this way, the brain is programmed so that people want to repeat these actions that make them feel good.

Substances that are addictive affect the brain's reward system. Instead of teaching people to repeat survival behaviors, though, they "teach" them to take more drugs. The way this happens varies from substance to substance. Some drugs, such as heroin* or LSD*, mimic the effects of a natural brain chemical. Others, such as PCP*, block the sending of messages between nerve cells. Still others, such as cocaine*, interfere with the molecules that carry brain chemicals back to the nerve cells that released them. Finally, some drugs cause brain chemicals to be released in larger

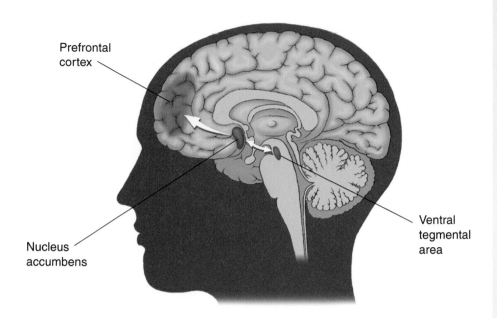

Prefrontal cortex

Nucleus accumbens

Ventral tegmental area

Addiction is believed to change the brain's pleasure circuits and pathways. A complex cascade of signals within the brain creates the craving that characterizes addiction. Thus, an addiction to a substance may be both psychological and physiological, as the body creates demands that are out of the person's control.

◀

amounts than normal. Methamphetamine, a type of amphetamine* also known as "speed," is one example. At first, drug use may seem fun, because it leads to feelings of pleasure or relaxation. Over time, though, drug use gradually changes the brain so that people need to take drugs just to feel normal.

Who Is at Risk of Addiction?

Addicts come in all shapes and sizes. The homeless man sleeping on the street may have an addiction, but so may the captain of the high school soccer team. Any person who abuses alcohol or other drugs is at risk of becoming addicted. For some people, however, the risk is especially high. For one thing, problems with drinking and drug use, just like heart disease or cancer, often run in families. Children whose parents are addicted to alcohol, for example, may be more likely than other people to have an alcohol or drug problem themselves.

People who have certain mental disorders also have a higher than average risk of addiction. This is not surprising, since it is thought that many mental disorders are caused in part by an imbalance in the same kinds of brain chemicals that drugs affect. People who suffer from depression, for example, may find that a certain drug lifts their mood for a while. The "self-medication" theory of addiction says that people learn to respond to a particular mood by taking a drug, in a misplaced effort to relieve their mental pain.

What Are Some Addictive Drugs?

People can become addicted to a wide range of substances, including alcohol, amphetamines, cocaine, heroin, inhalants*, LSD, marijuana*,

*amphetamines (am-FET-a-meenz) are stimulants, drugs that produce a temporary feeling of alertness, energy, and euphoria.

*inhalants (in-HAY-lunts) are substances that a person can sniff, or inhale, to get high.

*marijuana (mar-a-WA-na) is a mixture of dried, shredded flowers and leaves from the hemp plant that a person can smoke or eat to get high.

People who use cocaine often feel smart and powerful. Actually, a brain impaired by cocaine use is less active than a healthy brain. These positron emission tomography (PET) scans show areas of high brain activity in red and yellow. Note that brain activity is reduced in the cocaine user, especially in the frontal lobes (arrows) where ideas, thoughts, plans, and memories are created. *Photo Researchers, Inc.* ▶

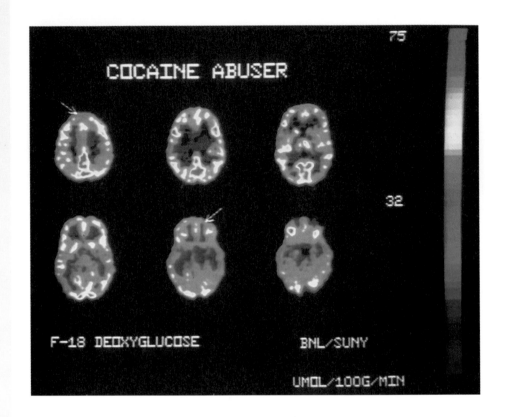

*__morphine__ (MOR-feen) is a narcotic, an addictive painkiller that produces a high.

*__sedatives__ (SAID-uh-tivs) are drugs that produce a calming effect or sleepiness.

*__hallucinations__ (ha-loo-si-NAY-shuns) are sensory perceptions that have no cause in the outside world. A person with hallucinations may see and hear things that are not really there.

morphine*, tobacco, PCP, and sedatives*, just to name a few commonly abused drugs.

Marijuana addiction   Some people believe that marijuana use is relatively safe, because it does not lead to addiction. However, regular marijuana users may become psychologically dependent on the drug. Some longtime, heavy users also can experience mild signs of physical dependence, including tolerance and withdrawal. Some studies suggest that marijuana affects the brain's reward system in much the same way as other addictive drugs.

Alcohol addiction   Alcoholism (AL-ko-hall-i-zm) is the common name for an addiction to alcohol. Some people with alcoholism develop a tolerance that lets them drink large amounts of alcohol without seeming drunk or passing out. Others have nasty withdrawal symptoms if they stop drinking. Delirium tremens (de-LEER-ee-um TRE-munz) is the name given to the most severe withdrawal symptoms seen in people who have alcoholism. These symptoms include confusion, disordered thoughts, and hallucinations*.

Tobacco addiction   Cigarette smoking is a very tough habit to overcome. This is because tobacco contains nicotine, a highly addictive substance that is added to tobacco when it is made into cigarettes. Smokers can build up a tolerance for nicotine, as shown by the fact that most smokers work up to smoking at least a pack a day by the age of 25. They also go through withdrawal when they are unable to smoke, which explains why many smokers rush to light up as soon as they leave a place where smoking is not allowed.

Caffeine addiction Among the most widely used mind-altering chemicals in the world is caffeine (ka-FEEN), a substance found in coffee, tea, colas, and many nonprescription medicines. It is no accident that coffee, a potent source of caffeine, is the favorite wake-up drink in so many homes. People often use caffeine for the temporary surge of energy it produces, much like the "buzz" that comes from some other drugs. Owing to tolerance, however, it eventually takes more and more caffeine to get this feeling. When daily coffee drinkers stop using caffeine, they may have withdrawal symptoms, such as headaches, fatigue, and irritability.

What Is an Addictive Disorder?

People also may develop harmful behavior patterns that share many of the same traits as dependence on alcohol or other drugs. Such behaviors sometimes are referred to as addictions too. Among the types of behavior that can be taken to an unhealthy extreme are gambling, sexual activity, and Internet use. When people say they have an addiction to gambling, for example, they mean that they have trouble controlling their desire to gamble, even when they experience harmful consequences, such as losing a lot of money.

Experts disagree about whether this kind of out-of-control behavior should be termed an addiction. Many doctors prefer to call it an impulse control disorder. People with an impulse control disorder are unable to curb their urge to do something that is harmful to themselves or others, even though they may try to resist and feel guilty for failing to do so. In everyday conversation, though, people often refer to excessive gambling, sexual behavior, and Internet use as addictions, since people with these problems act much like people who are addicted to alcohol or other drugs. Rather than responding to outside chemicals, however, such people may be responding in part to natural chemicals released inside the brain. Exciting activities, such as gambling and sexual behavior, can trigger the release of brain chemicals that have an arousing effect. This is similar to the effect that people get from taking cocaine or amphetamines.

Gambling addiction Gambling addiction, also sometimes called pathological (pa-tha-LAH-ji-kal) gambling, refers to out-of-control gambling with harmful consequences. Like people addicted to substances, gambling addicts may need to risk ever-increasing amounts of money to feel the same excitement they got from gambling a small amount at first. They also may become restless or cranky if they try to cut down or stop gambling, which makes it hard for them to quit. The continued gambling causes trouble at home, school, or work. Yet gambling addicts use

From Use to Misuse to Abuse to Addiction

Alcohol or drug use by teenagers typically moves through four stages as it goes from occasional use to full-blown addiction. The stages are:

- **Occasional use:** Teenagers at this stage typically use beer, marijuana, or inhalants on weekends with their friends. There are few obvious changes in behavior during the week.

- **Regular misuse:** Teenagers at this stage actively seek the high they get from drinking or using drugs. They may try stimulants (for example, amphetamines or cocaine) or hallucinogens (for example, LSD or PCP), and they may use drugs four or five times per week, even when they are alone. Grades start to slip, activities fall by the wayside, and old friends are replaced with new ones who also use alcohol or drugs.

- **Frequent abuse:** Teenagers at this stage can have mood swings that go from extreme highs to such lows that suicide becomes a concern. Many start to sell drugs to support their habit. As the drug use continues, lying, fighting, stealing, and school failure become problems.

- **Full-blown addiction:** Teenagers at this stage may need alcohol or drugs every day to fend off withdrawal. They will use whatever drug is handy and do whatever it takes to get high. Drug use is all they think about, and they may feel as if they have lost control. Guilt, shame, and depression are common emotions, and overdoses and medical problems may occur.

their habit as a way of escaping problems or feeling better, much the way someone else might use alcohol or drugs. They may find that much of their time is spent thinking about their next bet or scheming to get more money. They also may start lying to friends and family to hide how much they are gambling, or they may need to borrow money to cover their losses. As things get worse, they may even turn to stealing. Despite the problems, such people find it nearly impossible to stop gambling.

Sexual addiction Sexual feelings and desires are a normal, healthy part of life, but some people take these natural feelings to an unhealthy extreme, to the point where they are unable to control their sexual thoughts or behavior. Some people might spend hour after hour looking at pornography*, while others might have casual sex with partner after partner. In either case, there can be serious negative consequences. People who spend too much time looking at sexual pictures or videos may lose friends or drop out of other activities. Those who have numerous sex partners risk an unwanted pregnancy or a sexually transmitted disease (an infection, such as herpes or HIV, that can be passed from person to person by sexual contact).

Internet addiction A new problem in the computer age is seen among people who are unable to control their on-line behavior. Some people feel driven to "surf" websites or play computer games for hours on end, to the point where they lose interest in off-line activities. Others spend so much time "chatting" with on-line buddies that they have no time for real-world friends. Still others who already have trouble controlling their desire to gamble or look at pornography spend a lot of time at websites that cater to their frequent, strong cravings.

What Are the Signs of a Drug Addiction?

It is not always easy to tell when someone is suffering from an alcohol or drug addiction, since the person may go to great lengths to hide the problem. Nonetheless, there are usually signs that something is terribly wrong. Typical warning signs in young people include:

- getting drunk or high on a regular basis
- having to use more alcohol or drugs to get the same effect
- wanting to quit but being unable to do so
- lying about or hiding the alcohol or drug use
- avoiding friends in order to get drunk or high
- giving up other activities, such as homework or sports
- pressuring others to drink or use drugs
- taking risks, including having unsafe sex
- driving under the influence of alcohol or drugs
- getting into trouble with the law

* **pornography** is the depiction of sexual activity, in writing or in pictures or videos, that is meant to cause sexual excitement.

- being kicked out of school for a reason related to alcohol or drugs
- thinking that the only way to have fun is to drink or use drugs
- being unable to remember actions the night before while drunk or high
- feeling run-down, hopeless, or depressed.

What Are the Signs of an Addictive Disorder?

People with an addictive disorder may act much like those with alcohol or drug addiction. Typical warning signs include:

- taking part in the behavior more often or intensely than intended
- having to increase the behavior to get the same effect
- wanting to quit but being unable to do so
- feeling restless or cranky if the behavior stops
- continuing the behavior despite knowing that it causes real problems
- giving up other activities, such as homework or sports
- thinking about or planning for the behavior all the time
- spending a lot of time on the behavior and its aftereffects.

How Is an Addiction Diagnosed and Treated?

An addiction is a tough problem to beat, but it can be done. The first step is to seek professional help. To make a diagnosis, a physician or mental health professional, such as a psychologist, social worker, or counselor, will ask the person about past and present alcohol and drug use. If possible, the doctor or mental health professional also will talk to the person's family or friends. In addition, he or she will perform a full medical checkup and may order tests to check for diseases that are more common among addicts. For example, a person who injects drugs might be tested for HIV infection, which can be contracted by sharing needles with an infected person.

Once a diagnosis has been made, there are several treatment options. Medications can help control drug cravings and relieve withdrawal symptoms. These are not the same kinds of drugs that are involved in the addiction but rather medications that help lessen the addiction problem. Talk therapy can help people with addictions understand their own behavior, develop higher self-esteem, and cope better with stress. For most people, a combination of medication and talk therapy works best. Talk therapy can be done one-on-one with a therapist or in a group.

Many people do quite well being treated at a clinic while living at home, but others may need to spend a short time in a hospital. This is especially true if they have other mental disorders, are not motivated to change, have friends who still use alcohol or drugs, or have failed in past treatment efforts. Peer group self-help programs, such as Alcoholics Anonymous or Narcotics Anonymous, have become cornerstones of treatment for addiction problems.

Twelve 12-Step Groups

Since its founding in Akron, Ohio, in 1935, Alcoholics Anonymous has mushroomed to nearly 2 million members in more than 99,000 groups worldwide. Not surprisingly, dozens of other self-help groups have since tried to copy this successful model. They include:

- Chemically Dependent Anonymous, P.O. Box 4425, Annapolis, MD 21403. Telephone 800-CDA-HOPE. http://www.cdaweb.org
- Cocaine Anonymous, 3740 Overland Avenue, Suite C, Los Angeles, CA 90034-6337. Telephone 310-559-5833. http://www.ca.org
- Crystal Meth Anonymous, 8205 Santa Monica Blvd., PMB=114, West Hollywood, CA 90046-5977. Telephone 213-488-4455. http://www.crystalmeth.org

(continued)

- Debtors Anonymous, P.O. Box 920888, Needham, MA 02492-0009. Telephone 781-453-2743. http://www.debtorsanonymous.org

- Emotions Anonymous, P.O. Box 4245, St. Paul, MN 55104-0245. Telephone 651-647-9712. http://www.emotionsanonymous.org

- Food Addicts in Recovery Anonymous, 6 Pleasant Street, Suite 402, Malden, MA 02148. Telephone 781-321-9118. http://www.foodaddicts.org

- Gamblers Anonymous, P.O. Box 17173, Los Angeles, CA 90017. Telephone 213-386-8789. http://www.gamblersanonymous.org

- Marijuana Anonymous, P.O. Box 2912, Van Nuys, CA 91404. Telephone 800-766-6779. http://www.marijuana-anonymous.org

- Narcotics Anonymous, P.O. Box 9999, Van Nuys, CA 91409. Telephone 818-773-9999. http://www.na.org

- Nicotine Anonymous, 419 Main Street, PMB370, Huntington Beach, CA 92648. Telephone 866-536-4359. http://www.nicotine-anonymous.org

- Overeaters Anonymous, 6075 Zenith Court Northeast, Rio Rancho, NM 87124. Telephone 505-891-2664. http://www.overeatersanonymous.org

- Sexaholics Anonymous, P.O. Box 111910, Nashville, TN 37222. Telephone 615-331-6230. http://www.sa.org

Medications   Some medications block the effects of addictive drugs and relieve withdrawal symptoms. For example, methadone (METH-a-don) is a medication used to treat heroin withdrawal, while naltrexone (nal-TREK-zone) blocks the effects of heroin and related drugs. Other medications discourage the use of addictive drugs. For example, disulfiram (dy-SUL-fi-ram) works against alcohol use by causing severe nausea and other unpleasant symptoms when a person drinks alcohol.

Talk therapy   Several kinds of talk therapy (psychotherapy) are used to treat addiction. Cognitive (COG-ni-tiv) therapy targets the faulty thinking patterns that lead to alcohol and drug use. For example, people who think that alcohol protects them from pain may be helped to recognize the pain alcohol has caused them (such as loss of friends, work, self-esteem). People who use drinking as the only way to cope with problems may be helped to identify other ways to cope with problems. They are then helped to reconsider their old beliefs that alcohol is the only way to cope, and that drinking protects them from pain. By discovering that old beliefs are false, it is possible for them to decide what beliefs are more accurate. In this way, with time and effort, thinking patterns and false beliefs can change. Behavioral (bee-HAV-yor-al) therapy takes aim at negative forms of behavior, often by using a system of rewards and punishments to replace harmful behaviors with more positive ones. A teenager, for example, might get movie tickets for having a drug-free urine sample or lose the privilege of driving the car as a result of a setback. Behavioral therapy may also focus on identifying behaviors that keep a drug or alcohol problem in place (such as going to bars for recreation or spending time with friends who drink) and choosing behaviors that help beat the problem (going to the gym instead of a bar). Family therapy works on problems at home that may play a role in alcohol or drug abuse, such as conflict between family members. Family members may be taught to communicate better, or to solve problems more effectively.

Self-help groups   Self-help groups can be very helpful to people who are trying to deal with an addiction and to their family members. Many are 12-step groups, patterned on the 12 steps that are the guiding principles of Alcoholics Anonymous. Those who attend group meetings receive personal support from other people who are fighting the same addiction and winning.

Resources

Book

McLaughlin, Miriam Smith, and Sandra Peyser Hazouri. *Addiction: The "High" That Brings You Down*. Springfield, N.J.: Enslow Publishers, 1997.

Organizations

Alcoholics Anonymous, P.O. Box 459, New York, NY 10163. This oldest and largest 12-step group offers information about its program and referrals to local meetings.
Telephone 212-870-3400
http://www.alcoholics-anonymous.org

National Council on Alcoholism and Drug Dependence, 20 Exchange Place, Suite 2902, New York, NY 10005. This national organization provides information about alcohol and drug addiction and referrals to local support groups.
Telephone 800-NCA-CALL
http://www.ncadd.org

National Clearinghouse for Alcohol and Drug Information, P.O. Box 2345, Rockville, MD 20847-2345. This government clearinghouse is the world's largest resource for current information and materials on substance abuse and addiction.
Telephone 800-729-6686
http://www.health.org

National Institute on Alcohol Abuse and Alcoholism, 6000 Executive Boulevard, Bethesda, MD 20892-7003. This government institute provides in-depth information on alcohol abuse and addiction.
Telephone 301-443-3860
http://www.niaaa.nih.gov

National Institute on Drug Abuse, 6001 Executive Boulevard, Room 5213, Bethesda, MD 20892-9651. This government institute provides detailed information about drug abuse and addiction.
Telephone 301-443-1124
http://www.drugabuse.gov

Nemours Center for Children's Health Media, A. I. duPont Hospital for Children, 1600 Rockland Road, Wilmington, DE 19803. This organization is dedicated to issues of children's health. Their website has valuable information for children, teens, and parents on addiction and related topics.
http://www.kidshealth.org

▶ See also
Alcoholism
Hallucination
Substance Abuse
Therapy
Tobacco Addiction

Adjusting to Change *See* Anxiety and Anxiety Disorders; Death and Dying; Depression; Divorce; School Avoidance; Stress

Agoraphobia

Agoraphobia (a-go-ra-FO-bee-a) is an anxiety disorder that involves intense fear of having a panic (PA-nik) attack and avoidance of situations that a person fears may trigger a panic attack, such as leaving the home or being in a crowd. The effort to avoid such situations may greatly limit a person's life.

In Greek, the word agoraphobia means "fear of the marketplace." In English, the term is used to describe a disabling disorder that often leads people to fear being in crowds, standing in lines, going to shopping malls, or riding in cars, buses, or subways. In its most extreme form, the disorder can make people afraid of traveling beyond their neighborhoods or even stepping outside their homes. Put simply, agoraphobia is a fear of fear.

What Is Agoraphobia?

Agoraphobia refers to an intense, unreasonable, and long-lasting fear (a phobia) of panic attacks and avoidance of situations in which a panic attack might arise. A panic attack is a sudden surge of overwhelming terror that occurs unexpectedly and without good reason. The person is actually in no real danger. Although it is harmless, a panic attack can cause upsetting psychological symptoms, such as a feeling of unrealness and a fear of losing control, as well as unpleasant physical symptoms, such as a racing heart, sweating, trembling, shortness of breath, chest pain, upset stomach, and dizziness. People with agoraphobia have experienced panic attacks and are fearful about experiencing more attacks.

CHARLES DARWIN, AGORAPHOBIC

Charles Darwin (1809–1882), father of the theory of evolution, is one of the best-known figures in the history of science. Many people do not know, however, that Darwin suffered for much of his adult life from a strange illness that greatly limited his activities. Two modern scientists, writing in the *Journal of the American Medical Association,* suggested that this illness might have been agoraphobia. This would partly explain Darwin's lonely lifestyle and his trouble meeting with other people and speaking before groups.

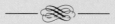

People with agoraphobia may limit themselves to being in places they think of as safe. Any movement beyond this safety zone leads to mounting worry and nervousness. They may worry about whether they could quickly escape from a certain place if they should begin to have a panic attack there. People with agoraphobia often avoid being on busy streets or in crowded classes or stores for fear that they might feel trapped if they start to have a panic attack. Gradually, the places that feel "safe" become fewer and fewer. Some people reach the point where they are too frightened even to leave their homes. Others still go out, but it causes great distress, and they may insist that family members or friends go with them. Such self-imposed limits can make it difficult for people to get on with their lives at school and work.

What Causes Agoraphobia?

Most people with agoraphobia experience the disorder after first having one or more panic attacks. Panic attacks usually strike unexpectedly, which makes it difficult for people to predict which situations will trigger them. This lack of predictability prompts people to worry about when the next attack will occur. It also teaches them to fear situations where attacks have happened in the past, even if this fear is unreasonable. As a result, people may begin avoiding such situations. Over time, avoidance actually can reinforce the person's phobia, making the condition worse.

What Are the Symptoms of Agoraphobia?

Agoraphobia typically starts between the ages of 18 and 35. Two-thirds of those affected are women. Most people with agoraphobia also have panic disorder, which means that they have repeated, unexpected panic attacks. A few do not have full-blown attacks, but they have similar symptoms of panic. Someone with agoraphobia may catastrophize (imagine the worst) about what could happen to them if they left home. For example, they may be afraid to leave home because they fear becoming dizzy, fainting, and then being left helpless on the ground. Without treatment, agoraphobia can cause misery for years.

How Is Agoraphobia Treated?

About one-third of people with panic disorder eventually go on to have agoraphobia, too. Treatment of panic disorder can help prevent agoraphobia. Once agoraphobia has set in, people still may be helped by the same kinds of medications and therapy used to treat panic disorder. People with agoraphobia may be helped by exposure therapy (a type of behavior therapy), in which they gradually are put in situations that frighten them until the fear begins to fade. Some therapists go to people's homes for the first few sessions, because someone with agoraphobia may not feel able to get to the therapist's office. Therapists who do exposure therapy also teach coping skills to help with anxiety. Exposure therapy may involve taking patients on short trips to shopping malls or other places that the patients have been avoiding. As people begin to spend more and more time in feared situations, using coping skills instead of avoidance, they may learn that they can handle their feelings after all.

Resources

Organizations

Anxiety Disorders Association of America, 11900 Parklawn Drive, Suite 100, Rockville, MD 20852. This nonprofit group promotes public awareness of agoraphobia and related disorders.
Telephone 301-231-9350
http://www.adaa.org

Anxiety Disorders Education Program, National Institute of Mental Health, 6001 Executive Boulevard, Room 8184, MSC 9663, Bethesda, MD 20892-9663. This government program provides reliable information about agoraphobia and related disorders.
Telephone 888-8ANXIETY
http://www.nimh.nih.gov/anxiety

KidsHealth.org is a website sponsored by the Nemours Foundation, created and maintained by the medical experts at A. I. duPont Hospital for Children, Wilmington, DE. It posts articles and information for kids, teens, and parents on a range of emotional concerns.
http://www.KidsHealth.org

▶ *See also*
Anxiety and Anxiety Disorders
Medications
Panic
Phobias
Therapy

KEYWORDS
for searching the Internet and other reference sources

Addiction

Alcohol dependence

Substance abuse

Alcoholism

Alcoholism (AL-ko-ha-li-zum) is a disease in which people crave alcohol and keep drinking even though it causes repeated problems in many parts of a person's life.

Jennifer had her first glass of champagne at a family wedding when she was 11. By the time she was 13, she was drinking beer with her friends on Saturday nights. At 15, she was locking herself in her room and drinking alone during the week, when she was supposed to be getting ready for school or doing her homework. At first, drinking seemed like an exciting thing to do. Before long, though, it became something she had to do just to get through the day. Jennifer was not old enough to get a driver's license, but she was already alcohol-dependent.

What Is Alcoholism?

Although many people do not think of it as one, alcohol is a drug. Alcoholism, also known as alcohol dependence, is really a drug addiction (a-DIK-shun), in which people have a strong craving to keep using alcohol even though it causes repeated problems at home, school, or work. The key traits of alcoholism are:

- **craving:** a strong need to drink
- **loss of control:** the inability to limit drinking
- **tolerance:** the need for ever-increasing amounts of alcohol in order to feel its effects
- **withdrawal:** physical symptoms that occur when alcohol use is stopped after a period of drinking.

Alcoholism has little to do with what kind of alcohol people drink, how long they have been drinking, or even how much they drink. What is important is the person's uncontrollable need for alcohol. This explains why it can be so hard for people with alcoholism to stop drinking, even if they try. They may feel the need for alcohol as strongly as other people feel the need for food and water. Although some people are able to break the grip of this powerful craving on their own, most need help to do so.

What Is Alcohol Abuse?

Alcohol abuse, like alcoholism, refers to an unhealthy pattern of alcohol use that leads to frequent, serious problems. Unlike alcoholism, it does not involve an extremely strong craving, a loss of control, or the physical signs of tolerance and withdrawal. In some ways, then, alcohol abuse is a less severe problem, but it still can have very serious effects. The key traits of alcohol abuse are:

- failing to meet responsibilities at home, school, or work, for example, neglecting chores at home or skipping classes due to drinking
- drinking in situations that are physically dangerous, for example, just before or while driving a car
- getting into alcohol-related trouble with the law, for example, being arrested for underage drinking, disorderly conduct, or DUI (driving under the influence)
- continuing to drink despite relationship problems that are caused or made worse by alcohol, for example, getting into arguments with parents or physical fights with friends or siblings.

Alcohol abuse can follow different patterns. Some people are binge drinkers, which means they drink only on certain days, such as on the weekend, when they have five or more drinks at one time. Binge drinkers

Fraternities Sober Up

College fraternity houses have long had an image as places where the alcohol flows freely. Even though not all fraternities deserve this reputation, when it is present, this hard-partying lifestyle has taken a terrible toll. For example:

- At Ohio Wesleyan University, a 20-year-old student died in a fraternity house fire. It has been reported that the student was drunk and may have been too confused to find his way out.
- At Clarkson University, 12 young men were charged in the death of a 17-year-old fraternity pledge (someone hoping to join). Reports indicated he had choked on his own vomit after drinking.

Deaths, injuries, assaults, and rapes are the dark side of too much drinking on campus. In addition, a study by researchers at the Harvard School of Public Health found that binge drinkers in college are 7 times as likely to miss classes and 10 times as likely to damage property as light drinkers. To combat these problems, many colleges now have alcohol-free fraternities, sororities, and dorms. They seem to be working. The Harvard study found that the number of college students choosing not to drink at all increased from 15 percent in 1993 to 19 percent in 1999.

often have accidents that hurt themselves or others or do things while drunk that they later regret. They also may go on to become heavy drinkers, which means they drink at this level on five or more days per month. Heavy drinkers, in turn, may go on to experience full-fledged alcoholism.

What Are the Short-Term Risks?

Alcohol dulls the senses, slows reaction time*, decreases coordination, and impairs judgment. It is little wonder that alcohol use is a major risk factor for accidents and injuries. Car crashes are the leading cause of death in 15- to 20-year-olds, and two of every five traffic deaths in this age group involve alcohol. Overall, people with alcoholism are nearly 5 times more likely than average to die in car crashes, 10 times more likely to be hurt in fires, and 16 times more likely to die in falls.

Alcohol robs people of their ability to think clearly. As a result, people are more likely to have unplanned sex when they have been drinking. This puts them at higher risk of unwanted pregnancy or sexually transmitted disease*. In addition, some boys still believe that it is okay to force a girl to have sex if she is drunk. As a result, girls who drink may run a greater risk of being raped by someone they know. Alcohol is involved in many cases of date rape.

What Are the Long-Term Risks?

Alcoholism not only disrupts people's lives but also destroys their health. Long-term, heavy drinking affects almost every organ in the body. The physical risks of alcoholism include:

- **Liver* disease:** More than 2 million Americans have an alcohol-related liver disease. Alcoholic hepatitis (he-pa-TY-tis) is inflammation of the liver, while alcoholic cirrhosis (si-RO-sis) is scarring of the liver. Alcohol-related liver disease can cause chronic illness and death.

- **Heart disease:** Long-term, heavy drinking raises the risk of high blood pressure, heart disease, and some kinds of stroke.

- **Cancer:** Long-term, heavy drinking also increases the risk of cancer of the mouth, throat, esophagus*, larynx*, stomach, pancreas*, liver, and possibly the colon* and rectum*. In addition, women who have two or more drinks per day have a slightly higher than average risk of breast cancer.

- **Pancreas disease:** Pancreatitis (pan-kree-a-TY-tis) is inflammation of the pancreas. It can cause severe abdominal pain, weight loss, and death.

- **Mental disorders:** Long-term, heavy use of alcohol can cause or worsen several mental disorders, especially depression and anxiety disorders.

*__reaction time__ is the time it takes a muscle or some other living tissue to respond to a stimulus.

*__sexually transmitted disease__ is an infection, such as the human immunodeficiency virus (HIV) or herpes, that can be passed from person to person by sexual contact.

*__liver__ is a large organ located in the upper abdomen that has many functions, including secreting the digestive fluid bile.

*__esophagus__ (eh-SAH-fa-gus) is the tube connecting the throat to the stomach.

*__larynx__ (LAYR-inks) is a structure in the throat, composed of muscle and cartilage and lined with a mucous membrane, that serves as the organ of voice.

*__pancreas__ is a large gland located in the upper abdomen that secretes various hormones and enzymes to help with digestion and metabolism.

*__colon__ is the part of the large intestine where stool is formed from waste.

*__rectum__ is the lower part of the large intestine, connecting the colon to the outside of the body. This is where stool is stored until is passes out of the body.

Alcohol also can interfere with the body's ability to absorb and use vitamins, especially the B vitamins. A lack of enough vitamins can damage the brain and cause problems with thought and memory. In severe cases, it can lead to Wernicke-Korsakoff (VER-ni-kee-KOR-sa-kof) syndrome, in which the ability to learn new information is seriously harmed.

How Are Women Affected?

Women get drunk more easily than men, even when differences in body weight are taken into account. This is because women's bodies contain less water per pound than men's bodies. Since alcohol mixes with body water, alcohol is closer to its full, undiluted strength in women than in men.

Women who drink during pregnancy can have children with a wide range of physical, mental, and behavioral problems. Fetal alcohol syndrome (FAS) is the most severe set of birth defects caused by alcohol. Children with FAS may have problems with eating, sleeping, vision, and hearing. They also may grow poorly and have birth defects of the heart, kidneys, skeleton, and other parts of the body. As children with FAS get older, they may have trouble following directions, learning to do simple things, and paying attention in school. They also may find it hard to get along with others and control their behavior. Since no one knows exactly how much alcohol it takes to cause birth defects, it is best not to drink any alcohol at all during pregnancy.

How Are Families Affected?

Living with or caring about a person with alcoholism can be very stressful. This is especially true for the 11 million children under age 18 in the United States who have an alcoholic parent. Alcohol use can lead to frequent arguments in the home, and it plays a role in the breakup of many marriages. In addition, alcohol use is a factor in more than half of all cases of family violence. It is not surprising that children of alcoholic parents are more likely to show signs of depression, anxiety, and low self-esteem than are other children. As they get older, they may have trouble in school, and they may tend to score lower on tests that measure verbal skills. They also may be more likely to have alcohol and drug problems of their own.

This does not mean that all children of alcoholic parents are doomed, however. Many do well and thrive, particularly if they have positive relationships with other people, such as friends in school, social groups, or at church, synagogue, or mosque. Support groups for family members and friends, such as Al-Anon and Alateen, also can help people learn to cope with someone else's drinking.

What Causes Alcoholism?

Millions of adults drink alcohol occasionally without any trouble. Yet as many as 1 in every 13 adults in the United States goes on to abuse alcohol or become alcohol-dependent. Alcohol problems are more common

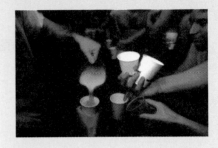

Students at a fraternity party crowd around a pitcher of beer. Binge drinking, or having several drinks in a row for the purpose of getting drunk, has become a growing problem on college campuses. Its effects can be serious, including alcohol poisoning, coma, and even death. *The Image Works*

News You Can Use on Booze

- Young people who start drinking before age 15 are four times more likely to become alcohol-dependent than those who delay drinking until age 21.

- The number of young people ages 12 through 17 who say they have drunk alcohol in the past month has dropped dramatically since the 1980s, from 41 percent in 1985 to 19 percent in 1998.

- Heavy or binge drinkers ages 12 to 17 are twice as likely to say their schoolwork is poor as are non-drinkers, and they are four to six times as likely to say they skip school or cut classes.

in men than in women, and they occur most often in young adults ages 18 through 29. Yet anyone of any age and either sex can be affected.

Many young people first start drinking as a way to escape their problems, feel accepted, or feel better about themselves. Those youngsters who move on to frequent or heavy drinking are more likely to be depressed, have low self-esteem, or feel as if they do not fit in. Pressure from friends and easy access to alcohol may make it more likely that drinking will get out of hand. Alcoholism also may tend to run in families. Children of alcoholic parents can be at risk for several reasons. They often live in stress-filled homes where heavy drinking might be seen as normal. In addition, the genetic* makeup of these children may raise their risk of alcoholism.

*genetic (je-NE-tik) pertains to genes, which are chemicals in the body that help determine a person's characteristics, such as hair or eye color. They are inherited from a person's parents.

What Are the Signs of Alcoholism?

Warning signs include:

- **Being preoccupied with drinking:** People with alcoholism generally are always thinking about their next drink.
- **Viewing alcohol as a cure-all:** People with alcoholism may drink to steady their nerves, treat a hangover, or "fix" almost any problem.
- **Needing to drink increasing amounts to feel high:** People with alcoholism often must drink ever-increasing amounts to get the desired effect.
- **Losing control over drinking:** Although they may try, people with alcoholism typically cannot limit themselves to one or two drinks.
- **Drinking alone:** Social drinkers enjoy the company of others. People who are alcohol-dependent enjoy the alcohol itself.
- **Needing to drink to feel normal:** People with alcoholism usually feel as if they must drink just to cope with their everyday lives.
- **Feeling guilty and making excuses:** People with alcoholism often blame their drinking on other people or on outside events.
- **Having blackouts:** People with alcoholism may be unable to remember what happened while they were drinking, which is sometimes called "alcohol amnesia."

How Is Alcoholism Treated?

Alcoholism is a treatable disease. Treatment often begins with detoxification, the process of safely getting all the alcohol out of a person's body. During the first days after drinking is stopped, people may be given medication by a physician to replace the alcohol and then gradually be weaned off the medication over a period of about a week. The goal is to reduce withdrawal symptoms and restore good health. Rest, a balanced diet, and plenty of fluids also are stressed.

Medications Once detoxification is complete, some people take medications to help prevent a return to drinking. Disulfiram (dy-SUL-fi-ram; Antabuse) can help deter alcohol use by causing several unpleasant symptoms when a person drinks alcohol, including severe nausea, vomiting, hot flushing, headache, and anxiety. Naltrexone (nal-TREK-zone; ReVia) is another medication that sometimes is given to people with alcoholism. Scientists think it may block the craving for more that these people usually feel after taking a first drink.

Therapy Various kinds of therapy are used to treat alcoholism. Therapy can help people identify the feelings and situations that trigger their drinking. It also can help them find new ways to cope that do not involve using alcohol. Therapy can be provided individually or in a group, and it can take place in a mental health center or a hospital. Social skills training teaches people to handle social situations better. Behavioral therapy helps people learn to control harmful behavior and the impulse to drink. Family therapy focuses on problems at home that may play a role in alcohol use, such as drinking by family members.

Self-help groups Most treatment programs include meetings of Alcoholics Anonymous or other self-help groups. People who take part in such groups get help and support from others who have faced the same problems. Membership is open to anyone with a desire to stop drinking. Alcoholics Anonymous has more than 50,000 groups with more than 1 million members in the United States alone.

How Well Does Treatment Work?

Alcoholism can be a tough addiction to beat, but treatment can be very helpful. Studies have shown that 7 of 10 alcohol-dependent people who get treatment have stopped or cut back on their drinking and improved their health within 6 months. The goal of treatment is to quit drinking entirely, but most people have at least one or two slips before they reach this goal. Such slips are common, and they do not mean that people have failed. They just mean that people must stop drinking again and get whatever help they need to give up the habit. The longer people go without drinking, the more likely it is that they will stay sober for good.

Resources

Organizations

Al-Anon/Alateen, 1600 Corporate Landing Parkway, Virginia Beach, VA 23454-5617. Al-Anon is an international self-help group for family

Don't Get Even. Get MADD.

MADD (Mothers Against Drunk Driving) is a national nonprofit group that aims to stop drunk driving and prevent underage drinking. It was founded by a group of California women in 1980 after a hit-and-run drunk driver killed a 13-year-old girl. The driver had been out of jail on bail for only two days for another hit-and-run crash, and he had three previous arrests (and two convictions) for drunk driving. The concerned women started a crusade to get drivers such as this one off the road. Today MADD has more than 600 chapters nationwide.

members and friends of people with alcoholism. Alateen is a group especially for teenagers affected by someone else's drinking.
Telephone 888-4AL-ANON
http://www.al-anon.alateen.org

Alcoholics Anonymous, Grand Central Station, P.O. Box 459, New York, NY 10163. This large, worldwide self-help group for alcoholics offers information about its program and referrals to local meetings.
Telephone 212-870-3400
http://www.alcoholics-anonymous.org

Mothers Against Drunk Driving (MADD), P.O. Box 541688, Dallas, TX 75354-1688. This nonprofit group works to stop drunk driving, support victims of this crime, and prevent underage drinking.
Telephone 800-GET-MADD
http://www.madd.org

National Association for Children of Alcoholics, 11426 Rockville Pike, Suite 100, Rockville, MD 20852. This organization works on behalf of children affected by a parent's alcohol or drug abuse. They offer videos and booklets on their website.
Telephone 888-55-4COAS
http://www.health.org/nacoa

National Council on Alcoholism and Drug Dependence, 20 Exchange Place, Suite 2902, New York, NY 10005. This national organization provides information about alcoholism and referrals to local groups.
Telephone 800-NCA-CALL
http://www.ncadd.org

National Clearinghouse for Alcohol and Drug Information, 11426-48 Rockville Pike, Suite 200, Rockville, MD 20852. This government clearinghouse offers current information and materials on alcohol abuse and alcoholism.
Telephone 800-729-6686
http://www.health.org

National Institute on Alcohol Abuse and Alcoholism, 6000 Executive Boulevard, Bethesda, MD 20892-7003. This government institute provides in-depth information on alcohol abuse and alcoholism.
Telephone 301-443-3860
http://www.niaaa.nih.gov

▶ *See also*
Addiction
Rape
Substance Abuse
Therapy

Alzheimer Disease

Alzheimer (ALTS-hy-mer) disease (commonly called Alzheimer's disease) is a condition in which abnormal structures (called plaques and tangles) form in the brain, accumulating over time and interfering with nerve cell connections. The disease leads to problems with memory and thinking and to changes in personality and behavior, called dementia (de-MEN-sha).

KEYWORDS
for searching the Internet and other reference sources

Dementia

Memory loss

Alzheimer *Not* Oldtimer's

Alzheimer disease is named after Alois Alzheimer, the German physician who first described it in the early part of the twentieth century. Some people mistakenly call this condition "oldtimer's disease." Their mistake reflects the fact that it usually affects people age 65 and older, with advancing age being the single biggest risk factor for the disease. (There is an early-onset form of Alzheimer disease that strikes middle-aged adults in their thirties, forties, or fifties, often affecting several members of the same family. This form of the disease is much less common.) Experts estimate that 1 in 10 to 1 in 20 Americans over age 65 have Alzheimer disease, which translates to about 4 million people. Since people are living

---

ALOIS ALZHEIMER

In 1907, the German physician Alois Alzheimer published an article on what he called a "new disease of the [brain] cortex." Little did he know that it would be named after him! In that article, he described the increasingly bizarre behavior of a 51-year-old patient and went on to describe what he found upon examining her brain after death. Here are Alzheimer's key observations, in his own words:

"The woman, 51 years of age, showed as her first symptom a jealousy towards her husband. Soon she showed a rapidly increasing amnesia; she became lost in her own apartment, carried objects about aimlessly, hid them, sometimes believed she was to be murdered, and had spells of unrestrained screaming. . . . The autopsy showed a diffusely atrophied brain . . . remarkable changes of the neurofibrillae. In place of a normal cell, one or several fibrillae, which ran parallel to each other, were altered in a similar fashion. Over the entire brain, and especially in the upper layers, miliary centers appear, which were caused by an unusual substance . . . The glia became fibrous, and many glia cells showed fatty deposits. . . . Apparently we are dealing with an unidentified illness."

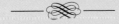

longer than ever, as many as 14 million Americans may have this disease by the year 2050.

In Alzheimer disease, structures called plaques and tangles form in the cerebral (se-REE-bral) cortex (KOR-teks), which is the outer surface of the brain, as well as in the brain matter just under the cortex. The cortex has several functional areas, including those involved with vision, hearing, speech understanding, and bodily awareness. These structures interfere with the normal functioning of the neurons (NU-rons), or nerve cells, and the transmission of messages between the brain and other parts of the body. Although these plaques and tangles occur to some extent with normal aging, they are much more prevalent in people who have Alzheimer disease. It is important to keep in mind that this disease is *not* a normal part of getting older.

At first, the condition usually hinders certain aspects of immediate memory. For example, a person might consistently forget where certain key possessions are, leave a boiling pot or kettle on the stove, or repeat the same stories. Gradually, symptoms worsen, affecting a greater portion of a person's memory and then, quite often, personality, decision-making abilities, and language skills. Everyday activities, such as working at a job, driving a car, keeping house, balancing a checkbook, and participating in social activities, become impossible. As the disease advances, people who have it seem less and less "like themselves," often showing drastic mood swings, unpredictable changes in temperament, inability to recognize loved ones, and increasing helplessness. At this point, people with Alzheimer disease usually need full-time care.

Causes, Diagnosis, and Treatment of Alzheimer Disease

Doctors are not sure what causes Alzheimer disease, and they do not have a simple test for diagnosing it. No treatments have proved effective in

These positron emission tomography (PET) scans show the dramatic difference in brain activity between a healthy person (*left*) and a person with Alzheimer disease (*right*). Brain activity, indicated by red and yellow, has been greatly reduced in the brain at right. *Photo Researchers, Inc.*

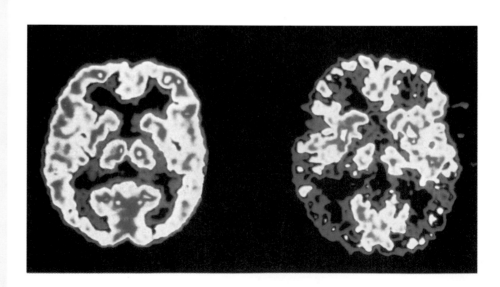

curing it. Neuroscience researchers are actively investigating these areas. They have discovered certain therapies that appear to help with the symptoms of Alzheimer disease. For example, the Food and Drug Administration has approved drugs that help slow memory loss and lessen other disease symptoms. These drugs increase the brain's level of acetycholine [a-see-til-KO-leen], a brain chemical involved in sending messages from nerve cell to nerve cell to allow the brain to function normally.

At present, Alzheimer disease is diagnosed based on a person's symptoms and by ruling out other possible causes. While there is no single test to show that a person has the disease, doctors now have access to technological methods that may prove very useful in diagnosing it. Using computerized tomography* scans and other special brain imaging techniques, doctors can examine the structure, blood flow, and metabolic activity* of the brain. These tests can help show the presence of Alzheimer disease.

The causes of Alzheimer disease largely remain a mystery, except in the less common early-onset form of the disease, which is clearly linked to genes*. For the more common form of the disease, researchers have not been able to trace a clear link to heredity or to other factors, such as dietary habits, occupation, personality type, or environmental factors. Researchers are working to identify how a person's genetic makeup and environmental factors might interact to cause this condition. At present, there is nothing a person can do to prevent Alzheimer disease, nor are there any tests available to predict whether someone will get the disease. Research in these areas may yield useful treatments for Alzheimer disease and maybe even a vaccine to prevent the disease.

Resources

Books

Klein, Norma. *Going Backwards*. New York: Scholastic, 1986. In this novel for young adults, family dynamics are strained when Grandmother Gustel, who has Alzheimer disease, moves in. Although Charles, a high school senior, tries to cope with his grandmother's disease, his father refuses to recognize the problem.

Wilkinson, Beth. *Coping When a Grandparent Has Alzheimer's Disease*. New York: Rosen Publishing Group, 1995.

Organizations

Alzheimer's Association, 919 North Michigan Avenue, Suite 1100, Chicago, IL 60611-1676. This health organization funds research into the causes, treatment, and prevention of Alzheimer disease and provides education and support to people affected with the disease and their families through a national network of chapters.

*computerized tomography (CT), also called computerized axial tomography, is a computer imaging technique using x-rays. These CT scans take images of "slices" of the body and brain (which do not involve actual cutting). Doctors can view these detailed images to find out what is going on inside a person.

*metabolic activity refers to the process in the body that converts food into energy and waste products.

*genes are chemicals in the body that help determine a person's characteristics, such as hair or eye color. They are inherited from a person's parents and are contained in the chromosomes, threadlike structures inside the cells of the body.

Telephone 800-272-3900
http://www.alz.org

Alzheimer's Disease Education and Referral Center, National Institute on Aging, National Institutes of Health, P.O Box 8250, Silver Spring, MD 20907-8250. This center, a service of the U.S. government, provides research updates and referrals on its website.
800-438-4380
http://www.alzheimers.org

Neuroscience for Kids is a website maintained by Associate Professor Eric Chudler at the University of Washington, Seattle. It features easy-to-understand information on a range of topics related to the brain and nervous system, including Alzheimer disease. The website gives an extensive bibliography of readings for children and teens.
http://faculty.washington.edu/chudler/alz.html

▶ *See also*
The Brain and Nervous System (Introduction)
Dementia
Memory

KEYWORDS
for searching the Internet and other reference sources

Brain injury

Concussion

Memory loss

Amnesia

Amnesia (am-NEE-zha) is loss of memory.

What would it be like to wake up one morning and not know who you are, not recognize your home or your parents, or not be able to account for your actions in the past days? This image of amnesia has been the basis of many movies and books. Amnesia is a gap in a person's memory. Although a short period of amnesia is fairly common, especially after a head injury, true amnesia is rarely as dramatic and extensive as it is portrayed by writers and filmmakers.

Types of Amnesia

There are three distinct phases to memory: registering the event in the brain, storing the information, and retrieving the information that has been stored. Problems in any of these phases may cause amnesia. The source of the problem can be either physical or psychological. The memory gap can be of events either before or after the trauma or other problem triggering the amnesia, and it may be temporary or permanent. There are several distinct types of amnesia:

■ Anterograde amnesia is the inability to learn new information. A person with this type of amnesia can accurately recall events in the past, before the trauma, but has marked difficulty remembering any new information for more than a few minutes.

- Retrograde amnesia is the partial or complete loss of memory of events that occurred before the trauma. New information, however, can be processed, stored, and recalled correctly.

- Transient global amnesia is a form of memory loss that appears suddenly and causes confusion, disorientation, and forgetfulness for 30 minutes to 24 hours. This type of memory loss normally clears up on its own, but a person experiencing transient global amnesia also may experience temporary retrograde amnesia.

What Causes Amnesia?

Most often, amnesia has a physical cause. The leading cause of amnesia is an injury to the head. For example, a hockey player who falls and hits his head hard on the ice may be unable to recall the events, or their sequence, immediately before he fell. A head injury that leads to temporary loss of consciousness or amnesia is called a concussion (kun-KUH-shun). Retrograde amnesia, either permanent or temporary, is very common in people who are in car accidents. People who have head injuries in a car accident rarely, if ever, remember the accident. While the body may heal, the retrograde amnesia usually is permanent.

There are other physical causes of amnesia, for example, when there is not enough blood flow to the brain (which is thought to be the usual cause of transient global amnesia), or when there is brain cell damage from long-term alcohol abuse. This condition, called Wernicke-Korsakoff (VER-ni-kee-KOR-sa-kof) syndrome, often produces anterograde amnesia. Malnutrition and brain infections are other physical conditions that may produce amnesia. People with Alzheimer disease frequently have amnesia, which is thought to be caused by physical changes in the brain. Treatment for amnesia involves treating the condition causing it, if possible.

When amnesia has psychological causes, it is called psychogenic (sy-ko-JEN-ik) amnesia. This type of amnesia is not common. It may occur when a person suffers a physically or emotionally overwhelming event or trauma (for example, witnessing the murder of a loved one). The memories of the traumatic event and the circumstances surrounding it are so upsetting that they are repressed. The repression is not done consciously, and it may be temporary or permanent. Treatment involves psychotherapy*. The use of hypnosis to recover lost memories is controversial since in some cases the "recovered" memory may not be real, but the result of suggestion by the hypnotist.

Resources

Article

"The Man Who Lost Himself." *World Press Review,* 44, no. 6 (June 1997): 36.

*psychotherapy (sy-ko-THER-a-pea) is the treatment of mental and behavioral disorders by support and insight to encourage healthy behavior patterns and personality growth.

KEYWORDS
for searching the Internet and other reference sources

Eating disorders

Food and nutrition

Weight loss

*****eating disorder** is a condition in which a person's eating behaviors and food habits are so unbalanced that they cause physical and emotional problems.

Organization

National Institute of Mental Health, 6001 Executive Boulevard, Room 8184, MSC 9663, Bethesda, MD 20892-9663. This government agency does research on amnesia and how the brain works and provides information to the public through pamphlets and their website.
Telephone 800-421-4211
http://www.nimh.nih.gov

Anger *See* Emotions

Anorexia

Anorexia (an-o-REK-see-a) is an eating disorder* involving excessive dieting, preoccupation with food, distorted body image, fear of getting fat, and rapid, significant weight loss. The disorder primarily affects young women.

Wendy has been taking ballet since she was 5. For as long as she can remember, her dream has been to dance professionally after she graduates from high school. This spring, the young dancer's company will perform the ballet *Swan Lake,* and Wendy hopes to be chosen for the lead part.

But since she turned 13 last summer, Wendy has noticed that her figure has started to round out. Constantly in front of the mirror in the dance studio, Wendy cannot help seeing every new curve of her body, and she feels self-conscious about how her growing breasts look in her skintight dancewear. She is worried about gaining weight. What if she becomes too heavy for her dance partner to lift? With try-outs for the spring ballet coming up soon, Wendy fears a tinier dancer will be chosen for the lead instead of her. Lately, she has been wishing for the body she had at 11: tiny and light, like the "perfect" ballerina she dreams of being.

For the past month, Wendy has been on a crash diet, keeping a strict record of everything she eats. She weighs herself morning and night. When there is time, she jogs after dance class. She is relieved to have lost some weight and wants to keep going. She has been allowing herself only the tiniest portions of food and has started to skip lunch altogether. Pleased with her weight loss so far, she decides to cut back to just a small salad for dinner and maybe just a yogurt for breakfast.

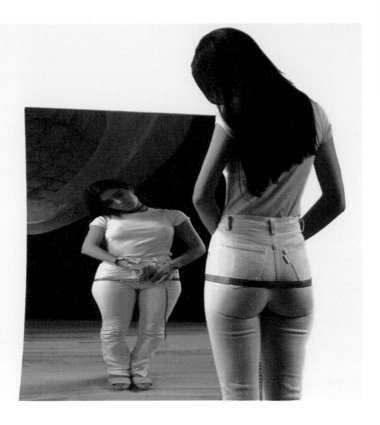

An anorexic person has a distorted perception of what her body actually looks like. She may lose a little weight from a normal diet, gain positive attention from people around her, and then become obsessed with losing more and more weight. But no matter how thin she gets, she still sees her body as unacceptable and unattractive. *Photo Researchers, Inc.*

Fear of Fat

No one sets out to have anorexia. It takes hold slowly and might start with a simple desire to lose a few pounds. However, in fully developed cases, people with anorexia are malnourished, often depressed, obsessed with food or exercise, and still are convinced that they are fat.

People with anorexia refuse to eat enough food to maintain normal healthy body weight. Because they fear getting fat, people with anorexia use extreme dieting to lose a lot of weight rapidly. They also may exercise excessively to burn off calories. People with anorexia lose at least 15 to 20 percent of their normal body weight. For example, a girl who starts out at 130 pounds might drop to 100 pounds. Anorexia involves a distorted awareness of the body. People with this condition become preoccupied with thinness and may continue to believe that they are fat even though others around them may see them as unnaturally thin. Over time, the weight that people with anorexia want so desperately to control can become frighteningly out of control for them.

Anorexia is much more common among girls (90 to 95 percent of cases), but boys can have it too. At least 1 in 100 young women in the United States have anorexia, and the disorder usually begins during adolescence. Girls who participate in activities that value thinness, such as dancing, gymnastics, or figure skating, are at higher risk than others for developing anorexia.

*****period**, or **menstruation** (men-stroo-AY-shun), refers to the monthly flow, or discharge, of the blood-enriched lining of the uterus that normally occurs in women who are physically mature enough to bear children. Most girls have their first period between the ages of 9 and 16. Because it usually occurs at four-week intervals, it is often called the "monthly period."

What Causes Anorexia?

No single factor causes anorexia. Emotional problems, family difficulties, social pressure, and biological variability all play a role. Contemporary society's glamorization of thinness influences many girls to diet excessively. Once started, some extreme dieting practices can be hard to stop. Girls who have a high need for perfection and control may see dieting as a way to be the prettiest, thinnest, and most perfect of their peers, or to live up their parents' expectations for perfection, or to look as perfect as models or stars they admire. Girls with anorexia tend to come from loving, highly controlled families. A girl who feels that she does not have enough independence may use control of eating as a way to assert herself. In other cases, anorexia may develop because of pressure to be extra-thin when certain sports or activities demand it.

What Can Happen When Someone Has Anorexia?

Anorexia can cause a number of serious medical problems, such as disturbed heart rhythms and vitamin and mineral deficiencies that can harm vital organs. With anorexia, the body is literally starving. Bone and muscle begin to waste away. Blood pressure and body temperature drop because the body cannot maintain them properly. Hair, nails, and skin become dry and brittle. Girls with anorexia often stop getting their periods*,

---

ATHLETES AND ANOREXIA

Girls and young women involved in sports that place a high value on thinness are three times more likely than others to develop anorexia or bulimia (bu-LEE-me-a; binge eating followed by vomiting or other methods of emptying the stomach). A 1992 study conducted by the American College of Sports Medicine estimated that as many as 62 percent of females involved in sports like gymnastics and figure skating struggled with eating disorders. Many well-known athletes have spoken out about their battles with eating disorders, including gymnasts and Olympic gold medal winners Nadia Comaneci and Kathy Rigby. Christy Henrich, who in 1989 was ranked the #2 gymnast in the United States, died from complications of anorexia in 1994 at the age of 22. The pressure to be thin does not appear to be easing up. The average gymnast in 1976 was 5'3" tall and weighed 105 pounds; the average gymnast in 1992 was 4'9" tall and weighed 88 pounds.

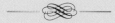

---

and overall body growth and development can begin to slow down. Without treatment, anorexia can cause irreversible damage to the body. It can lead to heart failure* and sometimes death. In the United States, about 1,000 young women die each year from complications of anorexia.

What Can Be Done About Anorexia?

There is help for people with anorexia, but it sometimes takes others to convince people with this problem that they need help. Family members or friends may ask about the weight loss. A girl with anorexia may be ashamed or self-conscious and may say she does not have a problem. Many girls with anorexia resist getting help because they do not want to gain weight. Seeking help sooner, rather than later, can be life-saving, but the distorted body image that is part of anorexia can make it hard for people with the condition to realize how dangerously thin they are.

Treatment for anorexia typically includes several parts and a few different health professionals. Treatment may begin with a medical visit to evaluate nutritional status and overall health. The doctor may ask about weight loss, order blood tests, and ask about the patient's eating habits and feelings about her body. Nutritional counseling helps with planning and following a healthy diet. Individual psychotherapy allows the person to talk about feelings and problems that led up to the anorexia, come up with new solutions, and work on body image. Group therapy brings together people with similar concerns to share their experiences and receive support. Medications are sometimes used to reduce anxiety* and depression*. If a person with anorexia is in a severe health crisis, she may have to be hospitalized to stabilize her medical condition and become better nourished before other aspects of treatment can begin.

Resources

Books

Berg, Frances M. *Afraid to Eat: Children and Teens in Weight Crisis.* Hettinger, ND: Healthy Weight Journal, 1997.

Brumberg, Joan Jacobs. *Fasting Girls: The History of Anorexia Nervosa.* New York: Vintage Books, 2000.

Levenkron, Steven. *Anatomy of Anorexia.* New York: W. W. Norton and Company, 2001.

Organizations

American Anorexia Bulimia Association, Inc., 165 West 46th Street, Suite 1108, New York, NY 10036.
Telephone 212-575-6200
http://aabainc.org

* **heart failure** is a medical term used to describe a condition in which a damaged heart cannot pump enough blood to meet the oxygen and nutrient demands of the body. People with heart failure may find it hard to exercise due to the insufficient blood flow, but many people live a long time with heart failure.

* **anxiety** can be experienced as a troubled feeling, a sense of dread, fear of the future, or distress over a possible threat to a person's physical or mental well-being.

* **depression** (de-PRESH-un) is a mental state characterized by feelings of sadness, despair, and discouragement.

Eating Disorders Awareness and Prevention, Inc. (EDAP), 603 Stewart Street, Suite 803, Seattle, WA 98101.
Telephone: (800) 931-2237 for toll-free information and referral hotline
http://www.edap.org

National Association of Anorexia Nervosa and Associated Disorders (ANAD), P.O. Box 7, Highland Park, IL 60035.
Telephone 807-831-3438
http://anad.org

TeensHealth.org, a website sponsored by the Nemours Foundation and the Alfred I. duPont Hospital for Children, Wilmington, DE, contains information about anorexia and other eating disorders.
http://www.teenshealth.org

▶ *See also*
Binge Eating Disorder
Body Dysmorphic Disorder
Body Image
Bulimia
Eating Disorders
Peer Pressure

KEYWORDS
for searching the Internet and other reference sources
Antisocial behaviors
Disruptive behaviors
Personality disorders

* **personality disorders** are a group of mental disorders characterized by long-term patterns of behavior that differ from those expected by society. People with personality disorders have patterns of emotional response, impulse control, and perception that differ from those of most people.

* **impulsive** means acting quickly before thinking about the effect of a certain action or behavior.

* **conduct disorder** is diagnosed in children and adolescents who have had serious problems with lying, stealing, and aggressive behavior for at least 6 months.

* **antisocial behaviors** are behaviors that differ significantly from the norms of society and are considered harmful to society.

Antisocial Personality Disorder

Antisocial personality disorder (APD) is an ongoing pattern of behavior in an adult that involves disregard for social rules and serious violation of the rights of others through aggressive, dishonest, reckless, and irresponsible acts.

What Is Antisocial Personality Disorder?

Antisocial personality disorder (APD) is one of the ten different types of personality disorders* that are currently classified by mental health experts. Like other personality disorders, APD refers to a personality style that consists of troubled ways of thinking, feeling, and behaving, and it is diagnosed only in adults (but the personality style and the problematic behavior it causes must have been present since adolescence). Of all the personality disorders, APD has been the focus of the most research and attention, perhaps because people with APD often cause harm to others and have a negative effect on society.

Adults with APD engage in aggressiveness or physical assaults, cheating, lying, or other behaviors for which they can get arrested. They are often impulsive* and reckless and disregard their own safety or the safety of others. People with APD tend to be poor planners, and they may ignore financial responsibilities like paying rent or other bills. They often have poor work records and many engage in impulsive criminal behavior or spousal abuse. To be diagnosed with APD, a person must have had symptoms of conduct disorder* since the age of 15, thus demonstrating a long-standing pattern of antisocial behaviors*.

APD was first described in the 1800s as a "defect of moral character" and as "moral insanity." The terms psychopath and sociopath have also been used to describe what is now called antisocial personality disorder. Those with APD seem to lack a conscience and fail to learn from consequences or punishment alone. They may fail to show remorse and may lack sympathy for those they have hurt. People with APD may experience most emotions at a shallow level.

What Causes Antisocial Personality Disorder?

Antisocial behavior tends to run in families. Researchers have tried to determine how much of this tendency is due to genetics and biology and how much is learned behavior. Some studies have identified certain brain problems and learning defects in people with APD. For example, researchers have found that areas of the brain that are involved in thinking ahead and in considering the consequences of one's actions may be different in people with APD. This finding lends evidence to the theory that an inherited brain problem may contribute to the poor planning and impulsivity that are characteristic of people with APD.

Other studies have found differences in the brains of people with APD that may contribute to disordered learning and attention. One series of experiments demonstrated that people with antisocial personalities did not experience normal anxiety before being given a shock and that they did not learn to avoid the shock like other subjects in the experiment did. This may explain why people with APD do not seem to learn from negative consequences or punishment.

Research that separates genetic from environmental factors (for example, studies of identical twins raised in different homes) has shown that genetic factors explain about half of antisocial behavior. Family environment or upbringing plays an important role as well. Experts currently believe that a combination of genetic inheritance and environmental factors lead to most cases of APD. In other words, some people seem to have a biological tendency to develop APD and the family environment will determine whether or not that tendency is fulfilled. People without the biological tendency for APD, regardless of the family environment in which they are raised, are not likely to develop APD as an adult (although they may have conduct disorder as a youth).

How Is Antisocial Personality Disorder Treated?

Treatment of APD presents a challenge because those with APD are unlikely to consider themselves as having a problem and are therefore unlikely to seek help. Without motivation to change one's own behavior, it is unlikely that any meaningful change will take place. Because people with APD tend to violate the rights of others, they often encounter the criminal justice system. Though they may be imprisoned, punishment alone usually fails to teach someone with APD to behave differently. Still, APD is a serious social problem. Some early interventions may help prevent APD from developing in those at risk, such as youth with severe conduct disorders and those who are juvenile offenders.

KEYWORDS
for searching the Internet and other reference sources

Generalized anxiety disorder

Obsessive-compulsive disorder

Panic disorder

Phobias

Separation anxiety disorder

Anxiety Attack

The percentage of people in the United States affected by anxiety disorders during a one-year period:

- all anxiety disorders: 13 percent

- phobias: 8 percent

- post-traumatic stress disorder: 4 percent

- generalized anxiety disorder: 3 percent

- obsessive-compulsive disorder: 2 percent

- panic disorder: 2 percent

These figures add up to more than 13 percent because some people have more than one kind of anxiety disorder.

Resources

Organizations

The Personality Disorders Foundation has a website that provides information about personality disorders.
http://pdf.uchc.edu/

The American Psychological Association has a website that provides information about personality disorders.
http://www.apa.org

Anxiety and Anxiety Disorders

Anxiety (ang-ZY-e-tee) is a feeling of fear, worry, or nervousness that occurs for no apparent reason. Anxiety disorders are conditions in which anxiety becomes so intense and long-lasting that it causes serious distress, and may lead to problems at home, school, or work.

On the first day of ninth grade, when Michelle started high school, she suddenly felt dizzy, sweaty, and short of breath when she walked down the hall toward her locker. For a few minutes, everything around her seemed strangely unreal. At first, Michelle thought it was just a little case of nerves. However, when the feelings returned the next day and the next, Michelle began to fear that she was losing control of her mind or that she had some terrible physical illness. In fact, Michelle was suffering from an anxiety disorder.

What Are Anxiety Disorders?

Everybody feels a little nervous now and then. Their palms may get sweaty when they take an important test, their heart may pound as they wait for the opening kickoff of a big game, or they may have butterflies in their stomach as they get ready for a first date. These feelings are perfectly normal. People with anxiety disorders, however, feel afraid, worried, or nervous even when there is no clear reason. Their feelings are intense and long lasting, and they may get worse over time. The feelings are very distressing to a person experiencing them, and can be so overwhelming that they can cause serious problems at home, school, or work.

Anxiety disorders are the most common of all mental disorders. All told, some type of anxiety disorder affects more than 19 million people in the United States. There are several different types of anxiety disorders.

Generalized anxiety disorder Generalized anxiety is a term for constant, intense worry and stress over a variety of everyday events and situations. People who experience generalized anxiety always expect the worst to happen, even when there is no real reason for thinking this way. For example, they may worry all the time about their grades or sports performance, even when they are successful students or athletes. They may worry about loved ones, about the future, school, health, safety, or upsetting things they imagine could happen. These feelings may be accompanied by physical symptoms, such as tiredness, chest pain, trembling, tight muscles, headache, or upset stomach. When someone has experienced these symptoms for 6 months or longer, a mental health professional uses the diagnosis generalized anxiety disorder to describe their condition.

Separation anxiety disorder   Separation anxiety is the normal fear that babies and young children feel when they are separated from their parents or approached by strangers. It is not uncommon for children to have mild separation anxiety on the first day of school in kindergarten or first grade, or the first day of overnight camp. Usually, this feeling goes away after a few days as a child gets used to a new situation, new friends, and new adults in charge. For most children, separation anxiety lessens with age and experience. In some children, however, this normal fear turns into separation anxiety disorder, which is extreme fearfulness anytime the children are away from their parents or home. Children with this disorder may call their parents at work often, be afraid to sleep over at friends' houses, or suffer extreme homesickness at camp. Separation anxiety disorder can result in frequent absences from school and avoidance of participation in normal social activities of childhood that involve being without their parents. Children with separation anxiety disorder tend to worry and they may be very afraid that their parents will get sick or be injured, or they may have frequent nightmares about getting lost.

Separation anxiety can carry over into the teenage years as well. Teenagers with separation anxiety may be uneasy about leaving home, and they sometimes start refusing to go to school. Extreme separation anxiety may be triggered by a change in school, or it may occur after a stressful event at home, such as a divorce, illness, or death in the family.

Panic disorder   Panic disorder is a disorder that involves repeated attacks of intense fear that strike often and without warning. People having a panic attack may feel as if things are unreal, or they may fear that they are going to die. Along with the fear, they may have physical symptoms, such as chest pain, a pounding heart, shortness of breath, dizziness, or an upset stomach.

Obsessive-compulsive disorder   Obsessive-compulsive (ub-SES-iv-kum-PUL-siv) disorder (OCD) is a condition in which people become trapped in a pattern of repeated, unwanted, upsetting thoughts, called obsessions (ob-SESH-unz), and behaviors, called compulsions (kom-PUL-shunz). The thoughts or behaviors seem impossible to control or stop.

Nothing to Fear

Not every fear is a phobia. Fears are not considered phobias unless they cause long-lasting, serious problems. Many fears are typical at different times of development. Common normal fears include:

- birth to 6 months: loss of physical support (fear of falling), loud noises, large fast-approaching objects, or sudden movement
- 7 to 12 months: strangers
- 1 to 5 years: loud noises, storms, animals, darkness, separation from parents
- 3 to 5 years: monsters, ghosts
- 6 to 12 years: injury, burglars, being sent to the principal, punishment, failure
- 12 to 18 years: tests in school, embarrassment

* **depression** (de-PRESH-un) is a mental state characterized by feelings of sadness, despair, and discouragement.

* **genes** are chemicals in the body that help determine a person's characteristics, such as hair or eye color. They are inherited from a person's parents and are contained in the chromosomes found in the cells of the body.

Examples of common obsessions include worrying constantly about germs, whether the house is locked, and if a loved one is safe. Examples of common compulsions include washing the hands repeatedly, checking the door lock over and over again, and saying something over and over to "keep a person safe."

Phobias   Phobias (FO-bee-uhz) are unrealistic, long-lasting fears of some object or situation. The fear can be so intense that people go to great lengths to avoid the object of their dread. There are three types of phobia problems that mental health professionals may diagnose. They are specific phobias, social phobia (also called social anxiety disorder), and agoraphobia (AG-or-uh-FO-bee-uh). People with specific phobias have an intense fear of specific objects or situations that pose little real threat, such as dogs, spiders, storms, water, or heights. People with social phobia have an extreme fear of being judged harshly, embarrassed, or criticized by others, which leads them to avoid social situations. People with agoraphobia are terrified of having a panic attack in a public situation from which it would be hard to escape, such as standing in a crowd. If left untreated, the anxiety can become so severe that people might refuse to leave the house.

Post-traumatic stress disorder   Post-traumatic stress disorder involves long-lasting symptoms that occur after people have been through an extremely stressful, life-threatening event, such as a rape, mugging, child abuse, tornado, or car crash. People with the disorder may relive the traumatic event again and again in strong memories or nightmares. They may have other symptoms such as depression*, anger, crankiness, and a lack of normal emotions, and they may be easily startled, unusually fearful, and have trouble paying attention.

What Causes Anxiety Disorders?

Genetics   There are probably several causes for anxiety disorders. Genetics may play a role in some cases. For example, research has shown that a twin is more likely to have obsessive-compulsive disorder if the other twin has it and if they are identical twins (twins that have identical genes*) rather than if they are fraternal twins (twins that do not have identical genes). Other twin studies have found a genetic component to panic disorder and social anxiety disorder.

Brain circuits   Some research has focused on pinpointing the exact brain areas and circuits involved in anxiety and fear, which are at the root of anxiety disorders. Scientists have shown that, when faced with danger, the body sends two sets of signals to different parts of the brain. One set goes straight to the amygdala (uh-MIG-duh-luh), a small structure deep inside the brain, which sets the body's automatic fear response in motion. This response readies the body to react to the threat. The heart starts to pound and send more blood to the muscles for quick action, while stress hormones and extra blood sugar are sent into the bloodstream to provide extra energy. The other set of signals takes a roundabout route to the cerebral cortex (suh-REE-brul KOR-teks), the thinking part of the brain. Thus, the body response is set in motion before the brain understands just what is wrong. As a built-in safety measure, this learned response is etched on the amygdala so the response will be quickly available for the next dangerous situation.

In people with anxiety disorders, an experience that feels scary, even one involving a normally safe object or situation, can create a deeply etched memory of fear. This memory can lead to the automatic physical symptoms of anxiety when the object or situation is experienced again. These symptoms, in turn, can make it hard to focus on anything else. Over time, people may start to feel anxiety in many situations. Studies have shown that memories stored in the amygdala may be hard to erase. However, people can gain control over their responses with experience and sometimes with psychotherapy*.

***psychotherapy** (sy-ko-THER-a-pee), or mental health counseling, involves talking about feelings with a trained professional. The counselor can help the person change thoughts, actions, or relationships that play a part in the illness.

Temperament   Another factor to take into account is a personality quality called temperament. Temperament refers to a person's inborn nature that consists of certain behavioral traits. To some extent, people's tendency to be shy or nervous may be inborn, simply part of their nature. Some research suggests that babies who are easily upset never fully learn how to soothe themselves early in life the way other children with calmer temperaments do. They may react more strongly to stressful or anxiety-provoking situations than people whose temperament makes them more adaptable. Some experts believe that people with an inhibited, cautious temperament may be more likely to have problems with anxiety.

Life experiences   Yet another factor that plays a role in some anxiety disorders is stress, especially when it occurs early in life. Scientists have found that when rat pups are separated from their mothers at an early age they have a much greater startle response to later stressful situations than rat pups that were not separated. In addition to separation from a parent, human children may be affected by stressful situations such as child abuse, family violence, or growing up in an unsafe neighborhood. Unsafe conditions or frightening experiences may teach children to be overcautious, to expect bad things, or to worry excessively about possible dangers. People with low self-esteem* also may be prone to developing anxiety disorders.

***self-esteem** is the value that people put on the mental image that they have of themselves.

What Are the Symptoms of Anxiety Disorders?

The fear response associated with all of the anxiety disorders can involve a number of physical symptoms. These include:

- pounding or racing heart

■ sweating

■ trembling

■ shortness of breath

■ choking feeling

■ chest pain

■ upset stomach

■ stomachache

■ dizziness

■ faintness

■ numbness

■ tingling

■ chills

Anxiety disorders also can lead to changes in the way a person feels, thinks, or behaves. For example, people with anxiety disorders might:

■ feel afraid and nervous

■ fear they are losing control or going crazy

■ fear they will die or get hurt

■ worry about a parent's injury or illness

■ worry about being away from home

■ worry about things before they happen

■ worry constantly about school or sports

■ refuse to go to school

■ be afraid to meet or talk to new people

■ avoid new situations

■ have trouble sleeping due to worry or fear

Without treatment, people may be driven to take extreme measures to avoid situations that trigger these unpleasant symptoms. They may refuse to join in many activities. Relationships with family and friends may suffer as a result. In addition, people who are always thinking about fears and worries are unable to concentrate on school, work, or sports. They may fail to do as well as they could in these areas.

How Are Anxiety Disorders Diagnosed and Treated?

Anxiety disorders often occur along with other mental disorders, such as depression, eating disorders*, or substance abuse*. They also may accompany physical illnesses. In such cases, these other disorders also must be treated. People with the symptoms of an anxiety disorder need a complete medical checkup to rule out other illnesses. They also need a

*eating disorders are conditions in which a person's eating behaviors and food habits are so unbalanced that they cause physical and emotional problems.

*substance abuse is the misuse of alcohol, tobacco, illegal drugs, prescription drugs, and other substances such as paint thinners or aerosol gases that change how the mind and body work.

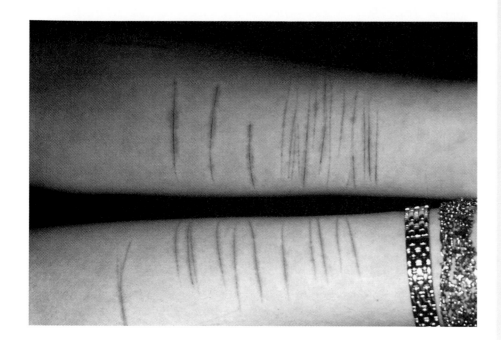

Self-injury and other behaviors that seem impossible to control are signs of an anxiety disorder. Cognitive-behavioral therapy and medication can help people learn how to change unwanted behaviors like cutting (intentionally cutting one's own skin with a blade or other sharp object), shown here, and how to create new ways of thinking about themselves and the stresses they encounter in their daily lives. *Photo Researchers, Inc.*

thorough psychological evaluation. The mental health professional will ask about symptoms and the problems that they cause. With children and teenagers, the professional generally will also talk to parents or even teachers.

Medications Medications cannot cure anxiety disorders, but they can be very helpful for relieving symptoms. Several kinds of medications are used to treat anxiety. Although these medications work well, they can be very dangerous if mixed with alcohol, and some can be habit forming. Increasingly, antidepressant medications originally developed to treat depression are becoming the more commonly prescribed anti-anxiety medicines as well. Finding the right medication and dose for a given person can take some time. Fortunately, though, if one medication does not work, there are several others that can be prescribed.

Psychotherapy Medications often are combined with psychotherapy, in which people talk about their feelings, experiences, and beliefs with a mental health professional. In therapy, a person can learn how to change the thoughts, actions, or relationships that play a part in their problems. There are many kinds of psychotherapy, but two kinds have been shown to work particularly well in treating anxiety disorders: cognitive (COG-nih-tiv) therapy and behavioral (be-HAY-vyor-ul) therapy. Often techniques from these two types of therapy are combined.

Behavioral techniques help people replace specific, unwanted behaviors with healthier behaviors. Behavioral approaches that may be used to treat anxiety include relaxation training and deep breathing, for example. People are taught to take slow, deep breaths to relax, because people with anxiety often take fast, shallow breaths that can trigger other physical symptoms, such as a racing heart and dizziness. Another behavioral technique, called exposure (ek-SPO-zhur) therapy, gradually brings people into contact with a feared object or situation so they can learn to control their fear response to what frightens them.

Cognitive-behavioral therapy helps people understand and change their thinking patterns so they can learn to react differently to situations that cause anxiety. This awareness of thinking patterns is combined with behavioral techniques. For example, someone who becomes dizzy during panic attacks and fears he is going to die may be asked to spin in a circle until he gets dizzy. When he becomes alarmed and starts thinking, "I'm going to die," he learns to replace that thought with another one, such as "It's just dizziness. I can handle it." Though anxiety disorders can be extremely distressing to those experiencing them, the good news is that these disorders respond very well to treatment.

Resources

Book

Bourne, Edmund J. *The Anxiety and Phobia Workbook*. Oakland, CA: New Harbinger Publications, 1995.

Organizations

Anxiety Disorders Association of America, 11900 Parklawn Drive, Suite 100, Rockville, MD 20852. This group is for people with a personal or professional interest in anxiety disorders. Telephone 301-231-9350
http://www.adaa.org

Anxiety Disorders Education Program, U.S. National Institute of Mental Health, 6001 Executive Boulevard, Room 8184, MSC 9663, Bethesda, MD 20892-9663. This government program provides a wide range of information about anxiety disorders. Telephone 888-8ANXIETY
http://www.nimh.nih.gov/anxiety

Asperger Disorder

Asperger disorder is a developmental condition in which a child does not learn to communicate and interact with others in a typical way. The condition, also called Asperger syndrome, is one of the pervasive developmental disorders, which is the group of conditions that includes autism (AW-tiz-um).

KEYWORDS
for searching the Internet and other reference sources

Autism

Brain disorders

Pervasive developmental disorder

Brian's Story

When Brian turned two years old, his parents were thrilled with his large vocabulary, which surpassed that of any other two-year-old they knew. Because Brian seemed so bright, they tried to ignore the fact that he spoke in a monotone, rarely made eye contact with them, and never wanted to play with the other children in his playgroup. When Brian became fixated on the weather channel on television, however, they had to admit that something might be wrong. When Brian's parents mentioned these behaviors to their pediatrician, she suspected that Brian had a form of autism called Asperger disorder.

What Is Asperger Disorder?

Asperger disorder is in the same group of developmental disorders as autism. Both autism and Asperger disorder are brain conditions that affect a person's ability to relate to others and to communicate normally with language. The main difference between children with Asperger disorder and children with autism is that intelligence and development of language is not delayed in children with Asperger disorder. In fact, children with Asperger disorder are often so clever with words that the Austrian doctor who first described the condition, Hans Asperger, called them "little professors." However, children with Asperger disorder often talk in a monotone, do not look people in the eye when they are talking, and may seem obsessed with odd or narrow interests. For example, they may memorize and recite train timetables or weather statistics but may have little idea of their usefulness.

Despite their intelligence and verbal abilities, children with Asperger disorder are socially atypical and unaware of what other people are thinking and feeling. They rarely if ever try to share their interests or enjoyment with people around them. Thus, they have difficulty making friends, and they may be teased or become socially isolated. People with Asperger disorder may also be hyperactive, irritable, anxious, or depressed.

What Causes Asperger Disorder?

Asperger disorder, like autism in general, results from some abnormality in the brain. However, no one knows exactly what the abnormality is or what causes it. Parents of a child with any form of pervasive development disorder, including Asperger disorder, are more likely to have another child with the same disorder, suggesting that genes* are involved. Some experts believe that the hereditary link is stronger in Asperger disorder than it is in classical autism.

The prevalence of Asperger disorder is not known. In some children, it is hard to distinguish Asperger disorder from milder forms of classical autism. However, it is believed that there are more males than females with Asperger disorder, and in one survey the male-to-female ratio was 4 to 1.

*__genes__ are chemicals in the body that help determine a person's characteristics, such as hair or eye color. They are inherited from a person's parents and are contained in the chromosomes found in the cells of the body.

How Is Asperger Disorder Treated?

Parents, teachers, and mental health professionals may all become involved in helping children with Asperger disorder. Behavioral training to assist in the learning of social skills is important. Children with Asperger disorder may attend special education classes and practice behaviors such as looking people in the eye while talking and trying to see things from another's point of view. They may also learn to read emotions such as anger or fear from the expressions on other people's faces, something that most children can do instinctively. Sometimes children with Asperger disorder are helped by special medications to treat associated problems like hyperactivity, anxiety* and depression*.

There is no cure for Asperger disorder. However, children with this condition, because they have greater verbal skills, often do better as they grow to adulthood than do children with autism. Although they may always be socially awkward, many children with Asperger disorder are able to go on to become well educated and to live and work independently.

Resources

Books

Attwood, Tony. *Asperger's Syndrome: A Guide for Parents and Professionals.* Philadelphia: Taylor and Francis, Inc., 1997.

Gagnon, Elisa, and Brenda Smith Miles. *This Is Asperger Syndrome.* Shawnee Mission, KS: Autism Asperger Publishing Company, 1999. Written for children 9 to 12, this book helps readers understand the behaviors and experiences of a child with Asperger disorder.

Willey, Liane H. *Pretending to Be Normal: Living with Asperger's Syndrome.* Philadelphia: Taylor and Francis, Inc., 1999. The author describes her own experiences as a person with Asperger disorder and as the mother of a daughter who also has the disorder.

Schnurr, Rosina G. *Asperger's Huh?: A Child's Perspective.* Gloucester, ON: Anisor Publishing, 1999. A book for children who have Asperger disorder.

*anxiety can be experienced as a troubled feeling, a sense of dread, fear of the future, or distress over a possible threat to a person's physical or mental well-being.

*depression (de-PRESH-un) is a mental state characterized by feelings of sadness, despair, and discouragement.

▶ *See also*

Autism

Birth Defects and Brain Development

Pervasive Developmental Disorders

Assessment   *See* Testing and Evaluation

Attention

Attention is the mental process in which a person concentrates awareness on a specific object, issue, or activity and excludes other potential stimuli* from the environment. While the human brain has amazing capabilities for processing information, it also has limited capacity. A person cannot attend to all the information being received through the five senses (sight, hearing, taste, smell, and touch) at any one time.

What Parts of the Brain Are Involved in Paying Attention?

Neuroscientists (nor-o-SY-in-tists), or scientists who study the brain and nervous system, believe that attention is largely a function of the brain's reticular activating (re-TIK-yoo-lur AK-ti-vay-ting) system, or RAS. This system includes a group of nerve fibers located in several parts of the brain, including the thalamus*, hypothalamus*, brain stem*, and cerebral cortex*. The RAS seems to account for the shifts in people's level of involvement with their surroundings, which ranges anywhere from full attention to sleep. When the system is fully operating, a person is awake, alert, and attentive; this would be the case when a person is listening to an interesting lecture or taking an important test. When the RAS is less active, a person is tired or inattentive. The highway signs urging drivers to "Stay Awake - Take a Break" actually are related to the RAS; it is much more difficult for people to pay attention when they are tired.

Within the RAS, the thalamus appears to play a key role in the moment-to-moment changes in the focus of attention. The thalami and cerebral cortex cooperate to register any incoming sensory signals, evaluate their contents, and mobilize brain resources in response to the demands made. Put simply, the thalami receive the messages that come through a person's senses and then relay the information to the proper receiving areas in the brain.

Chemical messengers known as neurotransmitters (nor-o-TRANZ-mit-erz) are also involved in the process of paying attention. In fact, all of the systems within the brain depend on chemicals that pass electrical signals from nerve cell to nerve cell. A test known as electroencephalography (e-LEK-tro-en-sef-uh-LAH-gru-fee), or EEG, can measure electrical signals within the brain. Two transmitter substances, noradrenaline (nor-uh-DREN-uh-lin) and dopamine (DOH-puh-meen), play important roles in helping people stay alert and attentive. The medicine methylphenidate (meth-il-FEN-ih-date; better known by its brand name, Ritalin®) is used to treat Attention Deficit Hyperactivity Disorder and is thought to work by regulating the levels of key neurotransmitters in the brain, particularly dopamine. After taking the medicine, people who

KEYWORDS
for searching the Internet
and other reference sources

Attention deficit disorder (ADD)

Hyperactivity

Neuroscience

Ritalin

***stimuli** (STIM-yoo-lie) are things in the environment that "excite" a person to function, become active, or respond. The singular form is stimulus.

***thalamus** (THAL-uh-mus) refers to a pair of large egg-shaped areas located in the middle of the brain just under the cerebral cortex. The plural form is thalami.

***hypothalamus** (hy-po-THAL-uh-mus) is a brain structure located deep within the brain that regulates automatic body functions such as heart rate, blood pressure, temperature, respiration, and the release of hormones.

***brain stem** connects the brain to the spinal cord. Twelve pairs of nerves branch off the brain stem and connect to the eyes, ears, nose, face, neck, and breathing and swallowing muscles. The brain stem is involved in motor functions, reflexes, and sensing.

***cerebral cortex** (suh-REE-brul KOR-teks) is the part of the brain that controls functions such as conscious thought, listening, and speaking.

have difficulty focusing their attention are better able to concentrate on a task.

This is an overly simplified explanation of a complex process. There are other parts of the brain and nervous system that play a role in the process of paying attention. For example, a group of structures in the middle of the brain compose the limbic (LIM-bik) system, which is linked

---

UNDERSTANDING ATTENTION: TWENTIETH-CENTURY MILESTONES

During the twentieth century, researchers developed a better understanding of what it really means to pay attention. A few key developments include:

- 1920s: A Russian scientist named Ivan Petrovich Pavlov observed some of the physical signs of attention in dogs and other animals, which came to be known as the orienting response. These signs included pricked-up ears, turning the head toward the stimulus, increased muscle tension, and other changes in the body. In his most famous experiment, Pavlov found that he could train dogs to associate the ringing of a bell with the delivery of food. Pavlov's discovery gave rise to a school of psychology known as behaviorism, which studies how behavior is caused by the brain's responses to external factors.

- 1950s: The theory of the bottleneck is used to describe the process of attention. Scientists theorize that the many signals entering the central nervous system are placed in temporary storage and then are analyzed for their importance. In this way, a person can filter out what needs attention and only allow those signals to pass through for further processing in the brain.

- 1990s: The development of new scanning technologies such as positron emission tomography (POZ-ih-tron e-MISH-un tuh-MOG-ruh-fee) (PET scan) and magnetic resonance imaging (mag-NE-tik REZ-uh-nans I-muh-jing) (MRI) allows researchers to watch the brain in action. For example, researchers at Duke University in North Carolina recently used a MRI scanner to take 480 snapshots per minute of the brain activity of several volunteers as they watched a computer-controlled television screen. The scans showed how areas of activity in the brain shift as the person shifts attention. Many other studies have used this technology to determine how different areas of the brain are involved in different activities.

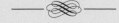

---

to various emotions and feelings such as fear, pleasure, and sadness. These structures are thought to play some role in how people decide to focus their attention. For example, when a student sits at a desk to read a school textbook, a variety of complex emotions may play a role in her decision to focus on the text: pleasure in the subject matter, fear of doing poorly on the next test, desire to perform well during class discussion, and so forth. To focus in on the task at hand, she must tune out all other stimuli, such as the other books scattered around the room, the sound of children playing outside, the color of the desk pad, and the ticking of the clock. Attention is not always under a person's control, however. If someone comes bursting into the room or turns on a stereo at full volume, the student's attention would likely be drawn away from the book. Thus, attention may be captured by an unexpected event rather than voluntarily directed toward it.

Do Television and Video Games Affect Attention?

Some experts have argued that watching too many fast-paced television programs and video games may actually increase the likelihood of attention problems. If the brain becomes accustomed to constant stimulation by rapidly changing visual effects, it may easily become impatient with tasks that require closer attention. Television also makes fewer demands on attention than do reading, studying, or playing a game. Without enough of these more challenging activities, the brain may "get out of shape."

However, the reverse may be true. Children and adults with limited attention resources may be attracted to intense stimulation and therefore may be captured by television or video games. Less intense activities may not hold the focus of individuals with attention deficits. More research is needed to better understand this issue.

Resources

Organizations

Neuroscience for Kids is an extensive and entertaining website maintained by Research Associate Professor Eric Chudler at the University of Washington, Seattle. It features easy-to-understand information on a range of topics related to the brain and nervous system, including attention.
http://faculty.washington.edu/chudler/neurok.html

KidsHealth.org from the Nemours Foundation posts information about attention deficit disorders and other issues concerning learning.
www.KidsHealth.org

▶ *See also*
Attention Deficit Hyperactivity Disorder

Brain Chemistry (Neurochemistry)

Attention Deficit Hyperactivity Disorder

Attention Deficit Hyperactivity (DEF-ih-sit hy-per-ak-TIV-ih-tee) Disorder, or ADHD, is a common developmental disorder that affects both children and adults, although it is usually diagnosed in childhood. ADHD affects a person's ability to study, learn, work, play, and even socialize with others. People with ADHD are less able to sit still, plan ahead, organize and finish tasks, and tune in fully to what is going on around them than are people without the disorder.

Kevin's Story

As a sixth-grader at a new middle school, Kevin was having a much harder time than he expected. Then again, school had never been easy for him. He often had trouble staying focused and controlling his impulse to talk out loud in class. Homework had always been a nightmare, too; he knew he had assignments to complete, but he forgot to write them down, often brought home the wrong books, and just could not sit still long enough to get anything done. Fortunately, Kevin's grade school teachers knew him well and worked with him on ways to stay focused and organized. From first through fifth grade, he always had one teacher for most of his subjects, one desk where he kept his books, and small classes. His parents and teachers were in constant communication, too. That had gotten him through most of the rough spots.

In the sixth grade, though, Kevin had a different teacher for every subject, a locker for his books and supplies, and a couple study periods during the day. He felt constantly overwhelmed and disorganized. Several of his teachers had already sent notes home expressing concern about disruptive behaviors such as calling out, walking around the room, and interrupting others. He could not keep track of his assignments and always felt like he was jumping from task to task.

After two bad report cards and many calls from concerned teachers, Kevin's parents took him to see his pediatrician. After examining Kevin and hearing about his problems in school, the pediatrician recommended that Kevin see a psychologist* for an evaluation. After meeting with Kevin's parents a few times, surveying his teachers and coaches, performing some special psychological tests, reading school reports, and even watching Kevin in the classroom, the psychologist confirmed what some of Kevin's teachers and his pediatrician suspected: Kevin had Attention Deficit Hyperactivity Disorder-Combined Type (or ADHD-Combined Type, meaning that he had problems with both inattention and hyperactivity). Because Kevin had learned ways to cope pretty well in grade school, the psychologist suggested that they all work together to develop new strategies that might help him deal with the more challenging environment of middle

KEYWORDS
for searching the Internet and other reference sources

Attention deficit disorder (ADD)

Hyperactivity

Impulsivity

Psychostimulant drugs

Ritalin

psychologist (sy-KOL-uh-jist) is a mental health professional who has specialized training in the diagnosis and treatment of emotional and behavioral conditions. Psychologists administer special tests to help them arrive at a diagnosis. Psychologists, like other mental health experts, also provide counseling services.

school. If those were not effective enough, then Kevin could try taking some medication that might help him stay more focused and attentive.

Just about every classroom in the United States has a student like Kevin. Experts believe that about 5 percent of students, or 1 in 20, have a form of ADHD. Boys are three to four times more likely than girls to be affected by ADHD. Of course, everyone has a hard time paying attention and staying focused now and then, but students with ADHD feel this way most of the time.

How Is Attention Deficit Hyperactivity Disorder Diagnosed?

Diagnosing ADHD is difficult because symptoms vary and there is no simple test that can determine whether someone has ADHD. In most cases, parents notice early on that their child is much less attentive or has less control over his behavior than other children. However, the disorder usually is not diagnosed until the child enters school and is expected to follow directions, cooperate with others, and be quiet at certain times.

To make the diagnosis, a psychologist or psychiatrist* looks for patterns of certain behaviors that have lasted for more than six months and interfere with two or more areas of a person's life (such as school and play, school and home, or home and work). In addition to interviewing the child and family members, the specialist may need to speak with others who know the child well, such as teachers and coaches. Former teachers may be asked to fill out an evaluation. Special tests may also be administered to clarify the diagnosis.

The behaviors that experts look for fall into three categories: inattention, hyperactivity, and impulsivity. Signs of inattention in a child include:

- failure to pay close attention to details
- finding it difficult to sustain attention in work and play
- not seeming to listen when spoken to directly
- not following through on instructions and failing to finish tasks
- having difficulty organizing tasks and activities
- avoiding, disliking, or seeming reluctant to engage in tasks that require concentration
- being easily distracted by unimportant sights and sounds
- losing things
- forgetting things

Hyperactivity refers to overly active behavior. Children experiencing hyperactivity might:

- fidget with their hands or feet
- squirm while seated

* **psychiatrist** (sy-KY-uh-trist) refers to a medical doctor who has completed specialized training in the diagnosis and treatment of mental illness. Psychiatrists diagnose and treat mental illnesses, prescribe medications, and provide mental health counseling.

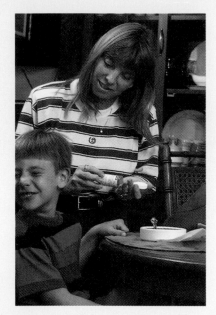

A mother gives her hyperactive son medication to help his behavior. *Stock Boston*

* **oppositional defiant disorder** (op-uh-ZIH-shun-ul de-FY-unt dis-OR-der) is a disruptive behavior disorder that can be diagnosed in children as young as preschoolers who demonstrate hostile or aggressive behavior and who refuse to follow rules.

* **depression** (de-PRESH-un) is a mental state characterized by feelings of sadness, despair, and discouragement.

* **anxiety** (ang-ZY-e-tee) can be experienced as a troubled feeling, a sense of dread, fear of the future, or distress over a possible threat to a person's physical or mental well-being.

* **neurotransmitters** (NUR-o-tranz-mit-erz) are brain chemicals that let brain cells communicate with each other and therefore allow the brain to function normally.

- leave their seat in the classroom and elsewhere
- run about or climb excessively
- have difficulty playing or engaging in leisure activities quietly
- seem on the go or act as if driven by a motor
- talk excessively

An impulsive child might:
- blurt out answers before questions have been completed
- interrupt or intrude on others
- have difficulty waiting his or her turn

Not everyone with ADHD has all of the above symptoms. There are three kinds of ADHD that are commonly recognized. People who have significant problems with attention but are not really hyperactive or impulsive are diagnosed with ADHD-Inattentive Type. Other children have problems mainly with hyperactivity and impulsivity. These individuals are diagnosed as having ADHD-Impulsive Hyperactive Type. Individuals with significant problems with impulsivity, hyperactivity, and attention are diagnosed with ADHD-Combined Type.

Children with ADHD may have other behavioral disorders as well. These may include oppositional defiant disorder*, depression*, anxiety*, and delays in learning speech and language.

What Causes ADHD?

Doctors and researchers are not sure why certain people have ADHD. There have been theories involving many possible causes, such as diet, head injuries, exposure to drugs before birth, and even family and home environment. However, none of these theories offers a satisfactory explanation for most cases of ADHD.

Researchers interested in learning about possible biological (by-uh-LOJ-ih-kul) causes of ADHD are looking at how the brains of people with ADHD might actually function differently than other people's brains. For example, using a special scanning test called a PET scan, positron emission tomography (POZ-ih-tron e-MISH-un tuh-MOG-ruh-fee), researchers can watch the brain as it works. The test lets them see how much glucose (GLOO-cose), a type of sugar, is used by the areas of the brain that inhibit impulses and control attention (glucose is the brain's main source of energy). Some studies have found that the areas of the brain that control attention use less glucose in people with ADHD; this means that these areas of the brain appear to be working less hard. Other researchers believe that ADHD has something to do with differences in the neurotransmitters* that deliver signals to the brain areas that control attention. Still, researchers are not sure why certain people's brains might function differently in this way. It does appear that children may inherit a tendency to develop ADHD. For example, children who have ADHD usually have at least one close relative with ADHD. In addition, if one of a pair of identical twins is diagnosed with ADHD, the other twin likely has ADHD as well.

How Is ADHD Treated?

Usually, ADHD is first treated with behavioral (be-HAY-vyor-ul) therapy. This involves working with a psychologist or psychotherapist* to learn ways of coping with the condition. The therapist can help people become more aware of their behavior, develop strategies for controlling it, and even help them practice how to deal with situations that caused problems in the past. A person also might find it helpful to participate in a support group with others in the same situation.

Parents and teachers are part of the treatment plan as well. Parents can learn how to establish more structure for the child, define limits more clearly, and be consistent with discipline, all of which are especially important for a child with ADHD. Teachers can provide predictable routines and structure in the classroom and try to keep the student away from distractions. Both parents and teachers can establish certain penalties and rewards to help the child make progress with behavior.

If these strategies are not effective enough in controlling the condition on their own, then a psychostimulant (SY-ko-STIM-yoo-lint) medication such as methylphenidate (meth-il-PHEN-uh-date; Ritalin, Concerta, Methylin, Metadate), dextroamphetamine (dex-tro-am-PHET-uh-meen; Dexedrine, Dextrastat), or mixed amphetamine salts (Adderall) might be prescribed. It may seem strange that an inattentive, overly active person would be treated with a stimulant (a drug that increases energy). However, these medications work by stimulating certain areas of the brain that make it possible for many people with ADHD to concentrate, behave more consistently, and take part in activities that were impossible before.

Why Is ADHD Diagnosed More Often Than in the Past?

More children than ever before are being diagnosed with ADHD-Predominantly Impulsive Hyperactive Type or ADHD-Predominantly Inattentive Type. In addition, the use of stimulant medications increased dramatically during the 1990s; according to one estimate, production of these medications increased by 700 percent between 1990 and 1997. There is some disagreement over why this is the case. Some people think that greater awareness of the condition is leading more parents to seek help for their children. Others believe that some cases of what is simply "bad behavior" are being misdiagnosed as ADHD. Some argue that parents may find it easier to accept that their child has a mental disorder rather than learn how to deal with unruly behavior or poor school performance due to other reasons. The debate continues, but experts agree that ADHD is a real condition that can have serious consequences if it is not diagnosed and managed appropriately.

* **psychotherapist** (sy-ko-THER-a-pist) is any mental health professional who works with people to help them change thoughts, actions, or relationships that play a part in their emotional or behavioral problems.

Can Food Cause Hyperactivity?

Anyone who drinks too much cola or coffee is likely to have a hard time concentrating, because caffeine can overstimulate the brain. At one time, mental health specialists believed that sugar and other food additives actually contributed to ADHD. As a result, parents were encouraged to stop serving children foods containing artificial flavorings, preservatives, and sugars. It was thought that this restricted diet could actually prevent or cure the symptoms of the condition. Researchers no longer believe that this is the case.

In the 1980s, the National Institutes of Health, the Federal agency responsible for biomedical research, held a major scientific conference to discuss the issue of diet and ADHD. After studying the data, the scientists concluded that the restricted diet seemed to help only a very small number of children with ADHD (mostly either young children or children with confirmed food allergies). Many books and websites still promote restricted diets and even vitamins as a cure for ADHD, but they are not backed by scientific evidence.

A boy with ADHD receives one-on-one instruction with his teacher. The method of teaching a child according to his or her own special way of learning is an effective way of managing ADHD. *Photo Researchers, Inc.* ▶

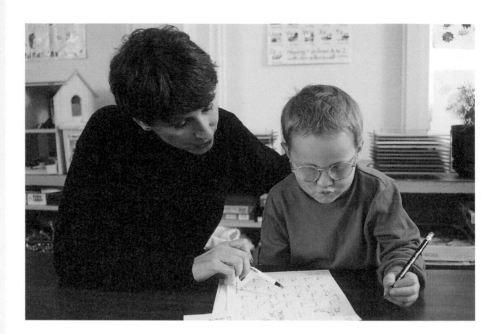

Living with ADHD

Living with ADHD can be difficult. Children and adults with ADHD may have a hard time keeping friends and performing well at school or work. While many individuals live well with ADHD, many may become lonely, depressed, and even use drugs or alcohol as an escape.

People with ADHD do not outgrow the condition. While they often become less hyperactive when they get older, people with ADHD may still have problems with restlessness and short attention span.

By using certain coping strategies, many people with ADHD learn to deal with the condition successfully and can achieve in school and thrive in rewarding careers. Many people are able to find the right kind of job for their strengths and abilities. For example, a person might be better suited for a position that offers variety and constant change rather than one that requires long periods at a desk.

The U.S. National Institute for Mental Health, the Federal agency for research on mental disorders, recommends the following strategies for living with ADHD:

- When necessary, ask the teacher or boss to repeat instructions instead of guessing about what was said.

- Break large assignments or job tasks into small, simple tasks. Set a deadline for each task and provide rewards for each completed task.

- Each day, make a list of what needs to be done. Plan the best order for doing each task, then make a schedule for doing them. Use a calendar or daily planner.

- Work in a quiet area. Do one thing at a time. Take short breaks.

- Write things down in a notebook with dividers. Write different kinds of information, like assignments, appointments, and phone numbers, in different sections. Keep the book on hand.
- Post reminders of things that need to be done.
- Store similar things together.
- Create a routine. Get ready for school or work at the same time, in the same way, every day.
- Exercise, eat a balanced diet, and get enough sleep.

Resources

Books

Barkley, Russell A. *Taking Charge of ADHD: The Complete, Authoritative Guide for Parents.* New York: Guilford Publications, Inc., 2000.

Quinn, Patricia O., and Judith M. Stern (eds.). *The Best of "BRAKES": An Activity Book for Kids with ADD and ADHD.* Washington, DC: American Psychological Association, 2000. This book provides a collection of tips, activities, games, puzzles, and other resources designed to help kids deal with ADD. This book is especially targeted at those between the ages of 8 and 13.

Organizations

CHADD (Children and Adults with Attention-Deficit/Hyperactivity Disorder), 8181 Professional Place, Suite 201, Landover, MD 20785. CHADD is a national organization for education, advocacy and support of people with ADHD.
http://www.chadd.org

Nemours Center for Children's Health Media, Alfred I. duPont Hospital for Children, 1600 Rockland Road, Wilmington, DE 19803. This organization is dedicated to issues of children's health and produces the KidsHealth website. Its website has articles about ADHD.
http://www.KidsHealth.org

United States National Institute of Mental Health (NIMH), 6001 Executive Blvd., Rm. 8184, MSC 9663, Bethesda, MD 20892-9663. The NIMH provides a booklet of information about ADHD at its website.
http://www.nimh.nih.gov

▶ *See also*

Attention

Brain Chemistry (Neurochemistry)

Impulsivity

Learning Disabilities

Oppositional Defiant Disorder

Autism

Autism (AW-tiz-um) is a brain disorder that affects a child's ability to develop normal communication skills and social responsiveness to other people. An infant with autism may seem to behave unusually from birth or may develop normally for a short time and then show autistic traits. To diagnose autism, symptoms must have been present before the child was 3 years old. Autism is part of a larger category of disorders called pervasive developmental disorders, all of which affect the brain's development.

KEYWORDS
for searching the Internet and other reference sources

Asperger disorder

Brain disorders

Pervasive developmental disorder

People who are shy are not very talkative and often look down or away when someone else talks to them. They also seem to spend a lot of the time by themselves. Still, they do talk to people some of the time, especially to family members and friends with whom they learn to feel comfortable, and they like to be around people some of the time.

Children with autism may appear to be shy, but shyness and autism are very different from each other. The symptoms of autism can range from mild to severe. Children with the most extreme forms of autism are almost totally isolated socially. Lacking the ability to relate normally to others, they seem always to prefer to be alone. Even within their own family, they seldom make eye contact or try to share their interests in toys or other objects. Many children with autism never learn to talk at all. If they do, they use language in unusual ways, such as by constantly repeating rhymes or jingles. They may refer to themselves by their own name, or as "you," instead of using "I" or "me." Sometimes they just repeat what someone has said to them, rather than replying in a meaningful way. Some children with autism may have above-average language skills, but often they do not use this ability to have conversations with others around them.

What Are Some Other Signs of Autism?

Children with autism often behave in unusual ways. Their activities are limited, and they may become very upset if there is some change in their environment or daily routine. For example, some may have temper tantrums if a piece of furniture in their room is moved or if they are put at a different place at the dinner table.

Characteristic behavior may include repetitive motor acts such as arm flapping, finger twisting, rocking, and walking on tiptoes. Some of these motions may be repeated for hours on end. Children with autism may also exhibit hyperactivity, fits of screaming, or self-injury, such as head banging. Often, children with autism fear harmless objects, such as a vacuum cleaner, but fail to perceive real dangers, such as crossing a busy highway. They may also be oversensitive to noises, lights, and odors, and

* **mental retardation** is a condition in which people have below average intelligence that limits their ability to function normally.

* **seizures** (SEE-zhurz) are "storms" in the brain that occur when the electrical patterns of the brain are interrupted by powerful, rapid bursts of electrical energy. This may cause a person to fall down, make jerky movements, or stare blankly into space.

they may dislike being touched. Many children with autism also have mental retardation*. About one in four people with autism may develop seizures* by the time they reach their teens.

How Common Is Autism?

Autism occurs worldwide in all cultures. The prevalence is usually said to be 2 to 5 per 10,000 people. However, it may affect as many as 20 per 10,000 (or 1 in 500) if Asperger disorder* and other pervasive development disorders are included. Prevalence estimates have tended to increase along with increased public awareness of autism and Asperger disorder. Rates of autism are 3 to 4 times higher in boys than in girls.

What Causes Autism?

Autism is not transmitted from one person to another like a cold, so it is impossible to catch it from someone else. However, no one knows what causes autism. While we now know this is not true, until the 1970s, autism was thought to be the result of a poor mother-child relationship in infancy. Since then, researchers have come to believe that autism is caused by abnormal development of the brain before birth. However, scientists do not yet know the exact nature of the abnormality.

Some studies have suggested that autism may result from defects in the action of brain neurotransmitters*. Other studies have indicated that brain cells and their connecting fibers may not grow properly in infants who develop autism. It is likely, however, that genes* have some role in causing autism. Parents who have one child with autism are more likely to have other children who develop the disorder (when compared to families who do not have children with autism). Identical twins (who share the same genes) have a high rate of concordance. In other words, if one twin has a condition, the other will likely have it too. If there is an autistic child in the family there is a higher rate of other developmental problems like language and learning disabilities in siblings. Also, autism is more common among people with the chromosomal disorder known as fragile X syndrome*.

How Is Autism Diagnosed and Treated?

There is no specific test for autism. Parents may first suspect that something is wrong if the child does not respond to them and dislikes cuddling or being held. Physicians need to rule out other disorders that have similar symptoms, such as deafness or mental retardation. To diagnose autism, doctors and psychologists* ask parents about the child's early development and observe how the child behaves, communicates, and relates to others.

Treatment is most effective when it is begun at an early age. Educational treatment is often intense, time-consuming, and very individualized in order to take into account the highly varied skills as well as disabilities present in children with autism. Behavioral treatments use

* **Asperger disorder** is a pervasive developmental disorder. Like autism, Asperger disorder is a developmental condition in which a child does not learn to communicate and interact socially with others in a typical way. Children with Asperger disorder have normal intelligence and generally good language development.

* **neurotransmitters** (NUR-o-tranz-mit-erz) are brain chemicals that let brain cells communicate with each other and therefore allow the brain to function normally.

* **genes** are chemicals in the body that help determine a person's characteristics, such as hair or eye color. They are inherited from a person's parents and are contained in the chromosomes found in the cells of the body.

* **fragile X syndrome** is a disorder associated with a faulty X chromosome (a chromosome is a structure inside the body's cells that contains DNA, which is the genetic material that helps determine characteristics such as hair and eye color; females have two X chromosomes whereas males have only one). Fragile X syndrome is associated with mental retardation, especially in males.

* **psychologists** (sy-KOL-uh-jists) are mental health professionals who have specialized training in the diagnosis and treatment of emotional and behavioral conditions. Psychologists administer special tests to help them arrive at a diagnosis. Psychologists, like other mental health experts, also provide counseling services.

The Oscar-winning film *Rain Man* (1988) tells the story of the relationship between two brothers, one of whom is autistic. Charlie (Tom Cruise, left), a selfish car salesman, sets out to find who his father left his fortune to after his father dies. His search leads him to discover that he has a long-lost older brother, Raymond (Dustin Hoffman), who is autistic and has been living in a mental institution. *Photofest* ▶

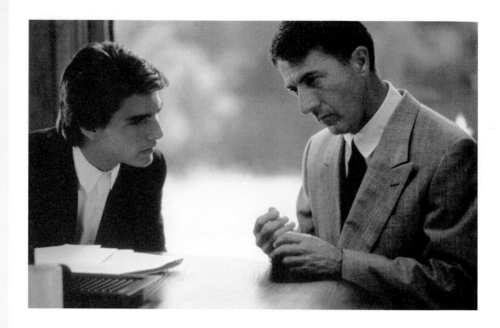

***anxiety** (ang-ZY-e-tee) can be experienced as a troubled feeling, a sense of dread, fear of the future, or distress over a possible threat to a person's physical or mental well-being.

rewards to establish new skills. Developing a communication system is key to treating autistic behavior. Special education programs tailored to the child's individual needs teach ways to better communicate and interact with others. For children with mild autism, educators reinforce existing skills and interests and build on them. Basic living skills, such as personal cleanliness and crossing the street, are also taught. Medications can decrease seizures, if present, and ease anxiety* and repetitive behaviors.

Living with Autism

Autism is not outgrown, and a child with the disorder usually will still be affected by it to some degree when he or she has grown up. With special education and communication training, many people with autism can learn to lead a more nearly normal life. Some with milder autism may even finish high school and go on to college. Many, however, will not be able to live and work independently and will always need special care.

Resources

Books

Janzen, Janice E. *Autism: Facts and Strategies for Parents.* San Diego: Academic Press, 2000.

Grandin, Temple. *Thinking in Pictures, and Other Reports from My Life with Autism.* New York: Random House, 1996.

Maurice, Catherine. *Let Me Hear Your Voice: A Family's Triumph over Autism.* New York: Random House, 1994.

Seroussi, Karyn. *Unraveling the Mystery of Autism and Pervasive Developmental Disorder: A Mother's Story of Research and Recovery.* New York: Simon and Schuster, 2000.

Organizations

Autism Society of America, 7910 Woodmont Avenue, Suite 300, Bethesda, MD 20814-3067.
Telephone 800-3AUTISM
http://www.autism-society.org

KidsHealth.org from the Nemours Foundation posts articles about autism at its website.
http://kidshealth.org/kid/health_problems/brain/autism.html
http://kidshealth.org/teen/health_problems/diseases/autism.html

▶ *See also*

Asperger Disorder

Birth Defects and Brain Development

Mental Retardation

Pervasive Developmental Disorder

B

Bedwetting (Enuresis)

Bedwetting is the involuntary release of urine into the bedclothes at night.

What Is Enuresis?

Enuresis (en-yoo-REE-sis) is the involuntary, unwanted release of urine either in the day or at night in people who are old enough (around ages 5 to 6) to have gained bladder* control. Bedwetting is a specific kind of enuresis that occurs at night during sleep. Most young children accidentally wet the bed occasionally, and this is normal. About 10 percent of six-year-olds still wet the bed, but only about 1 percent of adolescents experience enuresis. Bedwetting becomes a problem when it happens repeatedly in older children. In older children, bedwetting limits social activities and can be stressful and humiliating. It can contribute to psychological and emotional problems such as low self-esteem* and depression*.

Why Do People Wet the Bed?

Doctors are not exactly sure why some people experience problems with bladder control and others do not. They do know that bedwetting runs in families and that more boys than girls have this condition. Many children who wet the bed seem to sleep so deeply that they are not awakened by the urge to urinate. Recent research suggests that some people who wet the bed may produce less antidiuretic hormone (anti-di-u-RET-ik HOR-mone), or ADH, than do people who do not have enuresis. ADH regulates how concentrated the urine is. People generally produce more ADH at night, allowing them to create a smaller volume of more concentrated urine while they sleep. People who produce less ADH at night will produce more urine that is less concentrated (more diluted).

Bedwetting is sometimes related to medical problems such as infections of the urinary tract, sickle-cell anemia*, diabetes*, epilepsy*, or an improperly formed bladder. However, most people who wet the bed do not have medical problems and have normal-sized bladders. Occasionally bedwetting is linked to psychological problems, especially if a person has previously stayed dry at night. Stress from the birth of a sibling, divorce, or death in the family may all cause a (usually temporary) period of bedwetting, especially in younger children.

KEYWORDS
for searching the Internet
and other reference sources

Incontinence

Urinary tract

* **bladder** is the sac-like organ in which urine is stored until it is released during urination.

* **self-esteem** is the value that people put on the mental image that they have of themselves.

* **depression** (de-PRESH-un) is a mental state characterized by feelings of sadness, despair, and discouragement.

* **sickle-cell anemia** (SI-kul SELL uh-NEE-mee-uh) is a hereditary condition in which the red blood cells take on abnormal sickle (crescent) shapes and are unable to transport normal amounts of oxygen throughout the body. This disorder is found most commonly in people of African ancestry.

* **diabetes** (dy-a-BEE-teez) is a disorder that reduces the body's ability to control blood sugar levels.

* **epilepsy** (EP-i-lep-see) is a condition of the nervous system characterized by recurrent seizures that temporarily affect a person's awareness, movements, or sensations. Seizures occur when powerful, rapid bursts of electrical energy interrupt the normal electrical patterns of the brain.

How Is Bedwetting Treated?

Most children simply outgrow bedwetting. Bedwetting in older children can be treated in different ways depending on what is causing it. First, a doctor does a complete physical examination to determine if bedwetting is caused by a medical condition. If it is, the underlying condition is treated medically with drugs or corrective surgery. However, only a very small number of adolescents who experience bedwetting have an underlying medical condition that is responsible for the problem.

If the bedwetting appears to be caused by emotional or psychological stress or depression, seeing a mental health professional is the first step to resolving the problem. Counseling to help deal with the source of stress, combined with behavior modification techniques to bring about nighttime bladder control, are often very effective.

Most people wet the bed for no clear reason. These people are usually helped by behavioral strategies aimed at staying dry during the night. Behavioral modifications such as holding urine for a short while when there is an urge to urinate, rewards for dry nights, and relaxation techniques aimed at reducing stress sometimes help. The most effective behavioral technique, however, is the urine alarm. This is a pad with a bell or alarm attached to it. The pad is placed on the bed and the person sleeps on top of it. With this technique, an alarm rings at the first sign of wetness in a person's pajamas or sheets. The alarm awakens the person and allows him or her to get up and finish emptying the bladder. In time, the person's brain comes to recognize the sensation of a full bladder and wakes the person before urination occurs and the alarm goes off.

Nighttime dryness sometimes can also be achieved by the use of medication. Some medications work to affect urine concentration. Others seem to work by making it easier for a person to wake up when the bladder is full. Some medications are quite effective and work almost immediately while others may work over time. However, many people return to wetting the bed as soon as they stop taking the medication. As with all medicines, sometimes there are mild side effects to deal with as well.

Although bedwetting is not medically serious, it can have strong negative psychological effects on young people. It restricts their social lives and is embarrassing, upsetting, and frustrating. Fortunately most people can be helped to stay dry at night through a combination of the strategies mentioned above.

Resource

Organization

Nemours Center for Children's Health Media, Alfred I. duPont Hospital for Children, 1600 Rockland Road, Wilmington, DE 19803. This organization's KidsHealth website has articles about enuresis. http://www.KidsHealth.org

▶ *See also*
Depression
Self-Esteem
Stress

Binge Eating Disorder

Binge eating is out-of-control eating. A person with binge eating disorder exhibits a repetitive pattern of bingeing that often results in overweight or obesity*, "yo-yo dieting," and guilty or embarrassed feelings.

Eating for Comfort

Rebecca's parents sometimes got into fights that literally scared her out of the house. She often ended up at her neighbor's house, where she was treated to hot chocolate, cookies, and other goodies. Eating in the comfort of her neighbor's home always soothed Rebecca and lessened the pain she felt when her parents fought. Before long, Rebecca didn't bother going to her neighbor's house; she'd find a private place at home and eat whatever sweets she could find. She tried not to do it too often because it made her gain weight, but sometimes she felt she just couldn't stop. She was ashamed of what she did, but it took her mind off her problems.

What Is Binge Eating Disorder?

People who binge on a regular basis have binge eating disorder. Bingeing means eating abnormally large quantities of food (sometimes thousands of calories) in one sitting. Binge eating is sometimes referred to as compulsive overeating because the person feels little control to resist or stop overeating. People who binge often eat when they are not hungry. Women and girls are more likely to have binge eating disorder, but it can affect boys as well. The number of people with this disorder is estimated at 1 to 2 percent of men and women. As many as 30 percent of all women who seek medical treatment to lose weight have binge eating disorder.

Binge eating disorder is similar to another eating disorder called bulimia (bu-LEE-me-a). A person with bulimia binges and then purges. Purging means using vomiting, laxatives, and enemas to rid the body of food. A person with binge eating disorder binges but does not purge.

What Causes Binge Eating Disorder?

The causes of binge eating disorder are hard to pinpoint, but a number of factors are thought to contribute to the problem. People who have binge eating disorder are usually overweight and/or are constantly dieting. Preoccupied with food, they are caught in a cycle of dieting excessively, becoming too hungry, and then overeating. People who have trouble dealing with stress or painful emotions may use binge eating as comfort. Those who have a family history of obesity may be more likely to binge eat. The cultural preoccupation with thinness and dieting also plays an important role in binge eating and in other eating disorders. People who binge are often torn between their feelings of comfort with food, their wish to be thin, and the confusing messages about food and about thinness in the media.

KEYWORDS
for searching the Internet and other reference sources

Binge and purge

Food and nutrition

Compulsive overeating

Overweight

* **obesity** (o-BEE-si-tee) is an excess of body fat. People are considered obese if they weigh more than 30 percent above what is healthy for their height.

How Is Binge Eating Disorder Diagnosed and Treated?

People with binge eating disorder often seek help from a health care professional because they want to lose weight or because of concern about health problems related to obesity. A careful evaluation that involves questions about family and personal history, physical health, eating and dieting habits, psychological concerns, and personality issues may bring binge eating disorder to light.

Like other eating disorders, overcoming binge eating may take a long time, lots of commitment, and hard work. Treatment usually involves a number of professionals, such as a physician, a nutritionist, and/or a therapist. Treatments include counseling, change in eating and dieting habits, support groups, nutritional counseling, individual or group psychotherapy, and in some cases, medication.

Can Binge Eating Disorder Be Prevented?

According to Anorexia Nervosa and Related Eating Disorders, Inc. (ANRED), prevention involves becoming more aware of what triggers a binge and making choices that help to avoid a binge. They provide the following guidelines that may help prevent binge eating disorder:

- eating regularly and avoiding getting too hungry
- not avoiding good tasting food
- eating small or moderate amounts of favorite foods
- having satisfying experiences that do not involve food
- keeping tabs on feelings so they will not lead to binge eating
- being wary of temptations, such as "all you can eat" buffets

Resources

Organizations

Anorexia Nervosa and Related Eating Disorders, Inc. (ANRED), P.O. Box 5102, Eugene, OR 97405-0102.
Telephone 541-334-1144
http://www.anred.com

Eating Disorders Awareness and Prevention, Inc. (EDAP), 603 Stewart Street, Suite 803, Seattle, WA 98101.
Telephone (800) 931-2237 for toll-free information and referral hotline
http://www.edap.org

Overeaters Anonymous, 6075 Zenith Ct., N.E., Rio Rancho, NM 87124.
Telephone 505-891-2664
http://www.overeatersanonymous.org

▶ *See also*

Bulimia

Eating Disorders

Emotions

Obesity

Bipolar Disorder

Bipolar (by-POLE-ar) disorder is a condition in which periods of extreme euphoria* (yoo-FOR-ee-uh), called mania (MAY-nee-uh), alternate with periods of severe depression*. Bipolar disorder is sometimes also called manic (MAN-ik) depression.

What Is Bipolar Disorder?

Bipolar disorder is a type of depressive disorder*. People with bipolar disorder experience two (thus the prefix "bi") extremes in mood; they have periods of extreme happiness and boundless energy that are followed by periods of depression. Bipolar disorder can range from severe to mild. Different forms of bipolar disorder are distinguished from one another by the severity of mood extremes and how quickly mood swings take place. For example, full-blown bipolar disorder, or bipolar I, involves distinct manic episodes followed by depression. People with this form of bipolar disorder often experience trouble sleeping, changes in appetite, psychosis*, and thoughts of suicide. Another form of bipolar disorder called bipolar II affects some people. In bipolar II the mania is not extreme and the person does not lose touch with reality but does have periods of depression. Some people also experience mixed states where symptoms of mania and depression exist at the same time, and this form may be more common in children. Other people may experience a form of bipolar disorder in which there is a rapid cycling between "up" and "down" moods with few, if any, normal moods in between. Cyclorhythmia is a condition in which there are mood swings but with milder highs and lows.

Who Has Bipolar Disorder?

Ernest Hemingway, winner of the Nobel Prize in literature, showed signs of having bipolar disorder. So did presidents Abraham Lincoln and Theodore Roosevelt and the composer Ludwig von Beethoven. All of these men were intelligent, creative, successful individuals, but they all fought the two faces of bipolar disorder. At one moment they would be on top of the world, full of ideas and creative and physical energy. Then a few days, weeks, or months later they would be sunk in the despair and lethargy of depression.

Bipolar disorder affects about 1 out of every 100 people, or at least 2 million Americans. It affects people of all races, cultures, professions, and income levels. Men and women are affected at equal rates. Bipolar disorder tends to run in families and is believed to have an inherited genetic component. Studies on twins show that if one member of a pair of identical twins (twins who have identical genes*) has bipolar disorder, the other twin has about a 70 percent chance of also having the disorder. If one of a pair of fraternal twins (twins who do not have identical

KEYWORDS
for searching the Internet
and other reference sources

Depression

Mania

Manic-depressive illness

Mood disorders

* **euphoria** is an abnormally high mood with the tendency to be overactive and over-talkative, and to have racing thoughts and overinflated self-confidence.

* **depression** (de-PRESH-un) is a mental state characterized by feelings of sadness, despair, and discouragement.

* **depressive disorders** are mental disorders that involve long periods of excessive sadness and affect a person's feelings, thoughts, and behavior.

* **psychosis** (sy-KO-sis) refers to mental disorders in which the sense of reality is so impaired that a patient can not function normally. People with psychotic disorders may experience delusions (exaggerated beliefs that are contrary to fact), hallucinations (something that a person perceives as real but that is not actually caused by an outside event), incoherent speech, and agitated behavior.

* **genes** are chemicals in the body that help determine a person's characteristics, such as hair or eye color. They are inherited from a person's parents and are contained in the chromosomes found in the cells of the body.

75

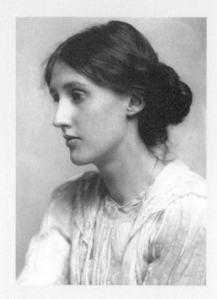

▲

Virginia Woolf (1882–1941), the British novelist and critic, suffered from bipolar disorder. She finally succumbed to her bouts of severe depression in 1941, when she committed suicide in Sussex, England. *Hulton-Deutsch Collection/Corbis*

genes, but do have many of the same genes) has bipolar disorder, the risk of the other twin having it is only 15 to 25 percent.

What are the Symptoms of Bipolar Disorder?

Bipolar disorder has two distinctive sets of symptoms.

Depression   During the depression phase, a person may experience:

- persistent feelings of sadness and anxiety
- feelings of worthlessness or hopelessness
- loss of interest in activities that were formerly enjoyable
- fatigue and decreased energy
- sleeping too much or too little; difficulty getting up or going to sleep
- eating too little or too much
- unexplained periods or restlessness, irritability, or crying
- difficulty concentrating or remembering things
- difficulty making decisions
- thoughts of suicide or suicide attempts
- increased difficulties in relationships with friends, family, teachers, or parents
- alcohol or substance abuse

Mania   During the manic or euphoric stage, a person may experience:

- great energy; ability to go with little sleep for days without feeling tired
- severe mood changes from extreme happiness or silliness to irritability or anger
- over-inflated self-confidence; unrealistic belief in one's own abilities
- increased activity, restlessness, distractibility, and the inability to stick to tasks
- racing, muddled thoughts that cannot be turned off
- decreased judgment of risk and increased reckless behavior
- substance abuse, especially cocaine, alcohol, and sleeping pills
- extremely aggressive behavior

How is Bipolar Disorder Diagnosed?

Bipolar disorder usually begins in early adulthood, although experts now recognize that younger children and teens may also have the disorder. Some children who are diagnosed with attention deficit hyperactivity disorder (ADHD)* may actually have bipolar disorder or both disorders. These children not only have symptoms of ADHD but often also have

*__Attention Deficit Hyperactivity Disorder (ADHD)__ is a condition that makes it hard for a person to pay attention, sit still, or think before acting.

symptoms such as significant and sustained tantrums, periods of anxiety*
(including separation anxiety*), periods of irritability, and mood changes.
With many children, mood states change rapidly and without warning.
Children with bipolar disorder are beginning to be researched by psychologists* and psychiatrists* who previously did not believe that such
disorders occur in early childhood.

Doctors often ask family members about the person's symptoms, as
people with bipolar disorder are often not aware of the changes they are
experiencing. People with bipolar disorder have had at least one period
of mania. Often after the first episode five or more years will pass before
another manic or a depressive period occurs. Despite the stretches of normal moods, bipolar disorder does not go away. Instead, the time between
mania and depression gets shorter and shorter, and the symptoms may
become more severe. Not infrequently, bipolar disorder can lead to psychosis or to suicide. About 19 percent of people who have required hospitalization for bipolar disorder commit suicide.

How Is Bipolar Disorder Treated?

Most people with severe mood swings can be helped by treatment. The
drug lithium has been one of the medications of choice for treating bipolar disorder, and it is often very effective. Other medications have also
have been helpful in controlling mood swings. These include various
antiseizure medications (for example, valproate and carbamazepine) and
antipsychotic medications. People with bipolar disorder need to continue
to take their medications even when they feel normal to prevent the re-
occurrence of mood swings.

Living with Bipolar Disorder

Living with a loved one who has bipolar disorder can be very hard on
family members.

Perhaps the most effective thing that family members can do is to help
the person with the disorder get treatment. Many family members find
joining a support group or participating in family therapy to be helpful in
understanding and managing the impact of this difficult problem.

People who are taking about suicide need emergency help. Many
telephone books list suicide and mental health crisis hotlines in their
Community Service sections, or help can be obtained by calling emergency services (911 in most communities).

Resources

Book

Steel, Danielle. *His Bright Light: The Story of Nick Traina.* New York:
Dell Publishing, 2000. Romance novelist Danielle Steel tells the true
story of her son's struggle with bipolar disorder.

* **anxiety** (ang-ZY-e-tee) can be experienced as a troubled feeling, a sense of dread, fear of the future, or distress over a possible threat to a person's physical or mental well-being.

* **separation anxiety** is the nor-mal fear that babies and young children feel when they are separated from their parents or approached by strangers.

* **psychologist** (sy-KOL-uh-jist) is a mental health professional who can do psychological testing and provide mental health counseling.

* **psychiatrist** (sy-KY-uh-trist) refers to a medical doctor who has completed specialized training in the diagnosis and treatment of mental illness. Psychiatrists can diagnose mental illnesses, provide men-tal health counseling, and pre-scribe medications.

KEYWORDS
for searching the Internet and other reference sources

Cerebral palsy

Congenital disorders

Cytomegalovirus (CMV)

Fetal alcohol syndrome

Genetic disorders

Phenylketonuria (PKU)

Rubella

Spina bifida

Teratogens

Toxoplasmosis

*__fetus__ (FEE-tus) in humans, is the unborn offspring in the period after it is an embryo, from 9 weeks after fertilization until birth.

*__embryo__ (EM-bree-o) in humans, the developing organism from the end of the second week after fertilization to the end of the eighth week.

*__toxins__ (TOK-sinz) are poisonous substances.

Organizations

The Child and Adolescent Bipolar Foundation (CABF), 1187 Wilmette Avenue, P.M.B. #331, Wilmette, IL 60091. CABF is an organization that provides information and support for families of children who have early-onset bipolar disorder.
Telephone 847-256-8525
http://www.bpkids.org

United States National Institute of Mental Health (NIMH), 6001 Executive Boulevard, Room 8184, MSC 9663, Bethesda, MD 20892-9663. NIMH is a government agency that provides information about bipolar disorder.
Telephone 800-421-4211
http://www.nimh.nih.gov

Birth Defects and Brain Development

Birth defects of the brain are a group of disorders that result from illness or injury to the brain and central nervous system of a developing fetus*. Birth defects can be inherited from a parent or acquired through the mother's contact with environmental factors such as drugs or infections. Birth defects of the brain result in problems that can range from mild to severe. They can affect one part or many parts of the central nervous system.

The Developing Fetus

Starting at conception, the developing embryo* is susceptible to many factors that affect development. During the first twelve weeks of development, the cells of the embryo and fetus are rapidly dividing and becoming the infant's muscles, bones, and organs. Exposure to disease or toxins* may disrupt the process of development and can result in birth defects and developmental problems in the infant.

Since rapid growth and organ formation occur during the first 12 weeks of development, that is when the embryo and fetus are most susceptible to injury or insult. The neural (NU-ral) tube, which develops into the spinal cord and the brain, begins to develop about 10 days after conception and continues to develop throughout the pregnancy. Because the mother and the developing fetus are connected, many things that the mother is exposed to or takes into her body can be passed to the fetus. If the mother becomes ill, takes medications, is exposed to toxins, or takes any drugs, the fetus may be affected. How severe the developmental problem that results will be depends on many factors including the type of illness or type or amount of toxin involved.

The developing fetus must also receive enough oxygen. Low levels of oxygen reaching the fetus result in what is called intrauterine hypoxia (hy-POX-ee-a). Because cells need oxygen to survive and grow, hypoxia can cause developmental problems in the central nervous system, especially in the early stages of development. Anything that disrupts development at this young age can cause effects that last throughout childhood and adulthood. These types of central nervous system defects are not generally correctable after birth.

When the developing brain is exposed to a toxin it is difficult to predict exactly which parts of the brain will be affected or how severely the brain will be damaged. Disorders of intrauterine brain and central nervous system development lead to congenital (con-JEN-it-al) disorders or birth defects. It is important to note that the cause of the majority of birth defects of the central nervous system is unknown or uncertain, that is, no specific genetic abnormality, or toxin, drug, infection, or other environmental factor can be identified.

What follows are descriptions of some of the most common types of central nervous system birth defects and some of the agents that may cause them.

Anencephaly

Anencephaly (an-en-SEF-a-lee) is a defect in the neural tube, which is the part of the developing fetus that forms the spinal cord and brain. During early development, the neural tube fails to close and results in a missing or malformed brain or spinal cord. A fetus with anencephaly is born with no brain or only the very basic parts of the brain that control processes like breathing. Anencephaly is always a fatal condition and the infant may be stillborn* or die within days or weeks of birth. The exact cause of this disorder is still not known. Some studies have suggested that a problem with the nutrition of the mother may be an important cause of this disorder. Lower than normal levels of the B vitamin folic acid in the mother may place the developing fetus at risk for anencephaly.

*__stillborn__ means a baby who is not alive at birth.

Spina Bifida

Spina bifida (SPY-na BIF-i-da) or myelomeningocele (MY-eh-lo-me-NING-oh-seel) is a congenital disorder of neural tube development where there is an opening in the spinal cord and the spinal column (backbone) of the developing fetus. Spina bifida is one of the most common birth defects that involve the nervous system and it may affect as many as 1 in 800 infants. As with anencephaly, deficiency of folic acid in the mother appears to be an important factor in the development of spina bifida. Because the spinal cord is not enclosed in the backbone, the infant has a high risk for meningitis, a serious infection of the spinal fluid, brain, and the lining covering the brain and spinal cord. Generally the affected person has a loss of body functions below the level of the opening in the

This infant was born with spina bifida. During fetal development, the cells of the neural tube differentiate to form the brain and spinal cord. Spina bifida ("split spine") is a neural tube defect in which the spinal column does not close completely before birth. *Custom Medical Stock Photos*

▶

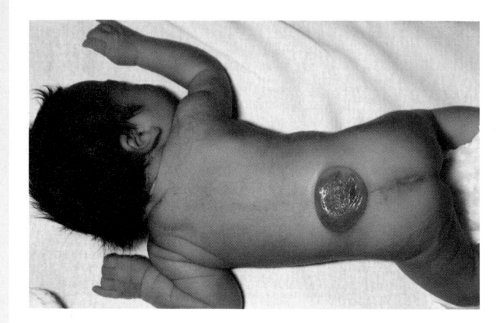

spinal cord. While surgery at birth will repair the opening, it will not change the loss of function. Children with spina bifida often do not walk unassisted and frequently have learning disabilities. Despite this, many children with spina bifida grow up to live productive lives.

Embryo Toxins

Embryo toxins are any substances that negatively affect or injure the embryo. In general, embryo toxins are called teratogens (tare-AT-o-jenz). Teratogens are substances that cause birth defects when the mother is exposed to them. Teratogens may include over-the-counter or prescription medicines, illegal drugs, common household chemicals, industrial waste, alcohol, or tobacco. It is important that the mother avoid teratogens while pregnant, especially during the first twelve weeks of pregnancy when the organs of the embryo and fetus are forming. Pregnant women or those seeking to become pregnant should consult with their physicians about which medications they can and cannot take.

Alcohol Alcohol is a teratogen that should be avoided during pregnancy. Mothers who drink during pregnancy put their child at risk for developing fetal alcohol syndrome (FAS). FAS can result in growth problems as well as mental and other physical congenital defects. Alcohol is a toxin that affects the developing central nervous system of the fetus. Children with fetal alcohol syndrome often show slow physical growth, delayed mental development that can be mild to severe, facial abnormalities, heart defects, and abnormalities of the skeleton. These children usually have mental retardation and frequently have behavior problems and hyperactivity.

Tobacco Nicotine from cigarette smoke is another teratogen that should be avoided during pregnancy. Nicotine from the mother's bloodstream is passed to the developing fetus. The nicotine affects the developing fetus and can contribute to a wide variety of problems, including low birth weight, birth defects, and sudden infant death syndrome (SIDS). Another problem caused by smoking is the lowering of blood oxygen content in the mother. When the mother's blood oxygen falls, the fetus also receives less oxygen, a condition called fetal hypoxia. This may contribute to the damaging effects of maternal smoking on the fetus.

Medications and Street Drugs Some drugs can act as teratogens and should be avoided during pregnancy. Illegal drugs such as amphetamines, cocaine, and heroin may affect the developing central nervous system of the fetus. In addition, these drugs may lead to other birth defects as well as addiction problems. Illegal drugs are not the only drugs that can cause problems. Prescription and over-the-counter medications can also affect the fetus. Pregnant mothers should consult with a physician about which medications are safe to take and which should be avoided.

Environmental hazards Exposure to household chemicals or other toxins in the environment may also contribute to impairment of the central nervous system of a fetus. In 1994 and 1995, a greater than expected number of infants along the Rio Grande in Texas and Mexico were born with anencephaly. While the exact cause was not found, it is suspected that pollution in the environment was involved. It is probably wise for pregnant women to avoid pesticides (such as weed killers) and insecticides. Some household cleaning chemicals contain substances that are teratogens and these should be avoided also.

Embryo Infections

Toxins in the environment are not the only things that affect the developing central nervous system. A number of infectious diseases may also affect the developing embryo. Some of these diseases may or may not affect the mother but can be passed to the fetus. Many of these diseases are caused by viruses, which are easily passed between the mother and fetus. Some infections that can have major effects on the fetus are:

Cytomegalovirus Cytomegalovirus (sy-to-MEG-a-lo-vy-rus; CMV) is a common virus that infects most people at some point in their lives. In some cases, the mother may pass the virus to the fetus through the placenta. In adults, CMV infections usually do not cause any significant symptoms. For the developing fetus, however, the infection can damage the brain. Children who had fetal CMV infections may have stunted growth, microcephaly (my-kro-SEF-a-lee; abnormally small brain and head size), and a number of other physical problems. Some of the symptoms may be treatable, but the central nervous system injury is permanent.

Syphilis Syphilis is a sexually transmitted bacterial disease that can be passed from mother to fetus. The risk of this occurring is 60 to 80 percent if the mother is infected and does not receive treatment. Early in the pregnancy, the developing central nervous system of the fetus

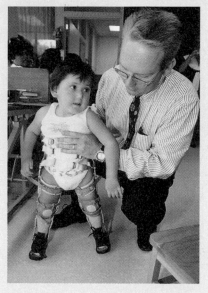

A doctor examines a child with spina bifida at a clinic near the Texas-Mexico border. The child's disorder is believed to have been caused by pollution in the area. *Annie Griffiths Belt/Corbis*

may be affected by the infection. At birth, some of these infants have meningitis (inflammation of the brain, spinal fluid, and lining covering the brain) or hydrocephalus (hy-dro-SEF-a-lus; excessive fluid within and surrounding the brain), and may have mental retardation as they grow older. Infants with the infection are treated with antibiotics to control the infection. This treatment may prevent additional damage to the nervous system but it does not reverse damage done to the developing brain before birth.

Rubella (German measles) Those who have received rubella vaccine are protected against infection. In the early stages of pregnancy, an unvaccinated, exposed mother can pass rubella to the developing fetus. The developing brain and central nervous system of the infant may be affected causing cerebral palsy and mental retardation, among other problems. There is no treatment that can reverse the brain damage rubella infection causes before birth.

Toxoplasmosis Toxoplasmosis (tok-so-plaz-MO-sis) is an infection caused by a parasite that is commonly found in undercooked meat and in cat stools. In most cases, there are no symptoms of the infection in healthy adults. However, the infection can be passed from the mother to the developing fetus. About 85 percent of infants born infected with toxoplasmosis show no symptoms at birth. Later, however, these children may develop learning disabilities, movement problems, mental retardation, and vision loss. Pregnant women should make sure that meat is cooked completely and they should avoid changing the cat litter box.

Metabolic Disorders

Metabolic (met-a-BOLL-ik) disorders are problems in the chemical reactions in the body involved with producing energy from food, and supporting the growth and function of the body's cells and tissues. When metabolic disorders occur during pregnancy or even during childhood, they may affect the developing central nervous system.

In conditions that affect the development of the central nervous system after birth, treatment for the condition may prevent problems such as mental retardation and other central nervous system problems. Two of the most common metabolic conditions that affect children are phenylketonuria (PKU) and hypothyroidism.

Phenylketonuria (PKU) Phenylketonuria (fen-il-kee-toe-NYOOR-ee-a) is an inherited genetic disorder that afflicts about 1 in 15,000 children. Children with this disorder are unable to chemically handle phenylalanine, an essential amino acid. If affected infants are not placed on a special diet soon after birth, they may develop seizures and permanent mental retardation. The diet for PKU restricts foods that contain phenylalanine.

Hypothyroidism Hypothyroidism is another metabolic condition that can affect the development of the brain and central nervous system. Hypothyroidism is a disease of the thyroid gland where there is an underproduction of thyroid hormones that are necessary for many body functions, including brain development in infants and children. Congenital hypothyroidism occurs in about 1 in 4,000 children, usually caused by failure of the thyroid gland to develop normally in the fetus. If it is left untreated, the infant's brain will not develop properly and the child will have slow physical growth and impaired mental abilities. Treatment with thyroid hormone (in pill form) started in the first few weeks of life will usually prevent developmental problems in the child.

Living with Birth Defects

Since currently there is no way to repair brain damage that occurs during early development, it is important to do what is possible to prevent these conditions. During pregnancy, the mother should take care of herself. She should avoid smoking, illegal drugs, and alcohol, taking medications without a doctor's approval, eating undercooked meat, cleaning the cat litter box, and exposure to toxic chemicals. She should eat a balanced diet and make sure she gets enough folic acid. That's a lot of things to think about when a woman is about to have a baby! Making frequent visits to the doctor when pregnant for advice on these issues is a good way to help give baby the best start possible.

 See also
Cerebral Palsy
Fetal Alcohol Syndrome
Genetics and Behavior
Mental Retardation

Body Dysmorphic Disorder

Body dysmorphic (dis-MORE-fik) disorder (BDD) is an extremely distressing, obsessive preoccupation with perceived flaws in one's appearance.

What Are Normal Concerns About Appearance?

Most people pay attention to their appearance. They may check themselves in the mirror, think about which clothes look nice on them, and try to look their best. Adolescents, whose bodies are changing dramatically, are notorious for paying special attention to their appearance. It is normal for adolescents to feel self-conscious about their looks at times, especially the appearance changes triggered by puberty*.

Jack feels self-conscious about his lack of body hair, while his friend Ben thinks that he has too much. Both boys feel a bit uncomfortable when they first get on the court for basketball practice because their uniforms reveal their legs, upper chest, and armpits. Terry feels self-conscious about having some acne* and did not want his girlfriend to take his picture at the class picnic. Anna finds that her legs seem to be growing faster than the rest of her body and felt hurt when someone teased her by calling her a beanpole. Nick is sure he has not grown at all this year and does not like being shorter than most of the girls in his seventh grade class. Luckily, the awkward body changes of adolescence almost always even out eventually.

KEYWORDS
for searching the Internet and other reference sources

Adolescence

Anxiety

Body image

Obsessions

Mood disorders

Puberty

Repetitive behaviors

* **puberty** (PU-ber-tee) is the period during which sexual maturity is attained.

* **acne** (AK-nee) is a condition in which pimples, blackheads, whiteheads, and sometimes deeper lumps occur on the skin.

Some self-criticism involves aspects of appearance that have nothing to do with puberty. Megan dislikes the freckled skin on her arms. Darlene wishes her hair were straight instead of kinky, while Angela wishes she had Darlene's waves. Andrea does not like her nose, and Paula wishes her lips were different. Jeanne thinks her complexion is too fair, and Derek thinks he is too dark-skinned.

Learning to like one's own body, coming to accept its imperfections, and growing to appreciate its unique beauty means having a healthy body image. Developing a healthy body image is an important task of adolescence.

What Are Extreme Concerns About Appearance?

Some people continue to have problems with body image long after adolescence is over. Body dysmorphic disorder (BDD) is a condition that involves extremely negative body image. BDD goes beyond self-criticism of one's features, concern with one's appearance, or poor body image. People who have BDD become overly preoccupied with what they see as flaws in their physical appearance, and they are often the only ones to perceive their features or characteristics as flaws. They may pick out tiny imperfections that others may not even notice and worry over these imperfections in a way that is out of proportion. Their self-criticism can leave them very distressed and too self-conscious to enjoy a full life. People with BDD are plagued by critical thoughts about their appearance and have a distorted body image that causes them to believe that they are ugly.

Marianne spent hours each day worrying about whether the skin on her hands was too wrinkly. She looked at them over and over, checking to see if the wrinkles were deeper than they had been the day before. She used all types of lotions and creams but still felt that her hands were too ugly to be seen. She never left the house without gloves, even in summer. She often called her sister to talk about the wrinkles, and her sister always said the same thing, "To me, your hands look the same as mine do, just like normal hands. I don't know why you let this bother you so much. I wish I knew what to say to make you stop getting so worked up over your hands."

Some experts estimate that BDD affects 1 to 2 percent of adults in the United States. Both males and females can have BDD. People with BDD, or "imagined ugliness", often stay at home and often become depressed* or isolated, and many experience anxiety*. Some have unnecessary plastic surgery* or go to great lengths to change or hide aspects of their appearance. Preoccupation with their appearance can leave them distracted and unable to enjoy activities with family and friends. Experts say that people with BDD often:

　　■　complain about their appearance, focusing on particular traits

* **depression** (de-PRESH-un) is a mental state characterized by feelings of sadness, despair, and discouragement.

* **anxiety** (ang-ZY-e-tee) can be experienced as a troubled feeling, a sense of dread, fear of the future, or distress over a possible threat to a person's physical or mental well-being.

* **plastic surgery** is the surgical repair, restoration, or improvement in the shape and appearance of body parts.

- look in the mirror frequently
- constantly fix, adjust, or hide their perceived flaws
- talk constantly about their perceived flaws
- ask others over and over for confirmation or reassurance about their appearance
- avoid situations where their flaws might be seen

What Causes Body Dysmorphic Disorder?

Though it may not be recognized and diagnosed until later, BDD usually begins before age 18. BDD usually starts during adolescence when the body is undergoing a lot of changes and when teenagers are forming their ideas about what is acceptable or desirable in physical appearance. Media images that emphasize perfection, as well as a person's own extremely high expectations or perfectionism about appearance, can be factors in the development of BDD. Harsh critical comments or ridicule about appearance by family or friends can be very destructive to body image and may plant the seeds for BDD.

In addition to social influences that may cause body image to be negative or distorted, biological factors may make certain people more likely to develop body dysmorphic disorder. Many experts believe that BDD is linked to obsessive-compulsive disorder (OCD). Obsessive-compulsive disorder causes people to become obsessed or extremely preoccupied with certain distressing thoughts. OCD also causes people to feel compelled to perform certain repetitive actions. BDD involves extreme preoccupation or obsession with appearance, harsh self-critical thoughts, and repeated checking or fixing of appearance. Viewed in this way, BDD may be one form of OCD.

How Is Body Dysmorphic Disorder Treated?

Because people with BDD are plagued by insecurity or self-consciousness and tend to isolate themselves, sometimes they alone know that they have this problem. Seeking treatment by a mental health professional can help relieve their distress. Treatment of BDD often involves psychotherapy that focuses on understanding the person's negative thoughts and opinions about his or her appearance, making needed adjustments in distorted thinking patterns and body image, and decreasing avoidance and repetitive thoughts and behaviors. Medications are sometimes used to relieve distress and to reduce anxiety or depression that can accompany BDD.

In some cases, a person's preoccupation with his or her appearance may actually be a symptom of another underlying disorder, such as an anxiety disorder*, an eating disorder*, or obsessive-compulsive disorder. Evaluation by a mental health professional can determine whether someone's BDD symptoms are part of a related problem. When that is the case, the person is treated for the other disorder as well.

* **anxiety disorders** (ang-ZY-e-tee dis-OR-derz) are a group of conditions that cause people to feel extreme fear or worry that sometimes is accompanied by symptoms such as dizziness, chest pain, or difficulty sleeping or concentrating.

* **eating disorder** is a condition in which a person's eating behaviors and food habits are so unbalanced that they cause physical and emotional problems.

Can Body Dysmorphic Disorder Be Prevented?

Experts say that teenagers can help prevent BDD by getting help with body image concerns early. While it is normal for adolescents to feel self-conscious about their changing looks, it is also important that they learn to like and accept their body and appearance. In time, many adolescents find that the very features they once wished were different are actually the ones that make their looks uniquely attractive. Concerns about appearance that get in the way of enjoying activities, being with friends, or that cause distress, anxiety, or depression may be a sign of body image problems. By paying the right kind of attention to such concerns early, mental health professionals can help prevent body image problems from becoming more serious.

Resources

Books

Phillips, Katharine A. *The Broken Mirror: Understanding and Treating Body Dysmorphic Disorder.* New York: Oxford University Press, 1998.

Walker, Pamela. *Everything You Need to Know about Body Dysmorphic Disorder: Dealing with a Distorted Body Image.* Brookshire, TX: Rosen Publishing Group, 1999.

Organization

Nemours Center for Children's Health Media, Alfred I. duPont Hospital for Children, 1600 Rockland Road, Wilmington, DE 19803. This organization is dedicated to issues of children's health and produces the KidsHealth website. Its website has articles about body image and body dysmorphic disorder.
http://www.KidsHealth.org

▶ *See also*

Anxiety and Anxiety Disorders

Body Image

Depression

Eating Disorders

Obsessive-Compulsive Disorder

KEYWORDS
for searching the Internet and other reference sources

Adolescence

Depression

Puberty

Self-image

Body Image

Body image is a person's impressions, thoughts, feelings, and opinions about his or her body.

"I'm fat." "I wish I had curly hair." "Why haven't I had a growth spurt yet?" "No one else in my class has diabetes." "Will I ever be strong enough to play on the football team?"

Most teenagers have similar questions and concerns about their bodies. They think a lot about their appearance, which seems in a constant state of change during adolescence. Everyone has an "image" of their body and appearance and how well it fits in with what they consider normal, acceptable, or attractive. For adolescents, body image is a big part of their total self-image.

Why Is Body Image So Important to Adolescents?

Teenagers' bodies are undergoing so many changes that it is easy to understand why they may be preoccupied with their appearance and their body image. Both boys and girls are experiencing growth spurts and sexual development. Girls' breasts and hips are enlarging, body hair is growing, and menstruation* is beginning. Boys' muscles are growing, their voices are getting deeper, and their testicles and penises are getting larger. Their features may be changing, and hormones may cause skin problems. It takes a while to get used to their new "image" or appearance.

Teenagers are very susceptible to criticism, teasing, or negative comments. Some teenagers lose confidence in their appearance if they receive negative or insulting comments about their looks, racial or ethnic features, physical abilities, or body changes associated with puberty*. With all of the focus on the body's appearance, teenagers may need to be reminded to give equal value to other important aspects of themselves, such as personality, inner strengths, mental aptitudes, and artistic and musical talents, which, along with body image, contribute to overall self-image.

What Leads to Body Image Problems?

Teenagers' body images are strongly affected by what they see on television and in the movies. Magazines are filled with pictures of thin and beautiful young women and lean and muscular young men. Teenagers are influenced by these images and may wish to look like their favorite models or stars. However, the degree of physical perfection that media images convey is largely an illusion created by makeup, hours of styling, special lighting, and photography. When people compare themselves to these perfect-looking images, they may become disappointed with their own appearance. Feeling the need to look perfect, or to have a perfect body, can lead to body image problems.

Body image problems affect both boys and girls, but they tend to bother girls more deeply than boys. One reason is that in American culture, girls' and women's worth and value traditionally have been linked closely to their physical attractiveness. Boys' appearance, while important, is not generally seen as their most important feature. Boys, however, often feel pressure to be tall, muscular, and strong.

Some teenagers have illnesses or disabilities that they cannot change. These things may challenge their body image at first. Teenagers who focus on what the body can do, rather than on what it cannot, learn that even with physical limitations, it is possible to develop a strong positive body image. Sometimes, overcoming limitations caused by a disability

* **menstruation** (men-stroo-AY-shun) is the discharge of the blood-enriched lining of the uterus. Menstruation normally occurs in females who are physically mature enough to bear children. Because it usually occurs at about four-week intervals, it is often called the "monthly period." Most girls have their first period between the age of 9 and 16.

* **puberty** (PU-ber-tee) is the period during which sexual maturity is attained.

What Does Perfect Mean?

Some girls are more influenced than others by the thinness craze. How much value a girl places on thinness may depend on how much value her cultural group gives it. One study of about 300 American eighth and ninth grade girls suggested that certain cultural differences might affect girls' body image ideals. The study compared the body image of girls of European ancestry with the body image of girls of African ancestry. Ninety percent of the girls of European ancestry in the study felt dissatisfied with their body weight and shape, whereas only thirty percent of the girls of African ancestry felt dissatisfied with their bodies! When asked to describe the "perfect girl," the descriptions by girls of European ancestry often focused on thinness as the key to popularity and happiness. For example, they

(continued)

described the perfect girl as someone who is 5'7" and 100 to 110 pounds (a trim, healthy body weight for someone 5'7" is about 125 pounds). Girls of African ancestry were more likely to emphasize the importance of personality and downplayed the importance of physical traits and thinness when they described the perfect girl. They described the perfect girl as someone who is smart, fun, easy to talk to, not conceited, and funny. They were more likely to describe beauty as an inner quality; in fact, two-thirds of them described beauty as the "right attitude." Their descriptions of the body weight and dimensions that they would like to have were more in line with healthy weights. Not surprisingly, studies have shown that there is lower incidence of anorexia and bulimia among girls of African ancestry than among girls of European ancestry.

* **depression** (de-PRESH-un) is a mental state characterized by feelings of sadness, despair, and discouragement.

* **eating disorders** are conditions in which a person's eating behaviors and food habits are so unbalanced that they cause physical and emotional problems.

* **psychotherapist** (sy-ko-THER-a-pist) is a mental health counselor who listens to people and helps them change thoughts, actions, or relationships that play a part in problems they may be experiencing.

Am I Too Fat?

Too much focus on physical appearance can create body image problems, especially for females. Even those of normal healthy body weight can feel fat when comparing themselves to super-thin

can create an unexpected boost to body image. For example, Tyrie, who has used a wheelchair since age nine, began to race competitively as an adolescent. The upper body strength and physical endurance he has developed by training for races has given him new confidence in his body's capabilities. He is proud of his muscular arms and chest, not to mention his medals. Even though he does not walk, his friends see him as one of the strongest guys in the tenth grade.

When Are Body Image Problems a Sign of Other Problems?

Some teenagers are satisfied with how they look and feel confident about their appearance. Others are more self-critical and always come up lacking when comparing their features with others. Extreme dissatisfaction with body image can lead to depression*, social isolation, or eating disorders*.

Sometimes body image can become distorted, and people may mistakenly believe themselves to be fat or ugly. These distorted or mistaken ideas can cause a person to feel extremely distressed, self-critical, and overly preoccupied with their physical imperfections. Someone who has a constant and distressing preoccupation with minor body "imperfections" may have a condition called body dysmorphic (dis-MORE-fik) disorder.

Some people develop a strong fear of gaining weight. They may begin to diet or exercise excessively, lose weight rapidly, and refuse to eat enough food to maintain a healthy weight. A person with this pattern may have an eating disorder called anorexia (an-o-REK-see-a). People with anorexia develop a distorted body image and see themselves as fat when they are not. Even though they may get dangerously underweight and malnourished, they continue to feel fat and refuse to eat.

Bulimia (bu-LEE-me-a) is another eating disorder that involves body image problems. People with bulimia have a distorted body image that causes them to be self-critical and to feel fat, and they place too much importance on weight and body shape. People with bulimia have episodes of out-of-control overeating, or binges, and then try to make up for them by making themselves vomit, by taking laxatives, or by exercising to excess to avoid gaining weight. People with excessive body image problems may need assistance from several mental health professionals including a physician, a psychotherapist*, and a nutritionist.

What Leads to a Good Body Image?

There are certain things that people cannot change about their appearance or physical capabilities, but having a good body image does not require a perfect body. People develop a healthy body image by taking care of their body, appreciating its capabilities, and accepting its imperfections. Positive body image is linked to positive self-image, self-confidence, and popularity.

Most teenagers can control their appearance to some extent; for example, they may choose haircuts or clothing that reflect how they see themselves. By doing so, they can create an outer image that pleases them.

Eating healthy foods and getting plenty of exercise can help teenagers develop strong, fit bodies of which they can be proud. Cutting down on junk foods helps them stay trim, and physical activities help them develop strength, coordination, and new capabilities. Healthy behaviors contribute to attractive appearance on the outside and add to positive inner feelings about body image.

Resources

Books

Shandler, Sara. *Ophelia Speaks: Adolescent Girls Write about Their Search for Self.* New York: HarperCollins, 1999.

Walker, Pamela. *Everything You Need to Know about Body Dysmorphic Disorder: Dealing with a Distorted Body Image.* Brookshire, TX: Rosen Publishing Group, 1999.

Organization

Nemours Center for Children's Health Media, Alfred I. duPont Hospital for Children, 1600 Rockland Road, Wilmington, DE 19803. This organization is dedicated to issues of children's health and produces the KidsHealth website. Its website has articles about body image and body dysmorphic disorder. http://www.KidsHealth.org

models and stars. Studies have found that 80 percent of adolescent girls feel fat, and up to 70 percent of adolescent girls are on a diet at any given time. Four out of five American women are dissatisfied with their appearance, and half of American women are on a diet. These attitudes and behaviors are showing up at younger ages. One study found that half of the girls in grades three through six want to be thinner, and 33 percent of them have already tried to lose weight. Extreme self-criticism about weight, dissatisfaction with body image, and the quest for perfection can lead to feelings of failure, unhealthy dieting, and serious eating disorders.

▶ *See also*
Anorexia
Body Dysmorphic Disorder
Bulimia
Eating Disorders
Obesity

Brain Chemistry (Neurochemistry)

The brain communicates with itself by sending out chemical information from one neuron, or nerve cell, to another. Brain chemistry is the sum of all the chemical messaging that takes place in the brain, which allows it to carry out its daily functions, such as generating movement, speaking, thinking, listening, regulating the systems of the body, and countless others.

Out of Balance: Hector's Story

Now a tenth-grader, Hector had been experiencing severe depression since he was in seventh grade. Everyone feels down or depressed every now and then, but Hector felt this way most of the time. He had a hard time making friends, he was not interested in his schoolwork, and he spent most of his time hanging out in his room alone. He had even thought about suicide. At first, his parents believed that this was just a phase he was going through, but then they became really concerned.

* **psychiatrist** refers to a medical doctor who has completed specialized training in the diagnosis and treatment of mental illness. Psychiatrists diagnose mental illnesses, provide mental health counseling, and can prescribe medications.

* **neurotransmitter** (NUR-o-tranz-mit-er) is a brain chemical that lets brain cells communicate with each other and therefore allows the brain to function properly. In other words, a neurotransmitter transmits (carries) a chemical message from neuron to neuron.

What was happening to their son, who had been generally upbeat and friendly until a few years earlier?

At the insistence of his parents and teachers, Hector started seeing a psychiatrist*, who tried to help him talk about what he was feeling. Based on her meetings with Hector, she decided to prescribe a type of medication known as an antidepressant. This medication increases the amount of a brain neurotransmitter* called serotonin (ser-ah-TO-nin), which is associated with feelings of well-being and control. The medicine, a selective serotonin reuptake inhibitor (SSRI), works by preventing (inhibiting) neurons from reabsorbing (reuptaking) the chemical messenger serotonin once it is released into the brain. As a result, there is more serotonin available, and this sometimes helps alleviate the symptoms of depression. If Hector's depression were being caused by too little serotonin, the medication likely would help him.

Sure enough, it did. Hector continued to see his psychiatrist while taking the medication. After about 6 months, his doctor decided to try taking Hector off the SSRI. Hector was afraid that his terrible feelings would return, but they did not. He found that talking through any problems with his doctor was enough to keep him on track.

A Cascade of Chemicals

Every day, researchers are learning more about the chemicals that the neurons (NUR-ons) in the human brain use to communicate with each other. They now know that all the feelings and emotions that people experience are produced through chemical changes in the brain. The "rush" of happiness that a person feels at getting a good grade on a test, winning the lottery, or reuniting with a loved one occur through complex chemical processes. So are emotions, such as sadness, grief, and stress. When the brain tells the body to do something, such as to sit down or run, this also sets a chemical process in motion. These "chemical communicators," or neurotransmitters, are the "words" that make up the language of the brain and the entire nervous system.

The billions of tiny neurons in the brain communicate with each other across small spaces called synapses (SIN-ap-siz). When one neuron is charged into action, it releases its chemical messenger, which then moves across the synapse to the next neuron, where it is accepted by a special receiving area, called a receptor, on the surface of the neuron. The chemical will be accepted only by receptors that recognize it, in a kind of "lock and key" system, that is, certain keys work only in certain locks. Once attached to a receptor site on another neuron, different neurotransmitters either trigger "go" signals that prompt the neuron to pass certain messages on to other cells or produce "stop" signals that prevent certain messages from being forwarded. (For an illustration of how neurotransmitters work, see "Medications.")

Any one neuron may be receiving many chemical messages, both positive and negative (stop and go), from the other neurons surrounding it.

These neurotransmitters may be "competing" to get the neuron to respond in different ways, or they may work together to produce a certain effect. Since all of this happens within a split second, the neurotransmitter must be cleared away quickly so that the same receptors can be activated again and again. This clearing away can happen in one of three ways. The chemical may be pumped back into the nerve ending it comes from, a process known as "reuptake," it may be destroyed by enzymes* near the receptor sites, or it may simply spread out into the surrounding area of the brain and be destroyed there.

Modifying Neurotransmission with Drugs

Many neurological (nur-a-LA-je-kal) conditions, ranging from emotional disorders, such as depression, to movement disorders, such as Parkinson disease, are associated with imbalances of certain neurotransmitters in the brain. Researchers have been able to develop many medications that work to correct these imbalances, improving people's symptoms and helping them lead more fulfilling lives. At the same time, many legal and illegal drugs, such as the nicotine in cigarettes and the street drugs heroin and cocaine, work by changing neurotransmitter levels. People report feeling "good" or "up" when they start taking these drugs, but soon the neurons in their brains become so accustomed to the change in chemical balance that it takes more of a drug to get that same feeling, and the brain starts to crave the substance. The result is chemical dependency or addiction. What happens when brain chemicals are modified is described in the three examples of neurotransmitters (serotonin, dopamine, and gamma-aminobutyric acid) below.

Serotonin Many studies have linked low levels of the neurotransmitter serotonin to depression, impulsive and aggressive forms of behavior, violence, and even suicide. The class of medications called SSRIs, like the one that was given to Hector, prevents the neurons that release this chemical from taking it back in once it is in the synapse. As a result, the person has more serotonin available to attach to receptors in the brain, which can ease the symptoms of depression, as it did for Hector.

An illegal drug known as "Ecstasy," or MDMA, also changes the level of serotonin in the brain, but much more radically. It causes the serotonin-releasing neurons to dump their contents all at once, which floods the brain with the chemical and produces feelings of extreme happiness and hyperactivity (excessive activity). This feeling comes with a price. Since Ecstasy uses up the brain's supply of serotonin, the person is likely to feel depressed when the immediate "rush" of the drug's effects ends after a few hours. This "down" period lasts until the brain can build its supply of serotonin back up to normal levels. Repeated use of Ecstasy may lead to depression or other problems over time, since the neurons can "bounce back" only so often.

* **enzymes** are natural substances that cause or speed up specific chemical reactions in living organisms, like the human body.

Up for Debate: Medicating Mental and Behavioral Disorders

Depression, social anxiety, excessive shyness, and hyperactivity are just some of the conditions that might be treated successfully with medications that alter neurotransmitter levels in the brain. Before these medications became available, people with these and other problems either had to live with them or worked with a psychiatrist or psychologist to deal with their feelings. Now we know that brain chemistry disorders can be treated, allowing more people to overcome much of their social difficulty.

Some experts fear that we are beginning to rely too heavily on these medications as a "quick fix." While the experts do not deny that there are some people who need drug treatment, they also argue that there are people who think that feeling down or socially awkward occasionally is the same thing as having a disorder. These people then ask their doctors for medications that should be reserved for people who are truly distressed. When symptoms interfere with a person's life to a large extent, medication is considered. In most cases, while medications can help to decrease symptoms, more complete and long-lasting relief is achieved through therapy that helps with behavior change. Normal variations in feelings in response to life's changes and challenges are to be expected. Other forms of intervention, such as behavioral therapy and exercise, should be considered as alternatives to medication or in addition to medication when symptoms create suffering and present undue difficulties.

(continued)

One of the hottest debates surrounds a condition known as attention deficit hyperactivity disorder (ADHD), which usually is diagnosed in childhood. Children with this condition have a hard time paying attention and sitting still, and they tend to be impulsive and overactive. More and more children are being diagnosed with ADHD, and many of them are taking medications that enhance the activity of the neurotransmitter dopamine. This helps the child be more alert, more focused, and therefore better able to stay "on task."

While most children (70 to 80 percent) with ADHD are helped by medication, some experts believe that some parents and doctors may be too hasty in labeling children with a diagnosis of ADHD to justify what is simply bad behavior and then medicating children who do not really need to be given drugs. They believe that medicine might be leading some parents and children away from other, potentially more helpful therapies. Others feel that children with ADHD have been under-diagnosed for many years and only more recently are being appropriately diagnosed and treated. There are no easy solutions to this problem, and the mental health and medical communities likely will be debating this issue for years to come.

* **schizophrenia** (skitz-o-FREE-nee-ah) is one of a large group of mental disorders in which a person loses touch with reality and is no longer able to think and act normally. People with this disorder may hear voices or see things that are not really there.

* **sympathetic nervous system** is the system of nerves that prepares the body for action by speeding up the heart and breathing rates and raising the blood pressure.

Dopamine   Neurons in the core of the brain release dopamine (DO-pa-meen), a neurotransmitter that affects processes that control movement, emotional response, and the ability to experience pleasure and pain. In people who have Parkinson disease, dopamine-transmitting neurons in this area of the brain die, which causes progressive loss of movement control. A medication called L-DOPA, which the brain can convert into dopamine, often helps control these symptoms. Some researchers have theorized that people with the mental disorder known as schizophrenia* are, in fact, overly sensitive to the dopamine in their brains. Some of these people seem to have been helped by medications that block dopamine receptors in the brain, thereby limiting the neurotransmitter's effect.

Another class of drugs known as amphetamines (am-FET-a-meenz) work by increasing the level of dopamine that neurons release and then preventing them from taking it back in through the reuptake process. These drugs have medical uses, such as the treatment of attention deficit hyperactivity disorder, but some people misuse amphetamines to help themselves stay awake or perform a task better.

Gamma-aminobutyric acid   Gamma-aminobutyric acid, or GABA, is the main neurotransmitter that works to inhibit the brain's neurons from acting. Research suggests that certain types of epilepsy, which is characterized by recurring seizures that affect a person's awareness and movements, may be the result of having too little GABA in the brain. The neuronal messaging system goes into overdrive, with tens of thousands of neurons sending messages intensely and simultaneously, which produces a seizure. Researchers believe that enzymes may be responsible for breaking down too much GABA, and they have developed medications that appear to help combat this process.

Hormones: Another Piece of the Brain Chemistry Puzzle

Norepinephrine (nor-e-pi-NE-frin) is a neurotransmitter that is involved in various arousal systems in the brain (systems that bring about alertness and attention) and in the sympathetic nervous system*. In the sympathetic nervous system, it is norepinephrine that causes the blood vessels to narrow, raising blood pressure, and speeds the breathing and heart rates. Norepinephrine also functions as a hormone when it is released by the adrenal glands located just above the kidneys, with similar results. Norepinephrine, epinephrine, and other hormones produced by the adrenal gland are involved in the "fight or flight" response of the body to stress.

Hormones are chemical substances that are sent into the bloodstream by the endocrine* (EN-do-krin) glands found throughout the body. They carry messages that produce certain effects in the body, much as the nervous system neurotransmitters do. In fact, there are many substances like norepinephrine that function both as neurotransmitters and hormones. This reflects the close relationship between these two body regulation systems. The brain plays an important role in regulating the release of hormones, and if hormone levels get out of balance (as neurotransmitter levels sometimes do), it can have an impact on how the brain functions and therefore on how a person feels.

Resources

Books

Powledge, Tabitha M. *Your Brain: How You Got It and How It Works.* New York: Charles Scribner's Sons, 1994.

Novitt-Moreno, Anne. *How Your Brain Works.* Emeryville, CA: Ziff-Davis Press, 1995.

Organizations

The website Neuroscience for Kids is a great resource for kids and teens about brain chemistry, structure, and function. It provides other resources and links as well.
http://faculty.washington.edu/chudler/neurok.html

Nemours Center for Children's Health Media, Alfred I. duPont Hospital for Children, 1600 Rockland Road, Wilmington, DE 19803. This organization is dedicated to issues of children's health and produces the KidsHealth website. Its website has articles about the brain, emotions, and behavior.
http://www.KidsHealth.org

Brain Injuries

Brain injuries usually result from impact or trauma to the brain that can lead to a variety of medical problems, depending on the nature of the injury.

Call a Doctor Right Away

Any significant impact or trauma to the head should be checked out by a doctor. Brain injuries may result from penetrating wounds or damage associated with impact. Penetrating wounds may be caused by foreign objects (for example, a bullet) or skull fragments that cause damage to brain tissue. Impact injuries might be the result of hitting the head with

* **endocrine** refers to the network of glands and other body tissues that produce and release (secrete) hormones into the bloodstream, where they travel to other parts of the body and act as chemical messengers.

▶ *See also*
Attention Deficit Hyperactivity Disorder

Brain and Nervous System (Introduction)

Depression

Medications

Schizophrenia

Stress

KEYWORDS
for searching the Internet and other reference sources

Brain damage

Concussion

Coma

Sports injury

*   **bacteria** (bak-TEER-ee-a) are round, spiral, or rod-shaped single-cell microorganisms with a distinct nucleus that commonly multiply by cell division. Some types may cause disease in humans, animals, or plants.

*   **hemorrhage** (HEM-o-rij) is bleeding usually due to damaged blood vessels.

*   **edema** (e-DEE-ma) is the abnormal accumulation of fluid in body tissues, such as the swelling that occurs after a sprained ankle or other injury.

force against a hard object, like the windshield of a car, or of being hit by a hard object, such as a baseball. Skull fractures may allow bacteria* access to the brain, leading to dangerous infections. The most common type of brain injury results from minor trauma. Such injuries usually do not involve loss of consciousness (being "knocked out"). More serious brain injuries may occur with or without a skull fracture as a result of impact trauma.

The brain is surrounded by a liquid called cerebrospinal (se-REE-bro-spy-nal) fluid (CSF). The CSF acts as a cushion to absorb some of the force of impact. Unfortunately, in the course of an impact injury to the head, the brain can shift, and tissue damage can occur, especially from rapidly speeding up or slowing down—much like what happens to Jell-O in a container that is dropped or suddenly yanked. The brain damage may be at the point of impact, opposite the point of impact, or spread across any of the areas of the brain. The delicate nerve tissues, the blood vessels, or the membranes surrounding the brain, called the meninges (men-NIN-jeez) may be torn or injured. The damage may result in abnormal brain activity, cerebral hemorrhage* or cerebral edema*. Because the skull is rigid and there is only limited room inside it, the swelling brain causes increasing pressure inside the skull, which can force brain tissue to press directly against the inside of the skull, resulting in more damage.

What Are the Causes of Brain Injury?

There are many causes of brain injury. One of the most common causes is motor vehicle accidents. Impact to the skull may be caused by the head striking the windshield or dashboard as well as by loose objects in the car. "Whiplash," a sudden, quick movement of the head back and forth (like cracking a whip), also can produce the kind of forces associated with impact. Head injuries also may result from falls from bicycles, skateboards, roller skates, or roller blades or during sporting events, particularly when a helmet is not worn. Head injuries also may result from slips, trips, or falls. Anytime there is trauma to the head, the possibility of brain injury is present, and a doctor should be consulted immediately if there is any change in level of consciousness, balance, ability to move, memory, or vision.

Not all brain injuries are the result of trauma. The brain can be damaged by lack of oxygen, as with drowning or near-drowning, or a particularly difficult birth. The brain can also be damaged through starvation, vitamin deficiencies, or certain other types of malnutrition. Toxins, such as heavy metals (like lead), can irreversably damage the brain. A wide variety of medical illnesses can also have an impact on the brain and central nervous system.

What Are the Signs and Symptoms of Brain Injury?

Brain injuries are difficult to diagnose, because there may be many different signs or symptoms that are present immediately after injury or that may

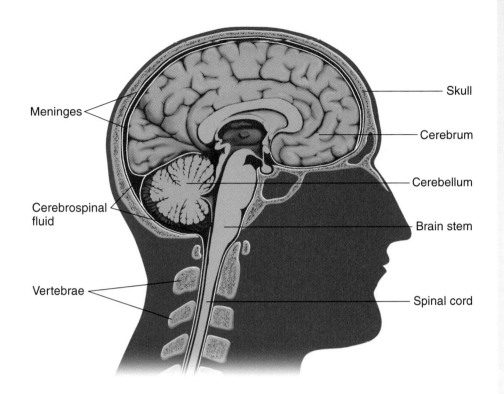

Meninges

Cerebrospinal fluid

Vertebrae

Skull

Cerebrum

Cerebellum

Brain stem

Spinal cord

Impact to the head may cause leakage of fluid and blood from blood vessels in the scalp, forming a painful lump. A stronger blow can tear the meninges, the protective membrane surrounding the brain, or injure the brain tissue itself. The bleeding and brain swelling this type of injury can produce may lead to increased pressure within the skull, resulting in a variety of problems including concussion and permanent brain damage.

not show up for hours or days. In the event of any type of head injury, it is important to gather as much information as possible about the accident. Anyone who witnessed the accident should provide details about exactly what happened and how the injured person acted after the accident.

Temporary amnesia (am-NEE-zha), or loss of memory, is common with many brain injuries. It is typical for the injured person not to remember what happened immediately before, during, and immediately after the accident. Brief periods of amnesia may occur during the recovery period after brain injuries. Longer-term amnesia is not common, except when a head injury is severe.

Brain injuries can affect a person cognitively (intellectually), physically, and emotionally. The following symptoms may be present at the time of the accident. While it is less common, some symptoms may appear hours, days, or even longer after the accident:

- Cognitive effects of brain injury may include short-term or long-term memory loss, inability to learn new information, trouble concentrating or staying focused, speech or communication difficulties, disorientation in space, problems in organizing aspects of daily living, impaired decision-making, and inability to perform more than one task at a time.

- Physical effects of brain injury may include seizures*, rigid limbs, muscle spasms, double vision*, dim vision, blindness, loss

* **seizures** (SEE-zhurz) are "storms" in the brain that occur when the electrical patterns of the brain are interrupted by powerful, rapid bursts of electrical energy. This may cause a person to fall down, make jerky movements, or stare blankly into space.

* **double vision** is a vision disorder that causes a person to see two images of a single object.

95

Steve Young, star quarterback for the San Francisco 49ers, is knocked to the ground during a football game. In 2000, after 13 years with the team, Young announced his retirement due to the series of head injuries he sustained on the field. *Associated Press/AP* ▶

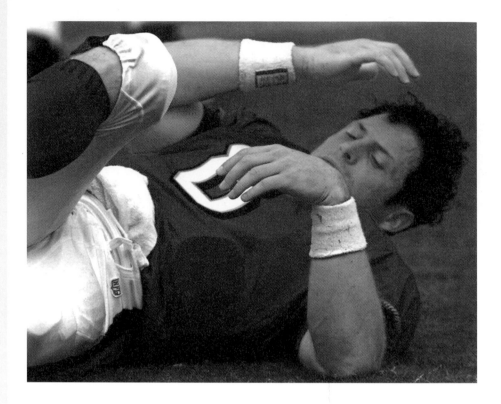

of the sense of taste or smell, slow or slurred speech, minor or severe headaches, balance problems, and tiredness.

▪ Emotional effects of brain injury may include anxiety (ang-ZY-e-tee), depression or mood swings, denial of having any problems, impulsive behavior, agitation (a-je-TAY-shun), and changes in personality.

What Are the Different Types of Brain Injury?

Minor Head Trauma   Anyone who suffers minor head trauma without loss of consciousness or other associated neurological* symptoms still should be watched closely. The injury may or may not be followed by symptoms such as vomiting, paleness of the skin, irritability, or sluggishness. If any of the symptoms last more than 6 hours or if they worsen, the symptoms may indicate a more severe injury. A doctor should be consulted immediately for an in-depth evaluation.

Skull fracture   A skull fracture, or injury to the bony structures protecting the brain, may or may not result in any neurological symptoms. In some cases the skull may have a noticeable depression (a "pushed in" appearance, like a dent), or there may be significant swelling or bleeding from the overlying scalp. Fractures may cause bruising or tearing of brain tissue, or blood vessels on the meninges. The injured person may

*__neurological__ (nur-a-LAH-je-kal) refers to the nervous system, a network of specialized tissue made of nerve cells, or neurons, that processes messages to and from different parts of the human body.

What Are the Long-Term Effects of Brain Injury?

Recovery from a minor brain injury, such as a concussion, usually takes a short period of time (3 to 6 months), and the recovery often is complete. For more serious injuries, degrees of recovery vary. Factors that predict good recovery are the patient's age (younger is better), duration of coma (longer is worse), presence of bleeding in the brain, and the site and amount of trauma to the head and brain. Patients who survive severe brain injury often face a long recovery process (years) and are left with permanent disabilities.

Rehabilitation programs help patients regain their cognitive and emotional faculties. During the rehabilitation process, it is common for patients to have lapses of memory, behavioral changes, emotional problems such as anxiety or depression, changes in sleep patterns, declines in intellectual ability, and seizures. Psychological counseling and brain injury support groups are available to help patients and families deal with the long-term rehabilitation process.

Patients who end up in a coma or a persistent vegetative state (PVS) usually have the most severe types of brain injury. In these types of injury, the cognitive centers of the brain are badly damaged while the brain stem that controls bodily functions remains intact. The PVS can last for many years. During the PVS, patients are not mentally aware of their surroundings but they still have basic reflexes and sleep cycles. Patients in a PVS that lasts longer than 3 months have a slight chance of some amount of recovery, while patients in a PVS for more than 6 months rarely recover.

How Can Brain Injury Be Prevented?

Most brain injuries are the result of accidents or falls. Wearing safety belts in cars and helmets when using wheeled vehicles, such as bicycles and skateboards, can prevent many of these injuries. Learning and observing safety practices is important. Wearing a safety belt in the front seat of a car prevents the wearer from hitting the dashboard, steering wheel, or windshield. Wearing seatbelts in the front seat or backseat keeps the wearer from being thrown around inside the vehicle or thrown out of the vehicle. Wearing a helmet while riding a bicycle or motorcycle or using a skateboard or skates helps protect the rider from injuries during falls. The helmets should be tight fitting and padded and have a chin strap. It is also important to wear helmets while playing contact sports such as football. Even in sports such as baseball, helmets should be worn whenever there is a possibility that the ball could strike the head.

Resources

Book

Levy, Allan M., and Mark L. Fuerst. *Sports Injury Handbook: Professional Advice for Amateur Athletes.* New York: John Wiley and Sons, 1993.

Sports-Related Brain Injury

Every year more than 750,000 people in the United States are injured while playing recreational sports. About 82,000 of these are traumatic brain injuries. Players of almost any sport can be injured, but those who play football, soccer, or ice hockey or those who wrestle or box may be most in danger of severe brain injuries. In just one playing season, as many as 10 percent of college football players and 20 percent of high school football players may have serious head injuries. Sports players who are hit in the head repeatedly, like boxers, may have permanent disabilities as the result of many injuries to the brain. The American Medical Association thinks that the danger is so grave that they have repeatedly called for a ban on boxing. Some professional boxers have a condition called "punch-drunk syndrome," which slurs their speech and makes them unsteady on their feet. Boxers who are punch-drunk also may have memory impairment and difficulties in concentrating or communicating. Muhammad Ali, three-time world heavyweight boxing champion and Olympic gold medalist, has parkinsonism, which may have resulted from his years in the ring. A person with parkinsonism usually has muscle rigidity, tremors, and twitches that may make it difficult to walk or even to talk. In severe cases, parkinsonism also may affect a person's mental abilities.

Covers head and neck injuries, with separate chapters on sports with the highest risk of concussion.

Organization

Head Injury Hotline, 212 Pioneer Building, Seattle, WA 98104-2221. This nonprofit organization is a clearinghouse for wide-ranging information on brain injury. They maintain a research library at their website and provide fact sheets as well as up-to-date news on health resources, support groups, rehabilitation facilities, and much more.
Telephone 206-621-8558
http://www.headinjury.com

Bulimia

Bulimia (bull-EE-me-a), sometimes referred to as the "binge-purge" disorder, involves repeated episodes of excessive eating (bingeing) followed by attempting to rid the body of the food by vomiting, using laxatives or enemas (purging), or exercising excessively.

Marlene's Perfect Figure

To her friends and family, Marlene had a perfectly fine figure, and she seemed confident and self-assured. But privately, Marlene suffered from bulimia and could not seem to stop bingeing and purging. Several times a week, she would eat whole batches of cookies, packages of candies, and as much bread and muffins as she could find. Her guilt and fear of overweight always led her to make herself vomit. Marlene stayed at a healthy weight for her size, but she was obsessed with her weight and body shape.

What Is Bulimia?

Eating disorders are habits or patterns of eating that are out of balance and may involve major health and emotional problems. Bulimia is a type of eating disorder in which a person binges, or consumes large quantities of food, and then purges, or attempts to rid the body of the food. When bingeing, people with bulimia often feel like they have little control over their behavior. After a binge, they feel guilty and fearful of becoming fat, so they try to rid the body of the food by vomiting or using laxatives or enemas. They may use diet pills or take drugs to reduce the volume of fluids in the body. Some people with bulimia also exercise excessively in order to burn up some of the calories eaten during binges. People with bulimia have a distorted body image*; even though many people with bulimia stay at a fairly healthy weight, they are fixated on body shape and weight and feel like they are fat.

KEYWORDS
for searching the Internet and other reference sources

Anorexia

Binge eating disorder

Binge and purge

Compulsive overeating

Eating disorders

*****body image** is a person's impressions, thoughts, feelings, and opinions about his or her body.

Most people who develop bulimia are girls and young women of European ancestry, although males and people of all ethnic groups can have it. Bulimia affects at least 1 to 3 percent of middle and high school girls and up to 5 percent of college-age women in the United States.

What Causes Bulimia?

Bulimia often starts out with dieting after a binge, but once the purging begins, the situation worsens. A person eats too much, feels guilty about it, and purges. The purging provides some immediate relief but is followed by shame and guilt. People with bulimia begin to believe that the only way to control their weight is to purge. They often feel intense social and cultural pressure to be thin. Family problems and conflict are also often present in the lives of people with bulimia. Poor self-esteem can also play a role. People with bulimia overemphasize the importance of body shape and size in their overall self-image.

What Are the Signs and Symptoms of Bulimia?

A person with bulimia can often hide it very well. A girl with bulimia is usually near a healthy weight but is preoccupied with eating and dieting. Bulimia and other eating disorders share many symptoms, such as fatigue, low blood pressure, dehydration, preoccupation with food, and secretiveness about eating. However, because of the purging, bulimia can be associated with additional, serious symptoms that include:

- tooth and other dental problems caused by stomach acids damaging tooth enamel
- rips or tears in the esophagus (the tube that runs from the throat to the stomach) from frequent vomiting
- other gastrointestinal problems
- imbalances in electrolytes (essential body chemicals and minerals) that can lead to heart and other health problems
- feelings of loss of control, shame, depression, irritability, withdrawal, and secretiveness

How Is Bulimia Diagnosed?

Like Marlene, people often keep their bulimia hidden from family, friends, and health care professionals. The shame and embarrassment about purging can be profound. Sometimes a dentist will notice damage to the tooth enamel. A health care professional might ask about a person's weight, diet, nutrition, and body image, and the responses may reveal an eating disorder. If concerned, a physician might order lab tests to study nutritional and medical status. A mental health professional may uncover bulimia when a person is treated for a different symptom, such as anxiety* or depression*.

* **anxiety** can be experienced as a troubled feeling, a sense of dread, fear of the future, or distress over a possible threat to a person's physical or mental well-being.

* **depression** (de-PRESH-un) is a mental state characterized by feelings of sadness, despair, and discouragement.

How Is Bulimia Treated?

Bulimia, like other eating disorders, is treated most effectively with a combination of therapies. The main treatment for bulimia is psychotherapy*. The focus of treatment is on changing eating behaviors and thinking patterns. To help a person overcome bulimia, a therapist will also address the person's distorted body image and fear of fat. Sometimes a physician will prescribe an antidepressant medication to relieve anxiety or depressive symptoms. Nutritional counseling, support groups, and family counseling can also be helpful.

Resources

Organizations

American Anorexia Bulimia Association, Inc., 165 West 46th Street, Suite 1108, New York, NY 10036.
Telephone 212-575-6200
http://aabainc.org

Eating Disorders Awareness and Prevention, Inc. (EDAP), 603 Stewart Street, Suite 803, Seattle, WA 98101.
Telephone: (800) 931-2237 for toll-free information and referral hotline
http://www.edap.org

National Association of Anorexia Nervosa and Associated Disorders (ANAD), P.O. Box 7, Highland Park, IL 60035.
Telephone 807-831-3438
http://anad.org

U.S. Food and Drug Administration (FDA) posts the fact sheet *On the Teen Scene: Eating Disorders Require Medical Attention* at its website.
http://www.fda.gov/opacom/catalog/eatdis.html

Bullying

Bullying is when a person repeatedly intimidates or acts aggressively toward those with less power or ability to defend themselves.

Sam looked at the clock and saw that it was almost lunchtime. He dreaded going to his locker, and he was kicking himself for putting his lunch there this morning. Sam knew Craig and Pete would be waiting for him at the lockers again. His face got red with anger and embarrassment remembering how yesterday, and the day before, they had pushed him against the lockers and grabbed his lunch, tossing it to each other high over his head so he could not get it back, taunting him about being short.

*psychotherapy (sy-ko-THER-a-pee), or mental health counseling, involves talking about feelings with a trained professional. The counselor can help the person change thoughts, actions, or relationships that play a part in the illness.

▶ See also

Anorexia

Binge Eating Disorder

Body Dysmorphic Disorder

Body Image

Eating Disorders

Peer Pressure

Self-Esteem

KEYWORDS
for searching the Internet and other reference sources

School shootings

Violence

He wished he would grow a foot taller like it seemed some of the sixth graders had done over the summer. He wished he had a black belt in karate. He wished his eyes did not fill up with tears when they pushed him and laughed. He wished these bullies would just leave him alone. Sam felt in his pocket to see if he had enough money to buy lunch in the cafeteria. He could hurry to catch up with Jack and Marc as soon as the bell rang, go straight to the cafeteria, and avoid the lockers altogether. Then he would just have to figure out how to steer clear of them on the bus ride home.

What Is Bullying?

Bullying is more than normal childhood conflict or occasional unkind words or actions between children; it is an early form of violence. Bullying is when a person gets singled out to be intimidated or picked on over and over again by someone who has more power. Bullying can be physical, verbal, or psychological.

About 1 out of every 10 children is bullied. That means that in an average elementary school classroom at least 2 or 3 children are being bullied. In some schools, more than half the students worry about being bullied. Children may avoid bathrooms, the cafeteria, or the playground for fear of being hurt, picked on, or humiliated by other children. Some children miss school days because of bullying. Others go to school feeling worried or sick and may have trouble concentrating because of it.

Who Are the Bullies?

Bullies can be boys or girls. Boys tend to bully with physical aggression and pick on those who are smaller or weaker than themselves. Girls are more likely to use mean gossip, unkind notes, or social forms of intimidation when they bully. Bullies are children who lack compassion and a sense of how other people feel. Bullies like to dominate others to feel powerful themselves. Many bullies have parents who have modeled aggression as a way to get what they want. Some bullies feel hurt or powerless inside because they have been bullied themselves. However, bullying is not a remedy for feeling powerless. Bullying gives only a false sense of power and usually costs a bully popularity, friendships, and more. As many as 1 of 4 children who are bullies in elementary school have a criminal record by age 30.

Who Gets Bullied?

While anyone can have trouble with a bully now and then, bullies tend to seek out those who are easiest to intimidate. Children who have few friends, cry easily, are timid or insecure, or have trouble sticking up for themselves are easy targets for bullies. Children who pester others, get easily upset, or lose self control may get bullied because the bully can get a big reaction from them. No one deserves to be bullied, and all children have a right to feel safe at school. Even children who do not get bullied are still bothered when they witness bullying in school.

A group of children bullies another student at school. Being physically surrounded and teased by a group can be especially frightening for the bullied child.
Jennie Woodcock; Reflections Photolibrary/Corbis

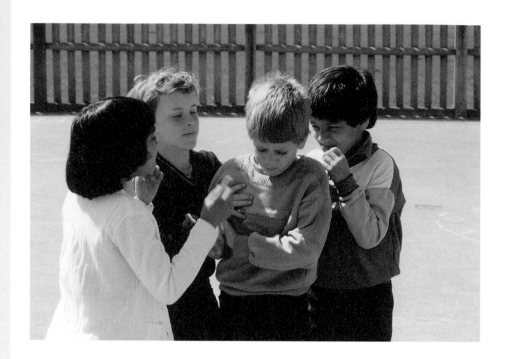

What Can Be Done About Bullying?

The most powerful tool to stop bullies is adult authority. Adults can help by knowing that bullying is not normal childhood behavior, by being on the lookout for it, and by taking steps to end it before it escalates. In many cases, the presence of an adult is enough to discourage bullying. Sometimes children do not let anyone know that they are being bullied because they are ashamed or because they do not think that adults will help. Adults need to let children know that they will listen and help if they are told about bullying. Many schools have started bully-proofing programs that make it clear that bullying is not tolerated. The goal of these programs is to take power away from bullies and to shift power to the larger group of caring, responsible children. Another goal is to teach children how to respond to bullying whether they are being bullied or are a bystander to bullying.

Resources

Books

Garrity, Carla, Kathryn Jens, William Porter, Nancy Sager, and Cam Short-Camilli. *Bully-Proofing Your School: A Comprehensive Approach for Elementary Schools.* Longmont, CO: Sopris West, 2000.

Kaufman, Gershen, Lev Raphael, and Pamela Espeland. *Stick Up For Yourself: Every Kid's Guide to Personal Power and Positive Self-Esteem.* Minneapolis: Free Spirit Publishing, 1999. For ages 8-13.

Romain, Trevor. *Bullies are a Pain in the Brain.* Minneapolis: Free Spirit Publishing, 1997. A light-hearted but practical guide for ages 8-13.

Organization

KidsHealth.org from the Nemours Foundation posts information about bullying and what to do about it.
http://KidsHealth.org/kid/watch/out/bullies.html
http://KidsHealth.org/teen/mind_matters/school/bullies.html

▶ *See also*
Conduct Disorder
Emotions
Fears
Oppositional Defiant Disorder
School Avoidance
Self-Esteem

C

Cerebral Palsy

Cerebral palsy (SER-uh-brul PAWL-zee) is a group of conditions characterized by a loss or limitation of movement or other nerve functions caused by brain injuries during fetal development or near the time of birth.

KEYWORDS
for searching the Internet
and other reference sources

Cerebellum

Cerebral cortex

Cerebrum

Movement disorders

Spastic syndromes

Marsha's Story

Marsha could not help comparing her baby to the others at the park. At ten months old, Sam could hardly sit up on his own, but most of the other babies Sam's age were crawling and pulling up to a standing position. Marsha also noticed that Sam often felt stiff when she picked him up. When Marsha took Sam to the doctor and described his symptoms, the doctor suspected that Sam had a form of cerebral palsy. Sam's doctor explained that cerebral palsy occurs when parts of the brain that control movement are injured or don't develop properly during pregnancy.

What Is Cerebral Palsy?

Cerebral palsy is not a single condition but instead identifies a group of movement disorders caused by a brain injury. Before birth or shortly after birth, developing brain tissue may be injured by trauma* or by diseases such as meningitis* or encephalitis*. Brain damage may also result from severe dehydration*, lack of oxygen, or a variety of other problems. In most cases, however, the cause of cerebral palsy is unknown.

In the United States, cerebral palsy occurs at a rate of about 5 cases per 2,000 births, and the rate is even higher in premature infants (about 5 percent of premature babies have cerebral palsy). Each year, 10,000 new cases of cerebral palsy are diagnosed in the United States.

What Are the Signs and Symptoms of Cerebral Palsy?

Cerebral palsy is divided into different types based on the symptoms that a person experiences. Spastic (SPAS-tik) syndromes are the most common form of cerebral palsy and account for about 70 percent of cases. People with spastic syndromes move in a stiff or jerky way. Spastic movements may affect one limb, one side of the body, both legs, or both arms and legs,

* **trauma** (TRAW-muh), in the broadest sense, refers to a wound or injury, whether psychological or physical. It occurs when a person experiences a sudden or violent injury (physical trauma) or encounters a situation that involves intense fear and loss of control (psychological trauma).

* **meningitis** (men-in-JY-tis) is an inflammation of the membranes that surround the brain and the spinal cord.

* **encephalitis** (en-sef-uh-LY-tis) is an inflammation of the brain that can range from mild to extremely serious. It is usually caused by one of many viruses.

* **dehydration** (dee-hy-DRAY-shun) is loss of fluid from the body.

*seizures (SEE-zhurz) are sudden episodes of involuntary (uncontrollable) body movements, changes in behavior or sensations, or loss of consciousness that result from bursts of abnormal electrical energy in the brain.

and the affected limbs are usually underdeveloped and have rigid muscles. In mild cases, the symptoms may only show during certain activities such as running. People with spastic syndromes also may experience seizures*, partial or full loss of movement (paralysis), sensory abnormalities, and speech, hearing, and vision problems. About 20 percent of people with cerebral palsy experience slow, writhing, involuntary muscle movements in the arms and legs. The symptoms usually increase with stress and disappear when the person is sleeping. Others (about 10 percent of people with cerebral palsy) have weakness, uncoordinated movements, and shaking; a person with this type of cerebral palsy has difficulty with rapid and fine movements. Some people with cerebral palsy experience a mixture of all of these symptoms.

How Is Cerebral Palsy Diagnosed and Treated?

Cerebral palsy is sometimes difficult to diagnose in infants. Clear diagnosis may be delayed until a child is about 2 years old. Children at risk for developing cerebral palsy, such as children who are born with very low birth weights (less than 2 pounds), should be watched closely.

Treatment for cerebral palsy is tailored to each individual's specific symptoms. Doctors and therapists work together to set up a treatment program to help the patient deal with the challenges of day-to-day living, such as getting dressed, grooming, and eating. Physical therapy can help people with cerebral palsy build strength and improve function in their limbs. Special equipment, such as leg braces, walkers, and wheelchairs, can provide mobility. Muscle relaxants may be used to reduce muscle tone and antiseizure medications may control seizures. Glasses and hearing aids may improve sight and hearing, and special education may help a child with cerebral palsy cope with learning problems.

Living with Cerebral Palsy

Cerebral palsy is a lifelong disorder. The extent of disability caused by cerebral palsy varies with the severity of the symptoms. Some people have mild forms that are barely noticeable; for example, a child might just walk and run with a limp. Other people have more severe symptoms; they might require a wheelchair to get around and have severe mental retardation. While long-term care such as institutionalization may be required in severe cases, many people with cerebral palsy lead full and happy lives. Most children with cerebral palsy do many of the things their friends do, such as go to school, go to summer camp, read, listen to music, talk on the phone, and play sports.

Resources

Organizations

Nemours Center for Children's Health Media, Alfred I. duPont Hospital for Children, 1600 Rockland Road, Wilmington, DE 19803. This

organization is dedicated to issues of children's health and produces the KidsHealth website. Its website has articles about cerebral palsy.
http://www.KidsHealth.org

United Cerebral Palsy, 1660 L Street NW, Suite 700, Washington, DC 20036.
http://www.ucpa.org

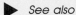

▶ *See also*
Birth Defects and Brain Development
Brain Injuries
Disability

Child Abuse *See* Abuse

Chronic Illness

A chronic illness is a mental or physical disorder that lasts for a long time, perhaps even a lifetime.

What Is Chronic Illness?

Chronic (KRAH-nik) illnesses are different from illnesses such as flu or chicken pox, where a person becomes sick for a short time and then returns to health. These short-term illnesses are called acute (a-KYOOT) illnesses. Unlike people with acute illnesses, people with chronic illnesses usually don't return to completely normal health. The illness does not go away, even when the symptoms are controlled.

What Are Different Types of Chronic Illness?

There are many types of illnesses that are chronic, each with its own symptoms, causes, and course. Some chronic illnesses affect people of any age or ethnic background, while others are more likely to appear in a particular age or ethnic group. Some chronic illnesses are present at birth, while others develop later in life. Chronic illnesses are sometimes inherited. Diseases that are inherited develop because a person has certain genes, the material in the body that helps determine physical and mental characteristics, such as hair and eye color. An example of an inherited chronic illness is sickle-cell anemia. This disease affects the blood's ability to carry oxygen through the body. Sickle-cell anemia is more likely to occur in people of African descent who carry the gene for the disease. Sometimes the symptoms of inherited chronic illnesses appear early in childhood. At other times, symptoms of an inherited chronic illness do not show up until much later in life.

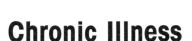

KEYWORDS
for searching the Internet and other reference sources

Asthma

Crohn's disease

Diabetes mellitus

Disability

Epilepsy

Fibromyalgia

Genetic disease

Hemophilia

Lupus

Sickle-cell anemia

* **bacteria** are round, spiral, or rod-shaped single-cell micro-organisms without a distinct nucleus that commonly multiply by cell division. Some types may cause disease in humans, animals, or plants.

* **viruses** are tiny infectious agents that lack independent metabolism (me-TA-bo-li-zum), the chemical processes by which living things produce and use energy. Viruses can reproduce only within the cells they infect.

* **muscular dystrophy** (DIS-tro-fee) is a group of inherited disorders in which there is a gradual deterioration and weakening of muscles.

* **cystic fibrosis** is an inherited condition in which certain glands produce very sticky mucus (MYOO-kus) that clogs the lungs, the intestines, and some other organs of the body, making it difficult to breathe and digest food properly.

* **multiple sclerosis** is an inflammatory disease of the nervous system that disrupts communication between the brain and other parts of the body, that can result in weakness, paralysis, blindness, and other symptoms.

* **Parkinson disease** is a disorder of the nervous system that causes shaking, rigid muscles, slow movements, and poor balance.

* **Alzheimer** (ALTS-hy-mer) **disease** is a condition that leads to gradually worsening loss of mental abilities, including memory, judgment, and abstract thinking, as well as changes in personality.

Some chronic illnesses are caused by environmental factors such as exposure to pollutants. Coal miners may breathe so much coal dust in the air that they begin to show symptoms of a chronic lung disorder called black lung disease. Bacteria* or viruses* also can cause chronic illnesses. For example, Lyme disease, a bacterial disease spread by the bite of ticks, causes an acute flulike illness at first, but it also can cause long-term joint, heart, and nervous system problems that may not show up for months or years. Some chronic illnesses are progressive. Progressive illnesses such as muscular dystrophy*, cystic fibrosis*, multiple sclerosis*, Parkinson disease*, or Alzheimer disease* can get worse as time passes.

How Is Chronic Illness Treated?

When doctors diagnose a chronic illness, they also recommend treatments that can relieve symptoms or keep the body functioning at its healthiest. Sometimes treatments involve medications the doctor will prescribe. Sometimes managing the illness also will depend on things the ill person can do to remain as healthy as possible, such as making changes in diet, quitting smoking, or exercising more. People with chronic illness seem to do best when they work as partners with their doctors to take an active role in caring for their health.

The symptoms of many chronic illnesses can be controlled with medication or changes in diet and activity. For example, people with diabetes (dy-a-BEE-teez) are unable to process sugars properly for use by the body. By taking insulin* or other medications and by eating properly, people with diabetes can lead very active, normal lives. Bobby Clarke, who played professional ice hockey for many years, is an example of a person with diabetes who has had a vigorous and demanding career, even though he takes insulin every day.

Some people with chronic illnesses have symptoms that appear only under certain conditions. For example, some people with asthma (AZ-ma), a chronic illness that affects the lungs, may experience difficulty breathing only when they exercise, breathe in pollutants, or are under stress. Others with asthma may need to take medications or use inhalers daily to prevent wheezing. When the symptoms of a chronic illness are not present or are minimal, the illness is said to be in remission (ree-MI-shun). Having an illness that is in remission is not the same as being cured, because the disease that causes the illness is still present.

Coping with Chronic Illness

Accepting that one must live with the limitations of a chronic illness can be emotionally difficult. How people react to the diagnosis of a chronic illness and how they cope depend partly on the nature of the illness, and the age and resilience of the person. The changes they believe the illness will make in their lives, and how the illness will change their family and social support, also influence how people cope. Many people go through a process of grieving for the health and freedom of activity that they have lost. They may pass through stages of denial, anger, depression, and worry when they find out that they have a chronic disease.

Self-image and self-esteem may suffer when a person must cope with a chronic illness, especially if that illness is painful or imposes limitations that interfere with social activities, school, or work. Chronic illness may be difficult for other family members, who frequently must take on additional responsibilities at home. Many chronic illnesses may get better or go into remission, only to reappear unexpectedly, sometimes with worse symptoms. Uncertainty about the course of the illness can be stressful. This uncertainty also may make planning for vacations or special activities difficult.

Support groups dedicated to specific illnesses are often effective in helping the person with a chronic illness and that person's caregivers make emotional and physical adjustments to the disease. Counseling and therapy for both the chronically ill person and caregivers or family members may help people find ways of dealing with the stress of chronic illness. Many people with chronic illness, even children, cope well with their condition and find ways of adjusting to their disease and leading full and meaningful lives.

Resources

Books

Huegel, Kelly. *Young People and Chronic Illness: True Stories, Help, and Hope.* Minneapolis: Free Spirit Publishing, 1998. True stories about teens with asthma, diabetes, lupus, hemophilia, Crohn's disease, and epilepsy, and strategies for how to cope with chronic illness.

Kaufman, Miriam. *Easy for You to Say: Q and As for Teens Living with Chronic Illness or Disability.* Toronto: Key Porter Books, 1995.

Organizations

Center for Disability Information and Referral, Indiana Institute on Disability and Community, 2853 East Tenth Street, Bloomington, IN 47408-2696. This organization focuses on the disability aspect of chronic illness. It provides referrals for all types of disabilities.
Telephone 812-855-9396
http://www.iidc.indiana.edu/~cedir

KidsHealth website has much valuable information for children, teens, and parents. Articles on muscular dystrophy, diabetes, and coping with chronic illness are available at their website.
http://www.KidsHealth.org

* **insulin** is a kind of hormone, or chemical produced in the body, that is crucial in controlling the level of glucose (sugar) in the blood and in helping the body use glucose to produce energy. When the body cannot produce or use insulin properly, a person must take insulin or other medications.

▶ *See also*
Depression
Disability
Self-Esteem
Stress

Cognitive Behavioral Therapy *See* Therapy

Conduct Disorder

When a child or adolescent shows an ongoing pattern of behavior that violates the rights of others and breaks social rules, he or she may be said to have conduct disorder.

Joe's Story

Joe always seems to pick fights on the school bus. He intimidates and bullies others and has few friends. Serving detention does not seem to help Joe learn to behave. Last year, in fifth grade, he was always in trouble for writing graffiti on school property, and he was suspended once for throwing rocks at a school bus. Though he was never caught, Joe stole money from the teachers' lounge and from the backpack of the girl who sat in front of him in English class. This year, he frequently cuts school. When he does not attend school, he hangs out behind the local convenience store smoking cigarettes he sneaks from his father's car.

What Is Conduct Disorder?

While all children and adolescents misbehave on occasion, some seem to do so all the time. Conduct disorder refers to serious and frequent antisocial behavior* in young people. Conduct disorder describes behaviors such as aggression or cruelty toward people or animals, bullying, threatening, physical fights, using weapons to hurt others, destroying property, fire-setting, lying, stealing, running away, and school truancy*. Someone who is diagnosed with conduct disorder has demonstrated at least three or more of these serious behaviors over the past year.

Young people with conduct disorder may act alone or in groups. Many youth involved in gang violence or other criminal or delinquent* behaviors have conduct disorder. When caught violating rules of conduct, antisocial youth often deny their guilt and may shift blame onto others. They often lack remorse for the deeds they have done and lack feeling for people or animals they may have hurt.

For some, conduct disordered behavior begins early in childhood. The earlier and more frequently the antisocial behavior occurs, the more likely it is to develop into more serious problems during adolescence. Others may not develop antisocial behaviors until adolescence; though still serious, their behavioral problems are sometimes more temporary. Most young people who have conduct disorder do not go on to have serious problems in adulthood, although for some it will lead to a lifelong problem with antisocial behavior. In adults, a pattern of aggressive and

---

* **antisocial behavior** is behavior that differs significantly from the norms of society and is considered harmful to society.

* **truancy** means staying out of school or work without permission.

* **delinquent** is a legal term that refers to a juvenile (someone under the age of 18) who has committed an illegal act. Delinquent behavior includes any behavior that would be considered a crime if committed by an adult as well as specific behaviors that are illegal for youth, such as school truancy, violating curfew, or running away.

antisocial behavior that disregards the rights of others may be diagnosed as antisocial personality disorder. All adults who have antisocial personality disorder have had symptoms of conduct disorder in their youth.

How Does Conduct Disorder Develop?

There are many different theories about what causes conduct disorder. There is no one single cause, and a number of factors seem to contribute to its development. Conduct disorder and related antisocial behaviors tend to run in families. This may be due in part to inherited genes that affect behavioral development, but there is strong evidence that antisocial behavior is learned and modeled in the family environment.

Genetics and behavior Many researchers have tried to determine how genetics and biology contribute to conduct disorder. Some studies have found that youth with conduct disorder may crave more stimulation, have trouble with self-awareness and with making goals, and lack skills for forethought and planning. Other studies have found that youth with conduct disorder have problems with social learning, which includes the skills needed to learn social rules and to interact well with others. Young people with conduct disorder also have less empathy than do others their age. Empathy is a type of emotional feeling for others; it involves the ability to see another person's point of view and to understand how someone else might feel in a given situation.

Children who have deficiencies in empathy, social learning, planning, and self-awareness may have a harder time developing behavioral controls, good problem-solving skills, and respect for others. Because they have fewer skills to solve problems in socially acceptable ways, they may be more likely to develop conduct problems. However, to what extent these deficiencies are part of a person's genetic make-up, or are tendencies that are learned by example and behavior in the family, remains unclear.

Learned behavior There is convincing evidence that aggression, the main ingredient of conduct disorder, is a learned behavior. People who observe others behaving in aggressive ways (and this includes watching aggression and violence on television, movies, and video games) are more likely to demonstrate the aggressive behaviors they have witnessed. Children who witness aggressive behaviors at home, such as physical fighting, pushing, and shoving, are at increased risk for developing conduct disorder. Children with conduct disorder often live in families in which there is a high level of conflict that takes physical form.

Certain parenting practices increase the risk that a child will develop conduct disorder. For example, parents who fail to provide enough supervision, consistent rules for behavior, and discipline contribute to conduct disorder. Parents who use overly harsh or abusive discipline also contribute to the development of conduct disorder.

Peers can also influence a child's behavior. Many young people with conduct disorder are rejected by their peers, which may make their conduct problems worse. Social rejection may also cause them to associate with other children with conduct problems; children and adolescents who have aggressive or delinquent peers are more likely to have conduct disorder.

How Is Conduct Disorder Treated?

Individual or group treatment for young people with conduct disorder often involves helping them to learn social skills they may be lacking, especially empathy and problem-solving skills. Good behaviors are rewarded and antisocial behaviors are punished. Parent training is an important ingredient in many treatment programs. It helps parents replace harsh and coercive parenting behaviors with consistent rules, appropriate consequences, and positive attention to children's good behaviors. Studies have demonstrated that these treatment methods can be effective in reducing antisocial behavior in youth with conduct disorder. Treatment works best when it begins soon after the child or adolescent has started to show antisocial behaviors and is more effective when the family also participates. Medication may also be used in some cases.

LEARNING TO BE AGGRESSIVE: ALBERT BANDURA'S EXPERIMENTS

In the 1960s, a social psychologist named Albert Bandura wanted to find out whether children would learn and perform aggressive behaviors simply by watching someone else behave in aggressive ways. Learning a certain behavior by watching someone else do it is called modeling, or observational learning. Bandura conducted a series of experiments that demonstrated that aggressive behavior is indeed learned simply by observation. Whether or not a child actually went on to behave aggressively depended on what happened to the person they observed. If a child saw that the other person was scolded or punished for acting aggressively, the child was not likely to perform the aggressive behavior, even though he or she had learned how. Children who saw that the other person's aggressive behavior was met with no consequence were more likely to perform the aggressive behavior they had observed as well as other aggressive behaviors.

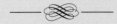

Resource

Book

Lewis, Barbara. *What Do You Stand For? A Kid's Guide to Building Character.* Minneapolis: Free Spirit Publishing, 1997. Helps teens learn ways to practice honesty, and develop empathy, tolerance, and respect. Ages 11 and up.

Consciousness

Consciousness is a person's awareness of his or her inner world, the most private place where thoughts and feelings are formed and impressions and experiences are processed.

Automatic Tasks Versus Conscious Choices

Here is a test: Try to write down all the steps you followed in getting dressed this morning. Did you put on your pants or your top first? Which shoe went on first? What steps did you take to tie your shoes? This is likely to be a tough test, because getting dressed, brushing teeth, or tying shoes are automatic tasks that can be done without much thought. Other examples of automatic tasks include riding a bike, playing a sport, and dialing a phone number from memory. These tasks may seem difficult when we learn them for the first time, but they soon become so familiar that we do not have to focus our conscious minds on them. Without even realizing it, we rely on learned routines to complete them efficiently.

Mindfulness

Automatic processing is not always enough for what someone needs to do. This is when the conscious mind takes over. Whether a person is mastering a new concept, focusing on a challenging book, writing a school paper, deciding how to spend the afternoon, or reacting to criticism from a friend, for example, that person is mindful, or conscious, of what he or she is thinking, feeling, saying, or doing. These and other tasks require the mind to be aware of the inside and the outside world, instead of relying on set automatic routines. It appears that "consciousness" gives human beings the awareness to be flexible in dealing with new situations and an ever-changing environment. Consciousness is a state of being aware and paying attention to thoughts, feelings, ideas, and actions at a given moment.

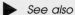

See also

Antisocial Personality Disorder

Bullying

Lying and Stealing

Oppositional Defiant Disorder

Peer Pressure

Personality

Personality Disorders

KEYWORDS
for searching the Internet and other reference sources

Brain

Learning

Nervous system

Cerebral Cortex

Generally, it is believed that the mechanisms of consciousness are controlled by the cerebral cortex, the upper wrinkled layer of the brain where higher functions, such as perception, memory, intelligence, and control of skilled movements, also are carried out. But it is not known whether scientists will ever be able to explain consciousness fully as a solely physical process carried out within the brain. This issue has been debated intensely over the years and likely will continue to be a topic of disagreement among experts. Consciousness has proved to be one of the most difficult functions to define, even though everyone experiences it.

Philosophy, Psychology, and Neuroscience: The "Hard Problem" of Consciousness

Scientists, physicians, and psychologists, who are specially trained to study the structure, function, and biology of the brain and nervous system, have made great strides in understanding how different brain regions and brain chemicals are involved in producing emotions such as anxiety, sadness, fear, and happiness. Using advanced brain imaging techniques, they also are gaining a better understanding of how different portions of the brain play a part in speaking, listening, processing information, and other activities.

Some researchers in the emerging field known as "consciousness studies" believe that one day we will understand consciousness more fully in this way as well. They include not only psychologists* and scientists but also some philosophers. Philosophy is the study of the nature of the mind and of the role of thought in how we experience and deal with the world around us, including ethics*, morality, decision making, motivation, and beliefs. These researchers believe that eventually we will be able to "map" the process we understand as consciousness within the brain, explaining it in terms of the connections and messaging among nerve cells of the brain. They believe that consciousness will come to be understood as the product of the sophisticated machinery of the human brain, just as emotions have begun to be understood in this way.

Other researchers disagree. They contend that the so-called hard problem of consciousness will remain something of a mystery. The "hard problem" of consciousness refers to the question of how the physical brain can give rise to the unique experiences that we each have in relation to the external world. These experts do not dispute the brain's role in taking in, processing, and interpreting concrete information from the outside world. For example, two people at the same concert hear the same music thanks to the inner ear's auditory nerve, which sends along impulses to the brain, where they are processed in the region that controls hearing. But this does not explain the inner aspect of thought and perception or the way the music "feels" for each person. If listeners were asked to share their innermost thoughts while hearing the music, they

psychologists (sy-KOL-o-jists) are mental health professionals who treat mental and behavioral disorders by support and insight to encourage healthy behavior patterns and personality growth. Psychologists also study the brain, behavior, emotions, and learning.

ethics is a guiding set of principles for conduct, a system of moral values.

likely would have very different responses based on personal experiences. For this reason, some experts contend that we will never be able to "locate" consciousness entirely within the structures and chemical processes of the brain. For them, it is too complex to explain consciousness fully in terms of gray matter and brain chemicals; instead, they argue that consciousness also draws on experiences and thoughts that are the essence of being human (and cannot be defined or measured).

The field of consciousness studies has brought together philosophers, psychologists, neuroscientists*, physicians, and other researchers to discuss this and other issues related to understanding consciousness. Their first major gathering was held in Tucson, Arizona, in 1994, and many meetings have been held since then. This is a young field of study and research, but it holds great promise for furthering our understanding of the mind.

Resource

Book

Brynie, Faith Hickman. *101 Questions Your Brain Has Asked About Itself But Couldn't Answer . . . Until Now.* Brookfield, CT: Millbrook Press, 1998. The book contains sections on learning memory, and even music and the brain.

*** neuroscientists** are scientists who study the nerves and nervous system, especially their relationship to learning and behavior.

▶ *See also*
The Brain and Nervous System (Introduction)

Brain Chemistry (Neurochemistry)

Hypnosis

Memory

Sleep

Conversion Disorder

Conversion disorder is a psychological condition in which a person loses abilities such as seeing, hearing, or speaking or becomes paralyzed, but no medical explanation can be found to explain the symptoms. Symptoms of conversion disorder often begin after some stressful experience, and they have traditionally been thought of as an expression of emotional conflict or need.

KEYWORDS
for searching the Internet and other reference sources

Factitious disorder

Hysteria

Malingering

Munchausen syndrome

Stress

What Is Conversion Disorder?

Conversion disorder is a mental disorder in which psychological symptoms are converted to physical symptoms, such as blindness, paralysis, or seizures. Unlike malingering, in which a person fakes an illness or injury, a person with conversion disorder does not intentionally produce symptoms.

Conversion disorder is rare, occurring in only about 1 to 3 out of 10,000 people. It is even less common in children younger than 10 years of age. Conversion disorder can be triggered by extreme psychological stress, such as injury, death of a loved one, or a dangerous situation. For

uterus (YOO-ter-us) in humans is the organ in females in which a fetus develops and grows during pregnancy.

psychoanalysis (sy-ko-a-NAL-i-sis) is a method of treating a person with psychological problems, based on the theories of Dr. Sigmund Freud. It involves sessions in which a therapist encourages a person to talk freely about personal experiences, and the psychoanalyst interprets the patient's ideas and dreams.

seizures (SEE-zhurz) can occur when the electrical patterns of the brain are interrupted by powerful, rapid bursts of electrical energy, which may cause a person to fall down, make jerky movements, or stare blankly into space.

example, in wartime, some soldiers undergoing heavy bombardment but not wounded were hospitalized because they could not walk or speak after the battle. Conversion disorder under these circumstances has been called shell shock and battle fatigue. In other circumstances, the purpose of conversion disorder appears to be to help the individual avoid or escape from a highly stressful situation.

What Causes Conversion Disorder?

The old term for conversion disorder was hysteria. Physicians in ancient Greece believed that hysteria only occurred in females and that it was caused by the uterus* wandering in the body (the Greek word for uterus is hystera). For centuries thereafter, people with hysteria were regarded as fakers or as imagining their symptoms. In the seventeenth century, some people with hysteria were thought to be involved with witchcraft and were burned at the stake.

The term conversion disorder came into use only in the late twentieth century. It is derived from the early work of the Austrian physician Sigmund Freud, the founder of psychoanalysis*. Freud believed that in times of extreme emotional stress, painful feelings or conflicts are repressed (kept from awareness or consciousness) and are converted into physical symptoms to relieve anxiety. Even in the twenty-first century, mental health experts do not all agree on the precise psychological mechanisms underlying conversion disorder. However, many mental health professionals see the benefits associated with the symptoms of conversion disorder, such as sympathy, care, and the avoidance of stressful situations, as significant to the disorder.

What Are the Symptoms of Conversion Disorder?

Sometimes people with conversion disorder have tremors or symptoms that resemble fainting spells or seizures*. There also may be loss of feeling in various parts of the body, or loss of the sense of smell, and symptoms may occur together. For instance, following an automobile accident a person may be unable to move or feel sensation in an arm or leg, even though no injury to the limb is apparent. Other people may have difficulty swallowing or feel like they have a lump in their throat. Interestingly, some people with conversion disorder may seem quite comfortable with their symptoms, even though they may be greatly handicapped by them.

How Is Conversion Disorder Diagnosed and Treated?

Possible medical, or physical, causes of a patient's symptoms need to be ruled out to establish the diagnosis of conversion disorder. Special instruments that measure electrical activity in the muscles and the brain can rule out some physical disorders. In addition, experienced physicians

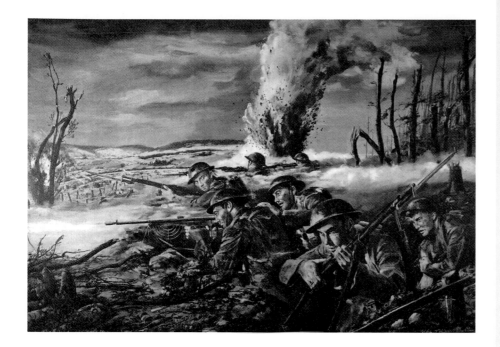

Symptoms of psychological and emotional pain may be converted to physical symptoms under conditions of extreme stress, such as war. During the First World War (1914–1918), soldiers with conversion disorder were said to have battle fatigue or shell shock. *The Granger Collection*

using close observation can often discover important diagnostic clues. For example, without realizing it a patient may momentarily use an arm or a leg that is supposed to be paralyzed. This clue would indicate that the symptom is psychological rather than physical, and might indicate conversion disorder. To rule out that the patient is just pretending to be ill, a mental health professional would need to perform a clinical interview to learn about the history of the individual and family, stressors that may be present, benefits the patient derives from the symptoms, and what factors may be sustaining the symptoms.

Conversion disorder is typically treated with psychotherapy*. The therapist attempts to help the patient understand whatever unconscious emotional conflicts or needs or gains may have given rise to the symptoms. In some instances, symptoms of the disorder may last for years. With treatment, however, the symptoms of conversion disorder frequently last for only brief periods.

* **psychotherapy** (sy-ko-THER-a-pea) is the treatment of mental and behavioral disorders by support and insight to encourage healthy behavior patterns and personality growth.

▶ *See also*
Hypochondria
Malingering
Munchausen Syndrome
Stress

D

Death and Dying

A person is dead when he or she stops breathing and the heart and brain permanently stop functioning. A dead person cannot see, hear, taste, touch, or smell and has no awareness or feelings.

Everyone on this earth shares two experiences: we are born and we die. Someone dies about every 20 seconds. Most of us know someone who has died. But we do not generally like to think about death or talk about death or even acknowledge that we all die. Around the world throughout the ages, death always has been a source of mystery and fear.

How Do We Understand Death?

Our reactions to death often depend on how someone has died and how old they were. The most easily understood are deaths at an old age, when a person's body simply wears out. But others die before their bodies wear out, and sometimes people die with no advance warning. Illness, injuries, natural catastrophes, and violence all can cause early death.

Sometimes people, including children, have to face their own deaths. They may have a terminal illness, a disease or condition that eventually will cause death. Psychologists and physicians who have worked with families in this situation believe that honesty and love from others are very important at this time. People with terminal illness and their families need to understand the effects of the illness and find ways to express their feelings about it. It helps to talk about it, enjoy time together, and help with caregiving.

What Is Grief?

Grief is the wide range of feelings that accompany a death, such as shock, sadness, anger, and confusion. Even when we know ahead of time that someone is going to die, it does not necessarily soften the impact. It still may be difficult to believe that the death has occurred and hard to imagine life without this special person. When the death is sudden and unexpected, the shock of the news may make it hard to come to grips with the reality. Such shock can take a while to fade. Most people need comfort and support while they grieve, either from their personal circle of family and friends or from clergy, therapists, or support groups.

KEYWORDS
for searching the Internet and other reference sources

Bereavement

Grief

Terminal illness

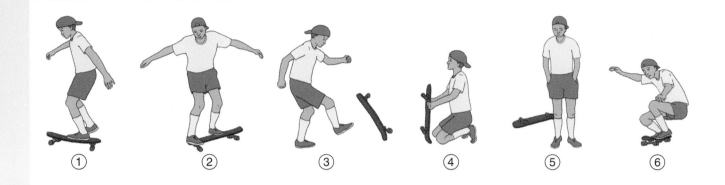

① ② ③ ④ ⑤ ⑥

▲

Adjusting to the terminal illness or death of a loved one is a gradual process, according to Elisabeth Kübler-Ross, author of the landmark *On Death and Dying* (1969). When normal life (1) is disrupted, people first go through a stage of denial (2), acting as if nothing in their lives has changed. Denial may be followed by anger (3) at the unwanted changes, and by praying or bargaining (4) such as "If I never fight with my sister again, Mom won't die." Sadness and depression occur when the loss sinks in (5). Acceptance comes when a loss has been mourned. Acceptance is not a happy feeling, but it does give people the strength to go on with their own lives (6).

How Do Children Cope with the Death of a Parent or Sibling?

When a sibling or parent dies, everyone in the family suffers. Very young children may not fully understand what has happened and that the death is permanent. Children feel many of the same feelings that adults do when someone dies: shock, sadness, or confusion. Children often personalize a death, asking, "Will it happen to me?" or "Did I cause this to happen to someone else?" A death can stir up fears: "Will I get cancer too?" or "Is it safe to drive?" A child may wonder how the death will alter his or her life: "Will Mom remarry now that Dad has died?" or "My brother died. Will we have to move?"

Sometimes it is hard for young people to understand their own feelings and reactions to death. Grief can cause people to lose interest in things that they normally enjoy, or they might avoid situations that used to involve the person who died. Reactions like these are normal. Finding someone to talk with (a family member, friend, or trusted adult) usually helps young people understand their feelings and eventually accept the death.

How Do Adults Cope with the Death of a Child?

As with the death of a parent or sibling, the death of a child causes extreme sadness and distress in a family. Whether the death came suddenly or gradually, parents often struggle with guilt that they could not prevent their child's death or even that they outlived their child. Sometimes, after a death, parents might feel the urge to move or change their lives to avoid situations that remind them of their dead child. Most experts say that this is not the best course. As the psychiatrist Elisabeth Kübler-Ross notes, it is usually healthier to face and acknowledge the pain, rather than avoid it.

How Do Rituals Help People Cope with Death?

Funerals, memorial services, and burials are generally held a short time after a death and sometimes on the anniversary of a death. These cere-

MUMMIES OF ANCIENT EGYPT

In ancient Egypt, there were elaborate rituals performed to preserve the body after death. This was done to make sure that the dead person would be connected to gods and spirits in the afterlife.

The first step was embalming, which involved removal of major body organs, drying the body, and wrapping it in linens and spices. The higher the individual's status in society, the more elaborate the ritual. The coffin was painted with a portrait of the person and filled with valuables, such as gems and prized possessions of the deceased, to be used in the afterlife. Cats, which were thought to be sacred, were sometimes mummified and buried with their owners.

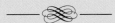

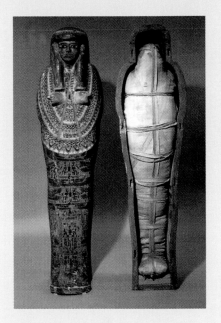

▲

An Egyptian mummy dating from about 1000 B.C., that shows the outer decoration of the coffin and wrapped body inside. *The Bridgeman Art Library*

monies are often sad and difficult to attend. But they help people to express their feelings, take comfort with others who are grieving, and pay tribute to a person's life. Funerals or other rituals—such as planting a memorial garden, writing, enjoying the person's interests—help people stay connected to the person even after the death.

What Happens After Death?

No one knows what happens after death, and people have many different beliefs about it. They might believe that people go to heaven when they die. Some people believe that a person's "soul" lives on and that the "spirit" goes somewhere else after death. Still others believe in rebirth or reincarnation, with the soul continuing its life in another person. Some people do not believe in a soul. Even in the face of these unknowns, most people take comfort in the natural cycle of life and death and find meaningful ways to enjoy the memories of people who have died.

Resources

Books

Brown, Laurie Krasny, and Marc Tolon Brown. *When Dinosaurs Die: A Guide to Understanding Death.* Boston: Little, Brown, 1998. A picture book written for younger children, but thorough and thoughtful enough to appeal to adolescents.

Dower, Laura. *I Will Remember You: What To Do When Someone You Love Dies: A Guidebook Through Grief for Teens.* New York: Scholastic, 2000. Personal stories from teens who have experienced loss, and hands-on creative exercises in coping.

Fitzgerald, Helen. *The Grieving Teen: A Guide for Teenagers and Their Friends.* New York: Simon and Schuster, 2000. A practical guide that answers questions and helps a teenager understand a range of situations involving dying and death.

Gootman, Marilyn. *When A Friend Dies: A Book for Teens About Grieving and Healing.* Minneapolis: Free Spirit Publishing, 1994. A sensitive guide to help teens cope with the death of a friend. For ages 11 and up.

Kübler-Ross, Elisabeth. *On Children and Death: How Children and Their Parents Can and Do Cope with Death.* New York: Simon and Schuster, 1997. A compassionate guide for families of dead or dying children.

Kübler-Ross, Elisabeth. *On Death and Dying: What the Dying Have to Teach Doctors, Nurses, Clergy, and Their Own Families.* New York: Simon and Schuster, 1997.

Trozzi, Maria, with Kathy Massimini. *Talking with Children About Loss: Words, Strategies, and Wisdom to Help Children Cope with Death, Divorce, and Other Difficult Times.* New York: Perigree, 1999. For adults, and suitable for older teen readers.

Organization

Nemours Center for Children's Health Media, A. I. duPont Hospital for Children, 1600 Rockland Road, Wilmington, DE 19803. This organization is dedicated to issues of children's health. Their website has articles on coping with death, with valuable links to support organizations. http://www.KidsHealth.org

► *See also*
Depression
Suicide

Delinquency *See* Conduct Disorders

Delusions

Delusions (dee-LOO-zhunz) are one or more false beliefs that a person holds despite either lack of evidence that the belief is true or clear evidence that the belief is not true.

Understanding Delusions

Imagine being completely convinced that someone is following you, to the point where you even call the police several times. Or imagine believing that your friend is spreading horrible rumors behind your

KEYWORDS
for searching the Internet and other reference sources

Delusional disorder

Schizophrenia

back, even though there is no reason to think she is. Or imagine thinking that you are about to release a new hit record, or that there is something physically wrong with you when your doctor has found otherwise.

These thoughts may sound ridiculous, but they help to illustrate what it means to be "delusional." It's normal for people to have occasional thoughts that, for example, a boss, teacher, or friend is "out to get them." Delusions are different, however. A person with delusions holds on to unfounded beliefs for a long period of time (at least more than a month) and absolutely believes that they are true in spite of evidence to the contrary.

Delusions often are classified into the following subtypes:

- erotomanic (air-ROT-oh-MAN-ik): People with erotomanic delusions falsely believe that someone is in love with them and make repeated attempts to establish contact through phone calls, letters, or stalking.

- grandiose (gran-dee-OSE): People with grandiose delusions falsely believe that they have a great talent or have made an important discovery. These so-called "delusions of grandeur" involve wild exaggeration of one's own importance, wealth, power, or talents.

- persecution: People with delusions of persecution may falsely believe that they are being plotted against, spied on, lied about, or harassed. They may repeatedly try to get justice through appeals to the court system and other government agencies.

- jealous: This type of delusion involves a false belief that a spouse or significant other is cheating, despite a lack of supporting evidence. People with jealous delusions sometimes resort to violence.

- somatic (so-MAT-tik): This type of delusion relates to a bodily function. For example, people with somatic delusions may falsely believe that they have a physical deformity, an unusual odor, or some kind of germ in their bodies.

Delusional Disorder Versus Schizophrenia

Delusions often are a symptom of serious psychotic (sy-KOT-ik) disorders, the most common being schizophrenia (skitz-oh-FREN-ee-uh). Besides delusions, other symptoms of schizophrenia include hallucinations*, disorganized thoughts and speech, and bizarre and inappropriate behavior. Typically, psychotic disorders affect people in late adolescence or early adulthood.

Not all delusions are caused by psychotic disorders, however. When a person has delusions, and the doctor can find no psychotic disorder that is to blame, the doctor may diagnose a delusional disorder. Unlike schizophrenia and other psychotic disorders, delusional disorder usually occurs in middle age (ages 35 to 55) or later adult life. Also, it generally

*hallucination (huh-LOO-sih-NAY-shun) is something that a person senses that is not caused by a real outside event. It can involve any of the senses: hearing, smell, sight, taste, or touch.

does not lead to severe problems with everyday functioning and thinking. Many people with delusional disorder can keep their jobs, and, on the whole, their personalities do not change. However, once delusions occur, the false beliefs often prove to be a long-term problem. Some people with delusions can become dangerous or violent, threatening harm to themselves or others.

Treatment

Treatment for delusions usually involves regular meetings with a doctor who specializes in treating mental disorders. People with delusions tend to resist treatment at first and deny that there is any problem. The doctor needs to establish a cooperative relationship with the person, listening to his or her thoughts, easing any fears, and suggesting ways of coping. Some medications, particularly those used to treat depression and psychotic disorders, may help as well. Hospitalization may be necessary if the person shows signs of dangerous behavior or suicidal tendencies as a reaction to the delusional beliefs.

Resource

Website

Internet Mental Health. This is an online mental health encyclopedia founded by a Canadian psychiatrist. It provides specific information about delusional disorder and schizophrenia.
http://www.mentalhealth.com/fr20.html

▶ *See also*
Psychosis
Schizophrenia

KEYWORDS
for searching the Internet and other reference sources

Brain tumor

Geriatrics

Head injuries

Huntington disease

Neurology

Parkinson disease

Dementia

Dementia (dee-MEN-shuh) is a decline in mental ability that usually progresses slowly, causing problems with thinking, memory, and judgment. It is most often seen in the elderly and is caused by deterioration in parts of the brain. A person with dementia eventually has difficulty with the activities of everyday living, such as balancing a checkbook, reading, and working.

Why Doesn't Grandpa Recognize Me?

As Jacob sat in the hospital waiting room, he reminisced about this same day last year; Grandpa had taken him to the Baltimore Oriole's home opener to celebrate his eleventh birthday. Since then, his grandfather had experienced a few small strokes, or blockages in the blood vessels that supply oxygen and nutrients to his brain. The resulting loss of oxygen caused damage to parts of Grandpa's brain, and now he could barely talk or make any decisions for himself. Grandpa was 70 years old, but he almost seemed like a little kid.

During today's visit, Grandpa did not seem to know that it was Jacob's twelfth birthday. In fact, Grandpa did not even seem to know who Jacob was. Seeing his grandfather in this state made Jacob very sad and a little bit angry. He did not understand why his grandfather did not recognize him. Grandpa's doctor saw Jacob sitting in the waiting room and knew he was upset. She sat beside him and explained that Grandpa did not recognize people because he had a condition called dementia, which was a result of the brain damage caused by the strokes. She said that only time would tell if Grandpa's condition would improve, but in the meantime Jacob should keep visiting him, talking to him, and including him in special occasions. She told Jacob that even though Grandpa might act differently in many ways, there was still a part of the old Grandpa inside, and that Jacob's presence could still bring enjoyment to him.

What Are the Symptoms of Dementia and Who Is Affected?

People who develop dementia typically experience changes in personality, frequent confusion, and a lack of energy. Thinking, reasoning, memory, and judgment are often affected, and a person with dementia might also have trouble with language and motor (movement) skills.

Dementia is mostly a disease of the elderly. It is estimated to affect more than 15 percent of people (about 1 in 7) over age 65 but as many as 40 percent of people (2 out of 5) over age 80. It is one of the most common reasons for nursing home admissions in the United States, and it is a condition that many older people fear. When dementia affects young people, it is usually the result of an injury or some other condition that causes brain damage.

What Causes Dementia?

Dementia can result from any damage that interferes with the normal functioning of the brain. This damage may be permanent or temporary, and it can have a variety of causes that are usually classified into three categories:

1. **Structural:** a problem with the structure of the brain.
2. **Infectious (in-FEK-shus):** a bacterium or virus causes an infection that interferes with brain function.
3. **Metabolic* or toxic:** a problem with the substances in the blood that are needed to nourish the brain.

Structural causes of dementia The most common cause of dementia is Alzheimer (ALZ-hy-mer) disease, a condition in which abnormal structures (called plaques and tangles) accumulate in the brain over

* **metabolic** (meh-tuh-BALL-ik) pertains to the process in the body (metabolism) that converts food into energy and waste products.

time and interfere with nerve cell connections. Alzheimer disease leads to a gradually worsening loss of mental abilities, including memory, judgment, and abstract thinking, as well as to changes in personality. This disease usually affects people over age 65, and doctors are not sure of the causes.

Successive strokes are the second most common cause of dementia. Strokes, or blockages in some of the blood vessels that feed the brain, gradually destroy areas of brain tissue that normally are fed by the blocked blood vessels. People who develop this condition often have a history of high blood pressure* and/or diabetes*.

Other structural causes of dementia include:

▪ A brain tumor, which is a mass of abnormal cells growing in the brain. As the tumor grows, it presses on certain areas of the brain and causes personality change and problems with thinking, movement, and other functions. Severe or repeated milder head injuries can lead to dementia, also.

▪ Parkinson disease is a slowly progressing, degenerative* disorder of the nervous system that leads to shaking, difficulties with movement, and muscle stiffness. About 15 to 20 percent of people who have it also develop dementia. Former Attorney General Janet Reno, boxer Muhammad Ali, and actor Michael J. Fox are three well-known people who have Parkinson disease.

▪ Huntington disease is a rare inherited disease in which people in midlife begin having occasional jerks or spasms that are caused by a gradual loss of brain cells. People with Huntington disease eventually develop uncontrolled movements and mental deterioration.

Dementia caused by infectious diseases   People who have Acquired Immunodeficiency Syndrome* (AIDS) sometimes experience dementia because the virus that causes AIDS can infect the brain. Another dementia-causing condition is Creutzfeldt-Jakob Disease (CJD), a very rare, rapidly progressing disease that affects the brain. Doctors are not sure what causes CJD, although in some cases it appears to have been passed from human to human by contaminated surgical instruments. One form of the disease has been found in humans who have eaten beef from a cow that has "mad cow disease". Yet another cause of dementia is viral encephalitis [en-sef-uh-LIGHT-us], an inflammation of the brain that can be caused by certain viruses, particularly those transmitted to humans by the bite of a mosquito.

Metabolic causes of dementia   Having too much or too little of certain substances in the body can damage the brain enough to cause dementia. For example, anoxia (too little oxygen reaching the brain), vita-

*high blood pressure, or hypertension, is a condition in which the pressure of the blood in the arteries is above normal. Arteries are the blood vessels that carry blood from the heart through the entire body.

*diabetes (dy-a-BEE-teez) is a condition in which the body is unable to take up and use sugar from the bloodstream normally to produce energy. It is caused by low levels of insulin (the hormone that controls this process) or the inability of the body to respond to insulin normally.

*degenerative (dee-JEN-er-uh-tiv) means progressive deterioration. A degenerative disease results in diminished function or impaired structure of a tissue or organ.

*Acquired Immunodeficiency Syndrome, or AIDS, is a viral disease that damages the immune system, leaving a person at high risk for many life-threatening infections.

min B12 deficiency, and hypoglycemia (hy-po-gly-SEE-mee-uh; a lower than normal amount of sugar in the bloodstream) are conditions that can lead to dementia if left untreated. People with severe alcoholism can also develop dementia, due to a condition known as Wernicke-Korsakoff syndrome. This syndrome occurs when a person's body has too little of a vitamin called thiamine, which plays a key role in helping the brain process sugar for energy; over time, a thiamine deficiency can cause mental confusion and memory loss. People who are malnourished or do not get enough of certain other nutrients from their diet have also been known to develop Wernicke-Korsakoff syndrome.

GET TO KNOW THE SCIENTISTS

Many dementia-causing conditions are named after the physicians or scientists who discovered them:

- Alois Alzheimer was the German physician who published an article on a "new disease of the cortex" (the outermost or "reasoning" portion of the brain) in 1907. The disease is now called Alzheimer disease.

- James Parkinson was the English physician who published "Essay on the Shaking Palsy" in 1817. This was one of the first articles on the disease now named for him.

- George Huntington was an American doctor from Ohio whose 1872 paper on hereditary chorea (kor-EE-uh; a condition of uncontrolled, rapid movements) made him famous because of its accurate and complete descriptions of this disease. The condition is now better known as Huntington chorea or Huntington disease.

- Hans Gerhard Creutzfeldt and Alfons Jakob were two German physicians who, in the 1920s, first described the brain disease now known by their names.

- Carl Wernicke was a German physician whose 1881 *Textbook of Brain Disorders* first described a nervous system condition caused by insufficient amounts of a vitamin known as thiamine.

- Sergei Korsakov was a nineteenth-century Russian psychiatrist who studied and described the connections among alcoholism, nerve inflammation, and mental symptoms.

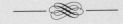

How Is Dementia Diagnosed and Is It Treatable?

The process of diagnosing dementia usually begins when the person and/or family members begin to notice that the person is experiencing increasing forgetfulness, lapses in memory, or problems with everyday tasks. The doctor may give the patient a mental status test by asking a series of questions that require memory of everyday events or by asking the patient to perform simple tasks like counting backwards. The doctor also will try to determine whether there is some underlying cause of the person's symptoms. Blood tests and scans of the brain can help the doctor see whether there is an imbalance of certain substances in the body or a structural problem in the brain. The doctor also will ask for a complete description of the person's symptoms, his or her family medical history, current medications, and about the presence of any other medical conditions (such as high blood pressure or diabetes).

In most cases, dementia cannot be cured; rather, it is more likely to worsen over time, especially when a progressive disease such as Alzheimer disease or Parkinson disease is the cause. However, in some cases the worsening of dementia can be slowed and sometimes the symptoms can actually improve if the underlying cause can be addressed. For example, controlling blood pressure and quitting smoking can slow or stop progressive dementia associated with blockages in blood vessels within the brain. Stopping excessive alcohol intake or correcting a vitamin deficiency can also help, if that is what is causing the problem.

When a Loved One Has Dementia

Dementia is especially hard on family members and loved ones who remember the person as he or she once was. The loss of memory, increased helplessness, and personality changes can be especially difficult to witness and accept. However, family and friends can play an important role in helping the person deal with dementia. The presence of familiar faces, regular exercise, and maintaining a bright, cheerful, familiar environment have been shown to help people with dementia. Caregivers can also help the person establish a routine, take part in low-stress activities, and get good nutrition and exercise on a regular basis. Large calendars and clocks can help the person keep track of the day and time. Reminders from family, friends, or other caregivers about what is going on, who they are, and where the person is can also be helpful.

Resources

Organizations

Alzheimer's Association, 919 North Michigan Avenue, Suite 1100, Chicago, IL 60611-1676. The Alzheimer's Association is a support organization for people with Alzheimer disease and their families.

Telephone 800-272-3900
http://www.alz.org

The American Geriatrics Society, The Empire State Building, 350 Fifth Avenue, Suite 801, New York, NY 10118. The American Geriatrics Society website features information on dementia and dementia-related conditions.
Telephone 212-308-1414
http://www.americangeriatrics.org

U.S. National Institute of Neurological Diseases and Stroke (NINDS), Bethesda, MD 20824. NINDS posts fact sheets about dementia and dementia-related conditions at its website; a keyword search for "dementia" calls up a range of information.
http://www.ninds.nih.gov

Family Caregiver Alliance, 690 Market Street, Suite 600, San Francisco, CA 94104. The Family Caregiver Alliance offers information helpful to people who are caring for loved ones with dementia.
Telephone 415-434-3388
http://www.caregiver.org

▶ *See also*
Alzheimer Disease
Brain Chemistry (Neurochemistry)
Brain Injuries

Depersonalization   *See* Dissociative Identity Disorder

Depression

Depression (de-PRESH-un) is a condition that causes people to feel long-lasting sadness and to lose interest in activities that normally give them pleasure. People with depression have continuing negative and pessimistic thoughts. They may experience changes in eating and sleeping patterns and in their ability to concentrate and make decisions.

More Than Ordinary Sadness

Everyone feels sad occasionally, especially after a loss or a setback. Feeling down for short periods is perfectly normal. However, when sadness lasts several weeks and starts to interfere with normal activities, such as studying, relationships with friends and family, attendance at school, or activities that are normally fun, then it is more than an ordinary variation in mood. It is depression.

KEYWORDS
for searching the Internet and other reference sources

Bipolar disorder

Dysthymia

Major depression

Mood disorders

Seasonal affective disorder

Depression is sometimes called an invisible disease, because it does not produce a rash or a fever or any other easily recognizable sign of a problem. In addition, many people are afraid or embarrassed to talk about how unhappy or hopeless they feel, mistakenly believing the feelings are a sign of weakness or a character flaw on their part. Sometimes those close to a person experiencing depression add to this mistaken belief by encouraging the person to simply "cheer up." Because it often goes unrecognized, depression often goes untreated, but it is just as important to treat depression as it is to treat illnesses like diabetes or asthma. Depression should be treated by a mental health professional. The good news is that 80 to 90 percent of people with depression can be helped by treatment, often within a few weeks. Left untreated, however, depression can get worse and last longer. This needlessly reduces a person's full participation in life. In severe cases, it can lead to suicide.

Who Gets Depressed?

Depression is a common illness that appears in several different forms. Up to 1 out of every 12 teenagers suffers from depression. In addition, about 1 out of every 10 adults experiences a period of depression in any given year. About one-fourth of all women and one-eighth of all men will experience at least one episode of depression during their lifetime.

Depression can be found in children, in elderly people, and in people of all ages in between. It affects people of all races, cultures, professions, and income levels. Women, however, experience depression about twice as often as men. The economic costs of depression in the United States, including lost wages, lost productivity, and treatment, are between $30 billion and $44 billion every year.

How Do People Know If They Are Depressed?

Depression differs from ordinary sadness or grief. With depression there is:

- a persistent feeling of sadness or emptiness that occurs daily and lasts longer than 2 weeks
- unhappiness or a feeling of worthlessness or guilt that interferes with normal activities
- loss of pleasure in activities that once were enjoyable, such as taking part in hobbies, listening to music, or going out with friends.

Not everyone experiences depression in the same way, but in addition to the symptoms listed above, other common changes that can occur include:

- eating too much or too little
- sleeping too much or too little; difficulty getting up or going to sleep
- unexplained periods or restlessness, irritability, or crying
- fatigue and decreased energy, even when getting enough sleep

- difficulty concentrating or remembering things
- difficulty making decisions
- increased interest in death
- thoughts of suicide

Preteens and teenagers experience many of these symptoms, but there are additional symptoms of depression that are common in young people. These include:

- ongoing physical problems, such as headaches, digestive problems, or persistent aches and pains that have no obvious physical explanation and do not respond to medical treatment
- increased absences from school or worsening school performance
- talking about or acting on the desire to run away from home
- unexplained outbursts of shouting, complaining, or crying
- increased irritability, anger, or hostility
- extreme sensitivity to failure or rejection
- being bored
- lack of interest in friends and a desire to isolate oneself
- increased difficulties in relationships with family, friends, or teachers
- alcohol or substance abuse
- reckless behavior
- abnormal fear of death

Because depression can involve physical symptoms, people with depression often consult their physician. This is very helpful since symptoms of depression can be symptoms of medical conditions as well. A medical check-up can determine if there is some medical reason for their symptoms, such as another disease or a side effect of medication. If these reasons are ruled out, a likely cause is depression. The physician may ask about feelings of sadness, hopelessness, or discouragement, loss of pleasure, and sleeping and eating problems to confirm a diagnosis of depression. The physicians then can discuss treatment options with the person, which may include a referral to a mental health professional for psychotherapy and, in some cases, medication.

What Causes Depression?

Experts are not exactly sure what causes depression. Depression is complex, but it appears to have mental, physical, genetic, and environmental components. These parts come together in different ways, making it difficult to pinpoint the exact cause of depression or predict who will become depressed and under what circumstances. One thing that is certain is that depression is not a weakness or a character flaw. It is not laziness or intentional bad

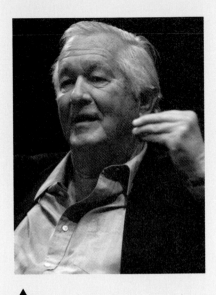

▲

In his autobiographical book *Darkness Visible*, William Styron explores the possible sources of his debilitating depression, his recovery, and the history of this illness which has affected many other artists and writers.
©Liaison/Newsmakers/OnlineUSA

behavior. People with depression cannot simply pull themselves together and drive out their sad and empty feelings, no matter how much the people around them encourage them to "snap out of it."

Mental components   Depression affects a person's thoughts, but it also seems that a person's thoughts can affect depression. Why this happens is not clear. Some experts believe that depression comes from anger that is not expressed, but is directed inward at oneself instead. Others believe that negative thoughts feed depression, and that people who think negative things about themselves, the world around them, and the future encourage and deepen the depression. Feelings of being helpless and of having no choices, even if in reality choices exist, also can be mental components of depression. People who have low self-esteem and perfectionists who set unrealistic goals for themselves also are prone to depression.

Physical components   Researchers have found a link between depression and an imbalance of certain chemicals in the brain, called neurotransmitters*. Brain imaging techniques show that areas of the brain responsible for moods, thinking, sleep, appetite, and behavior function differently in some people with depression. In addition to differences in brain chemistry, some medical illnesses, such as stroke*, heart attack, cancer, or diseases that cause long-lasting pain, can sometimes trigger depression. In women, hormonal changes that occur just after the birth of a child cause some new mothers to experience postpartum (post-PAHR-tum) depression, also called the "baby blues." For most women, this is a mild, short-lived problem that goes away on its own after a week or so. In a few cases, though, the problem is more severe and long-lasting, and treatment is required.

Genetic components   It appears that genetic (inherited) factors also cause vulnerability to some kinds of depression. This is demonstrated by the way that depression tends to run in families, and by twin research. Studies of twins have found that identical twins (twins who have the same genes*) are twice as likely to both experience major depression as are fraternal twins (twins who do not share all the same genes). Although a person with a parent, brother, or sister who has a depressive illness is more likely to become depressed than someone with no such family history, many people who have relatives with depression are not themselves depressed. For other people, depression seems to "come out of nowhere," with no family history of the condition. This indicates that while genetic factors certainly contribute to depression, other factors play a significant role in whether the depression actually develops.

Environmental components   The death of a loved one, a failure at school or on the job, the end of a romantic relationship, or many other kinds of losses can trigger an episode of depression in some people. Depression is different from the normal mourning process that follows a

*__neurotransmitter__ (NUR-o-transmit-er) is a chemical produced in and released by a nerve cell that helps transmit a nerve impulse or message to another cell.

*__stroke__ is a disorder in which an area of the brain is damaged due to sudden interruption of its blood supply. This is often caused by a blood clot blocking a blood vessel supplying the brain.

*__gene__ is a chemical found in the chromosomes in the body's cells that passes on information, such as eye color, height, or other characteristics, from parent to child.

loss. A person in mourning goes through distinct stages of psychological reaction to the loss, ending with the ability to accept the loss and resume normal functioning. With depression, the sadness continues over a long time with no progress being made toward acceptance of the change. There is no way to predict which environmental stresses will trigger depression in specific individuals.

Types of Depressive Illnesses

Depression can take a variety of forms. It may be mild, moderate, or severe. It may be mixed with periods of normal feelings or periods of abnormally heightened energy called manic (MAN-ik) periods, or depression may be continuous but low level. Some depressions occur seasonally. Although feelings of sadness, unworthiness, discouragement, and loss of interest in normally pleasant activities are common to all forms of depression, different depressive illnesses have different patterns of symptoms and are treated somewhat differently.

Major depression Major depression is a combination of the symptoms listed above that is serious and long-lasting enough to interfere with daily life. It is also called unipolar depression. Major depression is the leading cause of disability in the United States and worldwide, because it can become severe enough to leave people unable to work, concentrate, learn, or care for themselves or their family. If left untreated, major depression can last for months or longer. Some people have only one period of major depression in their lives. For many others, however, episodes of major depression come and go for years.

Dysthymia Dysthymia (dis-THI-mee-a) is the name given to a long-lasting depressed mood that is less severe than major depression, but which continues at a low level for a long time. People with dysthymia feel sad and show at least two other symptoms of depression for at least 2 years. Dysthymia often goes undiagnosed, because it is not disabling. However, it does leave people feeling sad and empty and keeps them from enjoying life and functioning at their best. Many people who have dysthymia also have episodes of major depression during their lives.

Bipolar disorder Bipolar (by-POLE-are) disorder used to be called manic-depressive illness. It has two faces. One face is major depression. The other is mania (MAY-nee-a), an unnaturally high mood in which a person may be overactive, overtalkative, or filled with tremendous energy. The severe lows of depression alternate with the extreme highs of the manic phase. Symptoms of mania include:

- great energy; ability to go with little sleep for days without feeling tired
- severe mood changes from extreme happiness or silliness to irritability or anger

- overinflated self-confidence; unrealistic belief in one's own abilities
- increased activity, restlessness, or distractibility; inability to stick to tasks
- racing, muddled thoughts that cannot be turned off
- impaired judgment of risk and increased reckless behavior.

For most people, the mood swings between depression and mania occur over a long period of time, sometimes years. If bipolar disorder is left untreated, though, the intervals between mood shifts tend to become shorter and shorter. In children, the cycle is usually quite short, sometimes occurring several times in a day.

Bipolar disorder is not as common as major depression. About 1 out of every 100 people has bipolar disorder, and unlike major depression, it occurs equally often in men and women. However, bipolar disorder appears to be more likely to run in families than major depression.

Adjustment disorder with depressed mood   It is not uncommon for people of all ages to respond to certain life stressors with emotional and behavioral symptoms. For example, someone may become depressed after losing a job or when a loved one has died. Another person may feel worried, anxious, or vulnerable after an injury or illness. A child or teen may have trouble concentrating in school or show some disruptive behavior in the months following his or her parents' divorce.

When symptoms are too mild to be diagnosed as another mental health condition and occur as a reaction to a specific known life situation, the condition is called an adjustment disorder. Because people may react to difficult life circumstances with a variety of different types of emotions and behaviors, there are many types of adjustment disorders.

When the main symptoms of an adjustment disorder are depressed mood and related changes in feelings and behavior, such as feeling hopeless and crying a lot, the condition is called adjustment disorder with depressed mood.

With adjustment disorder, the symptoms are temporary and disappear within 6 months after the source of stress has been removed.

Seasonal affective disorder (SAD)   SAD is a form of depression that comes and goes at the same time each year, usually starting with the onset of winter. People with seasonal affective disorder often experience fatigue and oversleeping, carbohydrate craving and weight gain, as well as an overly sad mood. More women have SAD than men, and children and teens can also experience SAD. SAD is linked to decreasing exposure to daylight that occurs naturally during the winter months. Studies have shown that when people with this form of depression travel south in winter, their symptoms improve, and when they travel north their symptoms worsen.

These findings have led to treatment with artificial light. With light therapy, people use bright "grow-light" type lights or special lightboxes for several hours each day. This therapy has shown good results, and research continues to investigate this form of depression.

How Is Depression Treated?

Treatment for depression depends on its type and severity. There are several approaches that can be used either alone or in combination. Current thinking suggests that medication combined with psychotherapy (sy-koe-THER-a-pea) is the most effective treatment for moderate to severe depression. The medication helps relieve the symptoms of depression, while the psychotherapy helps people change their negative thought patterns.

Medication   Antidepressant (an-tie-dee-PRESS-ant) medication can be prescribed by a psychiatrist (a medical doctor who specializes in mental disorders) or another physician. People usually must take a medication for several weeks before they notice changes in their mood, and they typically continue to take the drug for 6 to 9 months. Antidepressants are not habit-forming. Not every medication works for every person, however.

One group of antidepressants, introduced in the 1980s, is called selective serotonin (ser-o-TOE-nin) reuptake inhibitors (SSRIs). Serotonin is a neurotransmitter in the brain, and these drugs work by altering brain chemistry. They generally have fewer side effects than other drugs used to treat depression. Examples of SSRIs include fluoxetine (brand name Prozac), paroxetine (Paxil), and sertraline (Zoloft). Other types of antidepressants, including groups of drugs called monoamine oxidase inhibitors (MAOIs) and tricyclic antidepressants (TCAs), also can be helpful for some people.

Lithium (Eskalith, Lithobid) is a medication that can be very effective in treating bipolar disorder. However, lithium does not work for everyone. For these people, doctors sometimes prescribe another mood-stabilizing medication, such as carbamazepine (Tegretol) or divalproex sodium (Depakote).

St. John's wort (*Hypericum perforatum*) is an herb that is widely prescribed for mild depression in Europe. Although it is sold without a prescription in the United States, St. John's wort has not been approved by the U.S. Food and Drug Administration for the treatment of depression, because not enough controlled studies have been done to show whether it is safe and effective. Those studies are currently underway.

Psychotherapy   Psychotherapy, or "talking therapy," involves a therapeutic relationship between the depressed person and a psychiatrist, psychologist, or mental health counselor. Cognitive-behavioral (KOG-ni-tiv-be-HAVE-yor-ul) therapy (CBT) and interpersonal (in-ter-PER-son-al)

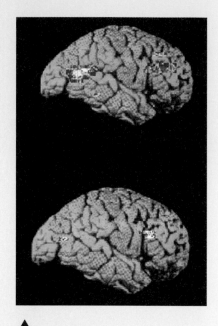

▲

Positron emission tomography (PET) records electrical activity inside the brain. With red and yellow showing brain activity, the brain of a depressed person at the top shows a decrease in activity compared to the brain of a person who has been treated for depression at the bottom. Treatment can improve metabolic acticity and blood flow in the brain. *Photo Researchers, Inc.*

therapy (IPT) have been shown to be particularly useful. CBT focuses on helping people change their thoughts and actions. IPT helps people focus on resolving problems in relationships that may be triggers for depression.

Electroconvulsive (e-LEK-troe-kon-VUL-siv) therapy (ECT)

ECT, popularly known as "shock therapy," is used to treat severe depression when immediate relief is needed. This treatment, which is performed by a physician, requires hospitalization and anesthesia to keep the person free of pain and injury. Carefully controlled electrical pulses are sent to the brain, causing a brief seizure. Although this treatment is controversial, it can be a lifesaver for someone who is suicidal and needs immediate relief.

Self-help groups   Many people experiencing depression find it helpful to join local support or self-help groups. These groups share information and tips for coping with depression. Some also offer support for close family members and friends.

Experiencing Depression

Sadly, about two-thirds of people who experience depression do not seek help. This is unfortunate, since the vast majority of people with depression can be helped to feel better in a relatively short time.

The best way to help someone with depression is to encourage that person to get professional help. If the depression is severe, encouragement may not be enough, however. It may be necessary to arrange a visit to a health care provider for them. Help is available through family physicians and health maintenance organizations, community mental health centers, hospitals, and mental health clinics. People who are talking about suicide need emergency care. Many telephone books list suicide and mental health crisis hotlines in their Community Service sections, or help can be obtained by calling emergency services (911 in most places).

Depression is not a sign of personal failure or something to be ashamed of. It does not mean that a person is "crazy." Depression is simply an illness that needs to be treated so that life will once more be enjoyable, purposeful, and worthwhile.

Resources

Book

Styron, William. *Darkness Visible: A Memoir of Madness.* New York: Random House, 1990. A short book by the author of *Sophie's Choice* about his battle with depression.

Organizations

American Psychiatric Association, 1400 K Street Northwest, Washington, DC 20005. A professional organization that provides information about depression on its website.
Telephone 888-357-7924
http://www.psych.org

National Depressive and Manic-Depressive Association, 730 North Franklin Street, Suite 501, Chicago, IL 60610-7204. A national support organization for people with depression and bipolar disorder.
Telephone 800-826-3632
http://www.ndmda.org/

U.S. National Institute of Mental Health, 6001 Executive Boulevard, Room 8148, MSC 9663, Bethesda, MD 20892-9663. A government agency that does research on depression and provides information to the public through pamphlets and a searchable website.
Telephone 800-421-4211
http://www.nimh.nih.gov

▶ *See also*
Anxiety
Bipolar Disorder
Brain Chemistry (Neurochemistry)
Electroconvulsive Therapy (ECT)
Genetics and Behavior
Medications
Seasonal Affective Disorder
Suicide
Therapy

Disability

Disability is a potentially limiting difference in the functioning of the human body. Disabilities can influence both the physical and mental well-being of a person, and they can have a strong impact on self-esteem and social adjustment.

KEYWORDS
for searching the Internet and other reference sources

Chronic illness

Congenital disorder

Handicap

Disability is a deviation from the normal range of functioning that places a limit on what a person can do or that imposes special conditions or needs that must be met to allow a person to function in the normal range or up to his or her full capacity. Disabilities can be mental, physical, psychological, or a combination of all three. The disability may be obvious to the casual observer, such as the loss of a leg, or invisible, such as a back injury. Some people prefer to refer to anyone whose range of function falls outside the norm as "differently abled," to stress that the condition is a difference rather than a lack of completeness. Many people with so-called disabilities do quite well meeting the challenges of life.

*genetic pertains to genes, which are the chemicals in the body that help determine physical and mental characteristics, such as hair or eye color. They are inherited from a person's parents.

*cystic fibrosis is an inherited disease of the body's mucus-producing glands that usually appears in early childhood. It mainly affects the respiratory and digestive systems and can lead to difficulty breathing and infection in the lungs because of an accumulation of abnormally thick mucus in the airways and lungs.

*rubella, also called German measles, is a viral infection that causes a rash and fever.

*fetal alcohol syndrome, which occurs if the fetus is exposed to alcohol, is a condition that can be associated with mental, physical, and behavioral differences. Oppositional behavioral problems, learning difficulties, mental retardation, and retarded growth can occur in the children of women who drink alcohol while they are pregnant.

Where Do Disabilities Come From?

People can be born with a disability. When this happens, it is called a congenital (kon-JEN-i-tal) disability. In many cases, the cause of a congenital disability is unknown. Some disabilities with known causes are:

- **Inherited disabilities:** Some disabilities are the result of genetic* disorders, for example, cystic fibrosis*.
- **Exposure of the mother to disease during pregnancy:** For example, a mother who has rubella* early in pregnancy may have a child who is deaf or who has other birth defects.
- **Exposure of the mother during pregnancy to alcohol, drugs, harmful medications, pollutants, or chemicals:** For example, if a mother drinks during pregnancy, she may have a child with fetal alcohol syndrome*.
- **Difficulties arising during the birth process:** Complications can arise during the delivery of a baby, for example, the loss of an adequate oxygen supply to the brain, which can lead to brain damage and mental retardation.

Some people hold superstitious beliefs that birth defects are punishment for the sins or evils done by the parents or that they occur because the mother has been cursed during pregnancy. Although these ideas are clearly false, people with disabilities and their families sometimes must confront these unfounded beliefs in themselves and in others.

Disabilities also can be acquired at any time after birth. Acquired disabilities commonly arise from accidents, illness, working conditions that expose a person to an unhealthy environment (such as coal miners who breathe in coal dust), or repetitive physical stresses (such as repeated heavy lifting).

Disability and Self-Image

Self-image is the mental picture we have of ourselves, including our external appearance, our intellectual abilities, our strengths, and our weaknesses. This mental picture begins to develop in infancy and continues to grow and change throughout life. People develop their mental pictures through their interactions with other people and the world around them. Self-esteem is strongly linked to self-image. Self-esteem is the value that people put on the mental image that they have of themselves.

Self-image and congenital disabilities Children who are born with a disability do not realize immediately that they are different from anyone else. Generally, children start to become aware of physical differences in human bodies, such as differences in hair and skin color, body size and shape, and gender, by their second year of life. Over time, children with disabilities realize that they are in some way different from most other people. At first this difference is neither good nor bad to them. Since congenitally disabled people may have never lived in a non-disabled body, they often feel complete, intact, and "okay" with the disability, even though the outside world may view them as different. Children whose parents accept them, support them, show pride in them and their abilities, and communicate factually and directly about the disability are more likely to develop good self-image and self-esteem.

When parents of children with disabilities encourage them to change and act more like "normal" people, hide their limitations, or dwell on things that they cannot do, the children may feel frustrated, unaccepted, and disappointed at not living up to their parents' expectations. When they are faced repeatedly with other people's negative reactions to their limitations, people with disabilities may come view themselves negatively and develop a poor self-image.

The conflict between "owning" a disability and making it part of oneself versus trying to get rid of the disability to become more like other people can be seen in the current debate in the deaf community about cochlear (KOK-lee-ar) implants. When these devices are installed surgically in a deaf person's inner ear, they allow some deaf people to hear, but not like "congenitally hearing" people do. On one side of the debate are people who were born deaf and who are comfortable with their deafness. They see deafness and deaf culture as part of their identity, and they do not want to change. On the other side are those deaf people who believe that it is in their best interest to enter the mainstream of hearing people, if that is possible.

Self-image and acquired disabilities

People who acquire disabilities later in life have a different experience from those who are born with a disability. These people have lost something that has played a part in the development of their self-image, whether it is an arm or leg or the ability to perform a particular activity. People with acquired disabilities tend to go through a grieving process similar to the grieving process for any other major life loss. Their emotions usually follow these stages: grief, denial, anger, depression, working out a new way to live, and acceptance of the disability. Unfortunately, some people get stuck on one or more of these steps and may never reach the last two steps.

Self-image and chronic illness

Chronic illness is a special kind of "disability." There are different kinds of chronic illnesses. Some illnesses, like diabetes*, often can be managed by the family doctor without hospitalization or pain. Others, such as back or neck injuries, can severely limit activities and may require treatment for pain with medications that may have some undesirable side effects. Progressive chronic illnesses, such as muscular dystrophy* or Alzheimer disease*, get worse with time and eventually can lead to death earlier than expected.

Some people with chronic illness may go through repeated periods of anger, sadness, and depression. They may become frustrated and angry

* **diabetes** (dy-a-BEE-teez) is a condition in which the body is unable to take up and use sugar from the bloodstream normally to produce energy. It is caused by low levels of insulin (the hormone that controls this process) or the inability of the body to respond to insulin normally.

* **muscular dystrophy** (DIS-tro-fee) is a group of inherited disorders that causes muscle weakening that worsens over time.

* **Alzheimer** (ALTS-hy-mer) **disease** is a condition that leads to gradually worsening loss of mental abilities, including memory, judgment, and thinking, as well as changes in personality and behavior.

In the middle of his career, artist Chuck Close became partially paralyzed due to a blood clot in his spinal column. To continue painting, he developed a technique that allowed him to work with his weakened hands from his wheelchair. He is still able to create the large, multicolored portraits for which he is known. *A/P Associated Press* ▶

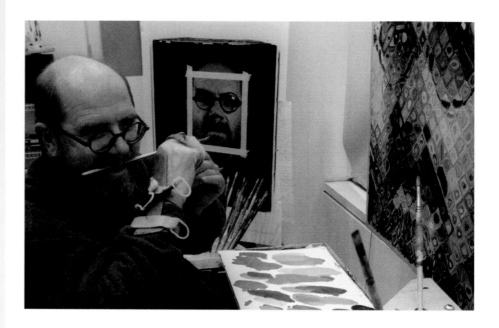

at their caregivers or feel inadequate and embarrassed by the extra burden they place on loved ones. Several studies have shown that males have more emotional problems when they are faced with chronic illness than females, although researchers are not sure why this is true. It should be stressed that chronic illness does not necessarily result in chronic problems with self-image. Most people with chronic illness would not consider themselves disabled, and generally, with good health care and family support, they deal effectively with their illnesses.

Disability and Health

Most physicians and mental health practitioners agree that there is a connection between mental health and physical well-being. In general, the better a person's self-image and self-esteem, the more able a person is to cope with life's ups and downs and the better a person feels both mentally and physically.

Many studies have found that people with disabilities experience psychological problems (especially depression and anxiety) and behavior problems at about twice the rate of the non-disabled population. Family members of people with disabilities are also more likely to experience emotional problems brought on by the extra responsibilities, financial burdens, and limitations of caring for someone with a disability. Though chronic illness and disability include the risk of psychological problems, most individuals and families learn to cope with these conditions.

In 1996, the American Academy of Pediatrics reviewed many studies of people with disabilities and concluded that certain risk factors increase the chance that people with disabilities will experience psychological problems. Other "protective" factors appear to decrease the chance that a person with a disability will have psychological problems.

Risk factors that increase the likelihood of psychological problems include:

- chronic illnesses that are painful, unpredictable (like seizures), or embarrassing
- "invisible" disabilities (because people may feel stressed by wondering if they should tell others about their limitations)
- disabilities that require a schedule of time-sensitive special treatments
- poor social skills and a rigid personality
- failure of loved ones and professionals to talk honestly with the person about the disability
- failure of parents to address sexuality in teens with disabilities
- allowing the disability to become the focus of family life
- fighting between the parents or break-up of the parents' marriage
- overprotectiveness on the part of parents or caregivers.

Factors that decrease the likelihood of psychological problems include:

- family acceptance of the disability
- strong bonds within the family that help the family work together
- open and direct communication about the nature of the disability and what to expect
- balancing of family needs with the needs of the disabled person
- good social skills and plenty of social interaction
- appropriate expectations of accomplishments
- a strong support network in the community.

Myths About People with Disabilities

Non-disabled people often are ignorant about the reality of life for a person with a disability. Some of the false beliefs people with disabilities frequently encounter include:

Myth: Disabled people are usually mentally retarded.

Reality: Most disabilities do not affect intelligence.

Myth: Disabled people are sick.

Reality: Illness is not the same as disability. Some people are disabled with chronic illness, while others are healthy.

Myth: People with disabilities can never have a good quality of life.

Reality: The quality of life mainly depends on the character of a person and society's acceptance of a person than on the disability itself.

Myth: People with disabilities need continuous supervision and cannot lead independent lives.

Reality: The degree of independence a person achieves depends on the nature of the disability, the person's education and training, and the accommodations that are available to make independent living physically possible.

Myth: People with disabilities are especially noble, brave, and courageous for coping with their handicaps.

Reality: There are all kinds of people with disabilities. Most disabled people carry on with their lives just as non-disabled people do.

People with Disabilities and the Community

The Americans with Disabilities Act is the federal law that is intended to integrate people with disabilities into mainstream life as much as possible. It requires that disabled people be provided with access to public and private spaces and with workplace accommodations and, whenever possible, that they be included in mainstream public education. Although physical accommodations, such as wheelchair-accessible restrooms or Braille instructions for the blind on automatic teller machines, are common in new buildings, many older facilities and private spaces still have not been renovated to accommodate people with physical disabilities.

Employers are increasingly willing to make workplace accommodations for people with physical disabilities, but they are still fearful of making such arrangements for people with emotional disabilities. The unemployment rate among disabled people, especially disabled women, is very high, and many people with disabilities are employed at jobs below

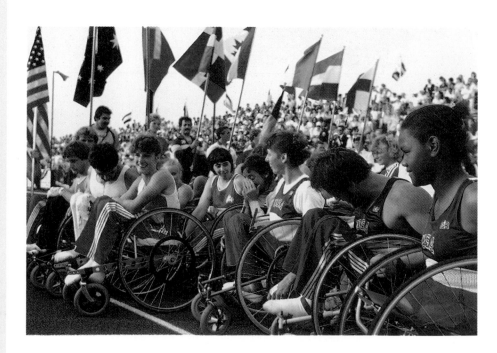

▶

Hundreds of wheelchair racers gather for the International Games for the Disabled, 1984. *Peter Arnold, Inc.*

their skill levels. Service industries hire more people with disabilities than any other type of employer. Ignorance on the part of the non-disabled is still the greatest barrier to achievement of their full potential for people with disabilities.

People with disabilities face some common challenges. At the same time, disabled people are also individuals with differing characters and needs. People who are born with a disability have self-image issues that are different from those of people who acquire a disability later in life. Someone who is confined to bed with a chronic (long-term) illness faces challenges that are different from someone who is healthy but who has a disability such as blindness or mental retardation.

Although researchers can draw a group picture of people who are disabled, this picture does not represent an individual with a disability any more accurately than a general picture of the "average American" represents a non-disabled person. Our society must learn to see people with disabilities as individuals, each with his or her own strengths, weaknesses, hopes, and dreams, before people with disabilities can achieve full equality.

Resources

Book

Kent, Deborah, and Kathryn A. Quinlan. *Extraordinary People with Disabilities.* New York: Children's Press, 1997. Profiles of more than 50 people with various disabilities.

Organizations

Center for Disability Information and Referral, Indiana Institute on Disability and Community, 2853 East Tenth Street, Bloomington, Indiana 47408-2696. This organization, which is associated with Indiana University, provides referrals for all types of disabilities. They also have an educational website for disabled and non-disabled children. Telephone 812-855-9396
http://www.iidc.indiana.edu/~cedir

disAbility Online, a website provided by the United States Department of Labor, addresses work and education-related disability issues. The site includes a state-by-state resource guide.
http://www.wdsc.org/disability

▶ *See also*
Body Image
Chronic Illness
Self-Esteem

Disruptive Behavior *See* Conduct Disorders; Oppositional Behavior

---

Dissociative Identity Disorder

Dissociative (di-SO-see-a-tiv) identity disorder (DID) is a severe mental disorder in which a person has two or more distinct sub-personalities that periodically take control of the person's behavior. Before 1994, DID was called multiple personality disorder (MPD).

*__amnesia__ (am-NEE-zha) is the loss of memory about one or more past experiences that is more than normal forgetfulness.

*__fugue__ (FYOOG) refers to a psychiatric condition in which people wander or travel and may appear to be functioning normally, but they are unable to remember their identity or details about their past.

*__depersonalization__ (de-per-son-al-i-ZAY-shun) is a mental condition in which people feel that they are living in a dream or are removed from their body and are watching themselves live.

What Is Dissociative Identity Disorder?

Dissociative identity disorder (DID) is the most complex of a group of disorders characterized by the process of dissociation (di-SO-see-ay-shun). Other dissociative disorders include amnesia*, fugue*, and depersonalization*. Dissociation is a defense mechanism that allows an individual to separate or "go away from" thoughts, memories, emotions, or events that are highly stressful. This process helps the individual deal with situations that would otherwise be intolerable. Because dissociation is an unconscious process, the person experiencing it is not aware of any personality changes that occur during an episode.

Mentally healthy people often experience mild forms of dissociation, such as daydreaming or getting lost in a book or a movie. Most people, especially adolescents, also find that different aspects of their personality tend to come out in certain situations or with certain groups of people. These changes in personality are normal.

DID, however, involves extreme and repeated dissociation that interferes with a person's normal functioning and can result in memory gaps and identity confusion. By repeatedly dissociating and blocking out painful or unpleasant memories, a person with DID develops two or more distinctly different, often colorful or dramatic, identities. People with DID may have between 10 and 15 sub-personalities, and some people may even have more than 100. Often these sub-personalities can differ in gender, style, voice, and psychological make-up. People with DID may discover unfamiliar articles in their homes that they have purchased while their behavior was controlled by a different sub-personality, and they may have conversations when one sub-personality is dominant that other sub-personalities cannot remember. Some life events and memories (particularly traumatic ones) are known to certain sub-personalities but remain unknown to others.

Is Dissociative Identity Disorder a Real Disorder?

The diagnosis of DID is the subject of controversy in the psychiatric community, Throughout history there are records of the occasional dissociated person who has behaved oddly. These people often have been described as "possessed," and later they have been unable to recall their behavior during the possession. In some cultures, these people are still considered possessed, and they are treated with exorcisms to drive out the demons that control them. However, prior to 1980, multiple personality disorder (MPD), as DID was then called, was considered to be a rare psychiatric disorder; only a few hundred cases in several centuries of recorded medical literature had been documented.

In 1956, a fictionalized story (later made into a movie) called *The Three Faces of Eve* helped introduce the public to the idea of MPD. In 1973, the subject was brought before the public again with a documentary, *Sybil*, which portrayed a woman with 16 different personalities. Since then, some psychiatrists have questioned the accuracy of the Sybil story. However, since about 1980 the number of people diagnosed with DID has increased sharply, and some psychiatrists estimate that as many as 1 and 3 percent of Americans may suffer from the disorder.

There are two different schools of thought about the DID:

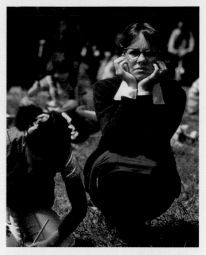

Sybil (1976), starring Sally Field, told the true story of a woman who was so severely abused as a child that she developed over 16 different personalities. This highly acclaimed television movie helped to raise the public's awareness of DID. *Photofest*

DID is a common and serious disorder   One group of psychiatric professionals recognizes DID as a common and serious psychiatric disorder. They believe that DID is caused by repeated severe physical, emotional, or sexual trauma or abuse in early childhood. Children find these experiences too terrible to remember, so they repress them and mentally "go away" in order to cope with daily life. Later, these traumatized children develop multiple sub-personalities to deal with the repressed memories. When under stress in adulthood, certain triggers cause the switching from one sub-personality to another as a way of coping. The sub-personalities may have different psychological problems and may even have different physical traits. They may even have distinctive handwriting or different allergies!

Psychiatrists who support DID as a common disorder point to the fact that child abuse is common, and because dissociation is a very effective coping tool for people who are powerless to change their situations, DID is therefore also likely to be genuine and common.

DID rarely develops independently   A second group of psychiatric professionals thinks that DID rarely develops on its own in a person. They believe that DID is unknowingly created by interactions between the therapist and the patient when patients are highly susceptible to the suggestions of the therapist. This group of psychiatrists believes that in some cases therapy causes patients to recover memories of abuse that did not really happen and to unconsciously invent sub-personalities. Because the abuse that is supposed to cause DID happens in early childhood, it is often impossible to confirm any trauma that the patient describes.

This doubting group of psychiatrists points out that symptoms of DID are detected by friends or family members only after therapy has begun. They note that DID is rarely seen in children, and that many children who survive stressful events such as extreme abuse, war, kidnapping, or genocide do not suffer from DID.

* **depression** (de-PRESH-un) is a mental state characterized by feelings of sadness, despair, and discouragement.

* **panic attacks** are periods of intense fear or discomfort with a feeling of doom and a desire to escape. During a panic attack, a person may shake, sweat, be short of breath, and experience chest pain.

* **anxiety** (ang-ZY-e-tee) can be experienced as a troubled feeling, a sense of dread, fear of the future, or distress over a possible threat to a person's physical or mental well-being.

* **phobias** (FO-be-as) are intense, persistent fears of a particular thing or situation.

* **hallucinations** (huh-LOO-sin-AY-shuns) are things that a person perceives as real but that are not actually caused by an outside event. They can involve any of the senses: hearing, smell, sight, taste, or touch.

* **eating disorders** are conditions in which a person's eating behaviors and food habits are so unbalanced that they cause physical and emotional problems.

* **schizophrenia** (skit-so-FRE-ne-a) is a serious mental disorder that causes people to experience hallucinations, delusions, and other confusing thoughts and behaviors, which distort their view of reality.

* **psychosis** (sy-KO-sis) refers to mental disorders in which the sense of reality is so impaired that a patient can not function normally. People with psychotic disorders may experience delusions, hallucinations, incoherent speech, and agitated behavior, but they usually are not aware of their altered mental state.

The validity of recovered memories is highly controversial. Psychiatrists are divided on whether recovered memories, especially those recovered under hypnosis, are real or if they have been unwittingly suggested to the person through therapy, news stories, or ideas they have gotten from relatives or loved ones. This complicates the issue of whether DID is caused by early childhood trauma and abuse. Almost all (98 to 99 percent) of people diagnosed with DID seem to have experienced severe trauma before age nine. However, only a small percentage of all people who experience documented childhood trauma develop DID.

How Is Dissociative Identity Disorder Diagnosed?

DID is difficult to diagnose. People with DID have distinct multiple sub-personalities, but within each sub-personality they tend to be consistent. To diagnose DID, a doctor must see two or more distinct sub-personalities that each become dominant for a period of time. Sometimes doctors use hypnosis to try to bring out different sub-personalities.

People with DID can also have many other symptoms. Almost every person who has been diagnosed with DID has been in the mental health system for a long time (an average of seven years in one study) and has had previous, presumably incorrect, diagnoses before a diagnosis of DID is made. People with DID usually show signs of other psychiatric and/or physical disorders, including amnesia, time loss, depression*, severe mood swings, sleep disorders, alcoholism, drug dependency, panic attacks*, anxiety*, phobias*, auditory and/or visual hallucinations*, eating disorders*, headaches, trances, and violence toward themselves or others. It takes careful evaluation over time to understand whether certain symptoms indicate DID or other conditions.

DID differs from schizophrenia* and psychosis*, although they all may share some symptoms. Schizophrenia is not a "split personality" (like the fictional Dr. Jekyll and Mr. Hyde), but a disorder of reality and thought. Unlike people with schizophrenia, people with DID are in full control of their thoughts, although they may be unable to remember large portions of their life when their behavior is being controlled by a different sub-personality. Unlike people with psychosis, who often have visual or auditory hallucinations, people with DID generally do not have bizarre, uncontrolled thoughts or serious problems in how they sense reality. Within each sub-personality a person with DID may function well.

How is Dissociative Identity Disorder Treated?

Therapists who believe that DID is brought about by childhood trauma use a technique called integrative psychotherapy*. This form of therapy involves recovering repressed or dissociated childhood memories and making them a part of a single personality in order to help the person become whole and reengage with the world. Often this process is emotionally painful because it involves facing past trauma. The use of hypnosis to recover memories of childhood trauma is controversial and not accepted by all mental health professionals. Therapists who believe that DID is unknowingly created in susceptible patients by well-meaning therapists believe that the correct treatment is to discontinue therapy. Both groups agree that medication does not often help the dissociation that occurs in people with DID, but it may help with other symptoms.

Resources

Book

Schreiber, Flora Rhea. *Sybil.* New York: Warner Books, 1974.

Organization

The National Alliance for the Mentally Ill (NAMI) is a nonprofit organization that provides education, support, and advocacy for people with severe mental illnesses and their families. NAMI's website provides information about many mental illnesses, including DID.
Telephone 800-950-NAMI
http:/www.nami.org

Divorce

Divorce is the legal ending of a marriage.

Divorce or the breakup of a nuclear family is an extremely stressful event for both the divorcing adults and their children. Although adults who are divorcing may feel relief that a difficult marriage is ending, children may feel frightened, confused, and uncertain about their futures.

Since the 1940s the divorce rate in the United States has risen steadily. In the 1940s, 14 percent of women who married eventually divorced. In contrast, it is expected that almost half of marriages that occurred in the year 2000 will end in divorce. As a result, more and more children are living in households headed by a single parent or in blended families with stepparents and stepsiblings.

What Happens During a Divorce

Divorce is a legal action that separates married partners. Divorce does not end the relationship between parents and their children, nor does it end parents' responsibility to care for or financially support their children. Under ideal circumstances, parents will peacefully agree on how to split up the family's money, property, and possessions and how to share responsibility for their children. Unfortunately, the divorcing adults

* **psychotherapy** (sy-ko-THER-a-pea) is the treatment of mental and behavioral disorders by support and insight to encourage healthy behavior patterns and personality growth.

▶ *See also*
Amnesia
Fugue
Hypnosis
Phobias
Psychosis
Schizophrenia
Stress

KEYWORDS
for searching the Internet and other reference sources

Stepfamily

often are bitter and angry and are unable to come to an agreement. When this is the case, the court usually steps in and makes decisions for them.

In the United States, each state has laws and guidelines for how money, property, and possessions are to be split by a divorcing couple. There are also guidelines for decisions that affect children. The courts can decide which parent the children will live with (called custody), who is financially responsible for the children (called child support), and how much time the children spend with the parent they do not live with (called visitation). The courts can even choose who may make medical or legal decisions for the children. Increasingly, courts are assigning joint custody, an arrangement in which divorcing parents share responsibility for their children equally.

Generally, the court makes decisions that are in the best interest of the children, but the interpretation of what is in a child's best interest varies greatly from judge to judge and court to court. Older children may be asked to give their opinions about issues such as custody or visitation, but judges are not required to consider a child's preferences. Young children rarely are consulted in this way.

How Children React to Divorce

Children are never responsible for their parents' divorce. How much children understand about divorce and how they react to it depends on their age and how well their parents explain the divorce process to them. Children under the age of 3 or 4 understand very little about the process of divorce, but they do recognize emotional distress and tension in the family. Young children may become confused, emotionally upset, and uncooperative as their lives change as the result of the divorce process.

Children who are ages 5 to 9 sometimes blame themselves for their parents' divorce and unrealistically believe that if they are "good," their parents will get back together. Their concerns center on very basic security issues: who will take care of them, whether they will have to move or change schools, where their toys will be kept, and whether their parents will leave them the way they left each other.

Preteens are likely to be angry, moody, and embarrassed by divorce. They may be intensely critical and resent or blame one or both parents. Preteens are old enough to worry about the financial effect of divorce and to be annoyed about extra household chores or childcare responsibilities that result from their changed circumstances. They also may worry about how their parents are coping.

Although they are capable of empathizing with their parents' feelings, teenagers still may feel angered by the divorce. They may be depressed and worry about questions such as whether they will be able to afford college. Teens may be confused because they are preparing to leave the family at a time when their family is "breaking up." Some teens turn to risky types of behavior, such as drinking or promiscuous sexual activity, to deal with their pain. Others become ultra responsible and step in to act as parents for younger siblings. Neither response is an emotionally healthy way of coping.

All children, regardless of age, feel loss during a divorce and go through a grieving process. Most children pass through normal periods of insecurity, guilt, depression, and anger. By having their children talk to a mental health professional, clergyman, or school counselor, parents can help young people work through these feelings. Joining a self-help group for children of divorcing parents can give children support and a safe place to talk about their feelings.

Some children have parents who break up without a legal divorce. These may include children whose mothers and fathers lived together but were unmarried or children living in households of two committed adults of the same gender. When these unmarried couples break up, there is no formal, legal divorce in most states because there was not a legal marriage, but children may feel the same grief or sense of loss that children experiencing a legal divorce feel.

Effects of Divorce

Many studies show that children of divorced couples are more likely to live in families experiencing poverty or difficult financial circumstances after the divorce. Stresses resulting from the life changes surrounding the divorce make children more vulnerable to physical and emotional illnesses, especially when parents continue to fight over custody issues. In general, children of divorced parents are more likely to have health problems, to participate in more risky and antisocial behavior, and to be at higher than average risk of school failure than are children from two-parent non-divorced families. In other words, divorce is very stressful for everyone.

Research is showing that there is much confusion and disruption during a divorce, and the effects can last much longer than previously thought. Some studies suggest that children of divorced parents have more difficulty establishing mature emotional relationships when they become adults. Although children of divorce are more likely to have these problems, the majority of children who experience divorce grow up happy, healthy, and emotionally stable.

Strategies for Coping with Divorce

Parents need to work hard to maintain a civil relationship with each other during and after the divorce. It is best that they never ask their children to take sides, carry messages from one parent to the other, or tattle on the ex-spouse. There are other things parents can do to help their children, among them:

- Talk honestly about the divorce without blaming.
- Explain what is likely to happen to the children during and after the divorce.

Talking about their relationship with a team of therapists can help couples cope with the emotional stress of getting a divorce. *PhotoEdit* ▶

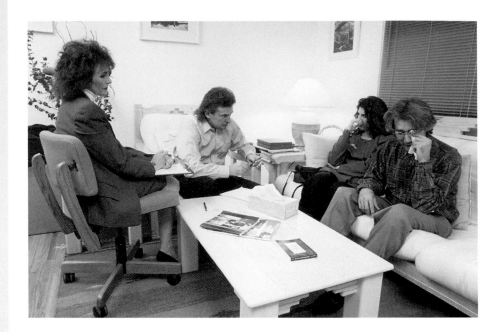

- Get counseling and support for themselves and their children.
- Keep the daily routine and participation in extracurricular activities as normal as possible.
- Discourage children's fantasies about the parents getting back together.
- Avoid making children feel guilty about wanting to spend time with the other parent.
- Encourage children to maintain established relationships with grandparents or other relatives on both sides of the family.

Divorce is an unsettling experience, and it is normal to feel grief for the family that has dissolved. While most people are able to pass through the grief, anger, and uncertainty to grow into happy, productive lives, the distress of the divorce process is real and needs to be met with appropriate support from family, friends and mental health counselors.

Resources

Books

Cleary, Beverly. *Dear Mr. Henshaw.* Ormond Beach, FL: Camelot, 2000. This book tells the story of Leigh, an 11-year-old boy who keeps a journal of his experiences and feelings, including those about his parents' divorce.

Rothchild, Gillian. *Dear Mom and Dad: What Kids of Divorce Really Want to Say to Their Parents.* New York: Pocket Books, 1999. A book for older children and their parents, focusing on the needs and emotions of children during divorce.

Schneider, Meg F., and Joan Zuckerberg. *Difficult Questions Kids Ask—and Are Afraid to Ask—About Divorce.* New York: Simon and Schuster, 1996. The question-and-answer format of this book addresses issues hidden behind children's asked and unasked questions about divorce.

Staal, Stephanie. *The Love They Lost: Living with the Legacy of Our Parents' Divorce.* New York: Delacorte Press, 2000. Stories of 120 people who have lived through the divorce of their parents.

Organizations

Rainbows, 2100 Golf Road, no. 370, Rolling Meadows, IL 60008-4231. An organization that offers peer support groups and training for children and adults grieving from a death, divorce, or painful family transition.
Telephone 800-266-3206 or 847-952-1770
http://www.rainbows.org

Stepfamily Foundation, Inc., 333 West End Avenue, New York, NY 10023. Provides telephone and in-person counseling from divorce through stepfamily formation.
Telephone 212-877-3244
http://www.stepfamily.org

▶ *See also*
Emotions
Families
Love and Intimacy

Domestic Violence *See* Abuse

Down Syndrome *See* Mental Retardation

E

Eating Disorders

Eating disorders are habits or patterns of eating that are out of balance and may involve major health and emotional problems.

KEYWORDS
for searching the Internet
and other reference sources

Anorexia nervosa

Binge eating disorder

Binge and purge

Bulimia nervosa

Compulsive overeating

Food and nutrition

Weight loss

What Are Eating Disorders?

Eating disorders are not merely unhealthy eating habits; they involve patterns of eating too little or too much, and they may cause a variety of physical and emotional problems. Eating disorders usually develop during adolescence and usually affect girls, although boys can also be affected. Eating disorders include anorexia (an-o-REK-see-a), bulimia (bull-EE-me-a), binge eating disorder, and obesity (o-BEE-si-tee).

Anorexia   Anorexia is an eating disorder that involves fear of becoming or being fat, intensive dieting or exercise, and a distorted body image. People with anorexia see themselves as fat even though they may be dangerously underweight. They severely restrict their food intake and/or exercise to extremes in order to lose weight. Someone may be diagnosed with anorexia if she refuses to eat enough food to maintain a healthy weight, and has lost more than 15 to 20 percent of her healthy weight. For example, a girl with anorexia whose healthy weight is 125 pounds might weigh 105 pounds. She might eat as little as 500 calories a day (most healthy teenagers eat 2,000 or more calories a day).

Bulimia   Sometimes referred to as the "binge-purge" disorder, bulimia involves repeated episodes of binge eating (consuming large quantities of food while feeling little control over the behavior) followed by purging (trying to rid the body of the food by vomiting or by using laxatives or enemas). Some people with bulimia also exercise excessively. In bulimia, self-image is overly tied to body shape and weight, and people with this disorder are dissatisfied with these aspects of their body. However, unlike those with anorexia, people with bulimia usually stay at a fairly healthy weight.

Binge eating disorder   Binge eating disorder involves out-of-control overeating but lacks the purging that is seen with bulimia. Binge eaters often are obese or constantly dieting and they often feels guilty after a binge. Painful emotions or stress may trigger binges.

Obesity   Obesity is an excess of body fat. People are considered overweight if extra body fat causes them to weigh 20 percent more than the healthy weight for their height and obese if they if they weigh more than 30 percent above what is healthy for their height.

Who Develops Eating Disorders?

Most teenagers are concerned about how they look. After all, their appearance is changing very quickly. Girls are developing breasts and their hips are becoming rounded and curvy. Boys' voices are deepening and body hair is increasing. Most teenagers have an ideal image in their minds about what they should look like, and images on television and in the movies reinforce the goal of thinness as perfection.

Many young people, particularly girls, go on diets to control their body weight. Dieting has been reported to start as early as elementary school. Dieting without guidance by a medical doctor can cause problems with growth and development for children and teens. Sometimes an earnest but misguided effort to control weight can evolve into an eating disorder.

Consider Diane, a 13-year-old seventh grader. Her diet began innocently enough. She thought she was 10 to 15 pounds overweight and switched her lunch from a sandwich and cookies to a salad. She lost a few pounds. She liked feeling thinner, got a lot of compliments, and pretty soon she reduced the salad at lunch to a carrot and a piece of cheese. Diane trimmed her dinner as well, telling her parents that she had eaten a big lunch and was not hungry. Before long, Diane had lost 20 pounds. But Diane was surprised that she did not feel happy; instead, she was obsessed with food and her weight (she still felt fat) and was embarrassed whenever anyone commented on her body. Diane continued dieting and also began to exercise two times a day to try to lose more weight.

Diane is not alone; experts say that more than five million American women and girls and one million men and boys suffer from eating disorders. About 1 in 100 girls between 12 and 18 years old has an eating disorder. As many as 1 in 10 college females has anorexia or bulimia. More than 1,000 young women die each year from the serious medical problems that develop because of eating disorders!

Young people who participate in sports that prize thinness are at particularly high risk of developing eating disorders. Female dancers, ice skaters, and gymnasts have a three times greater risk for developing an eating disorder than do girls not involved in such activities. Boys who participate in similar sports or in wrestling are also at higher risk. Girls who enter puberty early and girls who are overweight may also be more likely to develop eating disorders.

What Causes Eating Disorders?

There is no clear-cut, single cause for any of the eating disorders. Many factors seem to contribute, including influences from society and culture (such as the glorification of thinness by the mass media), emotional issues (such as a teenager's striving for perfection, exposure to intensely stressful situations, and fears of maturity, puberty, or sexuality), family factors (such as overly controlling parents, serious emotional conflicts, or problems expressing feelings), or poor childhood feeding and eating patterns. People who have an eating disorder usually do not set out to deliberately have this problem. Generally, eating disorders develop slowly, as do the signs and symptoms.

What Medical Complications Are Caused By Eating Disorders?

Eating disorders are serious problems and can cause a variety of medical complications. In anorexia, rapid weight loss can lead to blood chemical imbalances, failure to menstruate*, slow pulse, low blood pressure, and heart problems. In some cases, damage to vital organs is so serious that it can result in death. The frequent vomiting associated with bulimia can cause throat tears or sores, damaged tooth enamel, broken blood vessels in the eyes, and puffy cheeks from swollen salivary glands. With both anorexia and bulimia, bowel and intestinal problems can occur and serious vitamin and mineral deficiencies can cause serious and long-lasting problems. Binge eating often results in obesity, which in turn can lead to other health problems. People who are obese are at greater risk of developing diabetes*, heart disease*, high blood pressure*, osteoarthritis*, and other health problems.

How Do Doctors Diagnose Eating Disorders?

Teenagers with anorexia, bulimia, and binge eating disorder often try to hide the problem, so formal diagnosis can be delayed or difficult. Even when caring friends or family members ask about the weight loss or other symptoms, most teenagers with eating disorders are ashamed or embarrassed, especially by the purging that accompanies bulimia. Because of distorted body image, those with anorexia may not be able to recognize the seriousness of their extreme weight loss. Unbearable fear of being fat may cause people with anorexia to resist attempts to help them gain weight. A concerned health professional might ask questions about eating, body image, and exercise. Blood or other laboratory tests can help determine if a person's nutrition is adequate and if general body chemistry is balanced. A careful interview and health history may reveal concerns about body image or distorted opinions about body appearance.

A doctor can generally determine if adults are obese by measuring their body weight and height. Obesity in children can be similarly determined but these measurements should be considered more carefully because the child is still growing. Over the last decade, there has been a significant rise in obesity in children in the United States. This is likely in part a result of people eating more frequently in fast food restaurants, watching a lot of television, working or playing games on computers, and

*menstruate (MEN-stroo-ate) means to discharge the blood-enriched lining of the uterus. Menstruation occurs normally in females who are physically mature enough to bear children. Because it usually occurs at four-week intervals, it is often called the "monthly period." Most girls have their first period between the age of 9 and 16.

*diabetes (dy-a-BEE-teez) is a disorder that reduces the body's ability to control blood sugar.

*heart disease is a broad term that covers many conditions that prevent the heart from working properly to pump blood throughout the body.

*high blood pressure, or hypertension (hy-per-TEN-shun), is a condition in which the pressure of the blood in the arteries is above normal. Arteries are the blood vessels that carry blood from the heart through the entire body.

*osteoarthritis (os-tee-o-ar-THRY-tis) is a common disease that involves inflammation and pain in the joints (places where bones meet), especially those in the knees, hips, and lower back of older people.

Eating disorders have multiple causes, which may include social and cultural pressures, emotional issues, and family stressors. Chemical imbalances in the brain, shown here in cross-section, may also cause eating disorders. These imbalances affect the hypothalamus, which is believed to control appetite.

▶

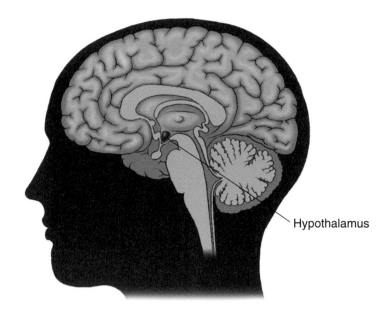

Hypothalamus

* **psychotherapy** (sy-ko-THER-a-pea) is the treatment of mental and behavioral disorders by support and insight to encourage healthy behavior patterns and personality growth.

* **calorie** (KAL-or-ee) is a unit of energy used to describe both the amount of energy in food and the amount of energy the body uses.

engaging in other activities that promote over-eating and a sedentary (sitting too much with little exercise) lifestyle.

How Are Eating Disorders Treated?

Overcoming eating disorders may take a long time and lots of commitment and hard work. Most teenagers with eating disorders need the assistance of mental health and other health care professionals to manage the problem. Anorexia, bulimia, and binge eating disorder are treated most successfully with a combination of therapies. Behavior change programs, monitoring of diet and eating patterns, individual or group psychotherapy*, support groups, nutritional counseling, family counseling, and sometimes medication may all be part of treatment.

People with obesity can be helped by doctor-recommended weight-loss programs that teach healthy habits. To lose weight, people must take in fewer calories* than they use, and the best way to control weight is through exercising and eating a balanced diet. In some cases, doctors may also treat severe obesity by prescribing very low-calorie diets or medications. In rare cases, doctors may advise a surgical procedure that either limits the amount of food the stomach can hold or causes food to bypass the stomach or part of the intestines.

Resources

Books

Bennett, Cherie. *Life in the Fat Lane*. New York: Random House, 1999. A novel about the high school experiences of an overweight girl.

Berg, Frances M. *Afraid to Eat: Children and Teens in Weight Crisis.* Hettinger, ND: Healthy Weight Journal, 1997.

Folkers, Gladys, and Jeanne Engelmann. *Taking Charge of My Mind and Body: A Girl's Guide to Outsmarting Alcohol, Drugs, Smoking, and Eating Problems.* Minneapolis: Free Spirit Publishing, Inc., 1997. For ages 11-18.

Siegel, Michele, Judith Brisman, and Margot Weinshel. *Surviving an Eating Disorder: Strategies for Family and Friends.* New York: Harper-Collins, 1997.

Organizations

U.S. Food and Drug Administration (FDA) posts the fact sheet *On the Teen Scene: Eating Disorders Require Medical Attention* at its website. http://www.fda.gov/opacom/catalog/eatdis.html

The American Psychological Association posts the fact sheet *How Therapy Helps Eating Disorders* at its website. http://helping.apa.org/therapy/eating.html

Eating Disorders Awareness and Prevention, Inc. (EDAP), 603 Stewart Street, Suite 803, Seattle, WA 98101. Telephone 800-931-2237 for toll-free information and referral hotline http://www.edap.org

www.KidsHealth.org, a website sponsored by the Nemours Foundation and the Alfred I. duPont Hospital for Children, Wilmington, DE, posts articles for kids, teens, and parents about eating disorders, obesity, nutrition, and related topics.

National Association of Anorexia Nervosa and Associated Disorders (ANAD), P.O. Box 7, Highland Park, IL 60035. Telephone 807-831-3438 http://anad.org

▶ *See also*
Anorexia
Anxiety and Anxiety Disorders
Binge Eating
Body Dysmorphic Disorder
Body Image
Bulimia
Depression
Emotions
Obesity
Peer Pressure
Stress

Electroconvulsive Therapy

Electroconvulsive (e-LEK-tro-kon-VUL-siv) therapy (ECT) is a form of treatment for certain severe psychiatric disorders that involves applying a mild electrical shock to each side of the skull. ECT is performed by a physician while the patient is monitored closely and kept pain-free.

KEYWORDS
for searching the Internet and other reference sources

Convulsions

Tonic-clonic seizure

What Is ECT?

ECT is a form of treatment for certain severe psychiatric disorders that involves using electrical shock. In ECT, a physician applies a mild electrical shock (20 to 30 milliamps) to each side of the patient's skull near

***anesthesia** (an-es-THEE-zha) is a state in which a person is temporarily unable to feel pain while under the influence of a medication.

***tonic-clonic seizure** (TON-ik-KLON-ik SEE-zhur) is an episode in which a person usually loses consciousness, stiffens due to muscle contractions, and lets out a loud cry as air is forced through the vocal cords during the tonic phase. In the clonic phase, the muscles of the body contract and relax rhythmically, which causes the body to thrash about.

On the Horizon

Transcranial magnetic stimulation (TMS) is a new, painless treatment that uses magnetic pulses to stimulate brain activity. In some early studies, TMS appeared to work against depression. About one-third of the patients treated with TMS experienced temporary, mild headaches after the treatment, but there seemed to be no other side effects. If TMS is shown to be as effective as ECT, it may become another treatment option for severe depression in the future.

the area of the temples. The procedure is done under anesthesia*, and the patient is monitored carefully. The shock is applied until the patient experiences a tonic-clonic seizure*. Normally, this would produce strong muscle contractions, causing the body to thrash about. However, the patient also is given a medication to relax the muscles, which prevents this kind of whole-body response. Instead, the seizure occurs just within the brain, where it lasts for a minute or so.

Who Benefits From ECT?

In the United States, about 100,000 people each year receive ECT. The types of mental disorders that are treated with ECT include schizophrenia, severe depression, mania, and delusional states. ECT is particularly effective as a short-term therapy for sudden, severe episodes of depression associated with suicidal tendencies. Because medications take several days or more to have an effect on severe depression, in some cases ECT is a way to provide immediate relief and protection from suicidal intent. About 60 to 70 percent of people who receive ECT experience some benefits. ECT is used with both children and adults.

Why Is ECT Controversial?

Despite its proven benefits, ECT is still somewhat controversial. The debate about its use today is based in part on the treatment's history.

Earliest treatments ECT was first tried in Italy in 1938. It soon was used to treat mental disorders that were resistant to other types of treatment. However, in the early days of ECT, few considerations were given to the patient's overall health. In addition, many people experienced pain from the shock itself or injuries from the whole-body seizures that resulted. Nevertheless, ECT was found to be an effective treatment for conditions such as severe depression, acute psychosis, and mania.

Modern treatments Modern improvements have made ECT a much safer and more comfortable experience for the patient. These improvements include the use of medications to produce a pain-free state and prevent violent muscle contractions. In 1999, the U.S. Surgeon General's report on mental health concluded that ECT was a safe and effective treatment for certain severe mental disorders when used according to current standards of care. Even so, the states of California, Texas, and Tennessee still prohibit the use of ECT with children and adolescents.

Media portrayals Some of the lingering debate about ECT is based on its portrayal in movies, television shows, and novels. In the movie *One Flew Over the Cuckoo's Nest*, for example, ECT was used as a punishment for unwanted behavior. Unfortunately, this kind of depiction often frightens people unnecessarily, keeping them from using a treatment that can be highly effective and even lifesaving.

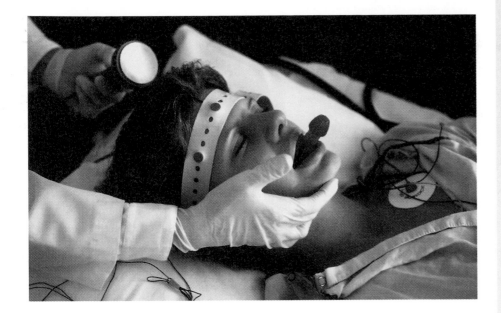

How Does ECT Work?

Scientists do not know for sure how ECT works, although research now is being done to find answers to this question. Most of the research is focused on ECT's effect on part of the brain called the hypothalamus*, which, among its many functions, regulates emotional expression and controls the endocrine glands. Changes in endocrine* function are often seen after ECT treatments.

What Happens During ECT Treatment?

ECT is performed in a hospital setting under the careful guidance of a physician. First the patient is given anesthesia and muscle-relaxing medications. Then the patient receives a mild electrical shock to each side of the skull. Thanks to the medications, the patient feels no pain, and the body does not convulse. Once the procedure is over, the patient awakens after 5 to 10 minutes, much as someone would after minor surgery. ECT generally is given in a series of 6 to 12 treatments over a period of a few weeks.

Many people experience some memory loss after ECT. Usually, this loss is temporary, affecting mainly memories of events from the days, weeks, or months just before or during the series of treatments. In most cases, the memories return within several weeks after the completion of ECT.

Resource

Organization

American Psychiatric Association (APA), 1400 K Street Northwest, Washington, DC 20005. A professional organization for psychiatrists,

* **hypothalamus** (HY-po-THAL-a-mus) is part of the brain that controls (among other things) the autonomic nervous system*, the endocrine glands, basic drives such as hunger, thirst, and aggressive and sexual drives. The hypothalamus also regulates emotional expression.

* **autonomic nervous system** is a branch of the peripheral nervous system that controls various involuntary body activities, such as body temperature, metabolism, heart rate, blood pressure, breathing, and digestion. The autonomic nervous system has two parts—the sympathetic and parasympathetic branches.

* **endocrine** (EN-do-krin) refers to a group of glands, such as the thyroid, adrenal, and pituitary glands, and the hormones they produce. The endocrine glands secrete their hormones into the bloodstream, and the hormones travel to the various organs in the body that they affect. Certain hormones have effects on mood and sometimes are involved in symptoms such as irritability, emotional swings, fatigue, insomnia, depression, suspiciousness, and apathy.

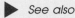 *See also*

Bipolar Disorder

Depression

Schizophrenia

Suicide

KEYWORDS
*for searching the Internet
and other reference sources*

Feelings

Mood

Mood disorders

Stress

physicians who specialize in treating mental disorders. Psychiatrists perform ECT treatments, and information about the treatments can be found on the APA website.
Telephone 888-357-7924
http://www.psych.org

Emotions

Emotions are specific and intense psychological and physical reactions to a particular event.

One morning Mandy waited for the light to change so that she could cross the street to school. As the light in her direction turned green, she stepped off the curb. Suddenly, Mandy froze as a car shot right past her through the red light and crashed into a car already in the intersection. Mandy was not hurt. The car that went through the red light was not that close to her, but she felt terrified, then weak and shaky. She was so upset that she started to cry. That morning at school, whenever Mandy thought about the accident she had seen she felt nervous and shaky. By lunchtime, when she talked to her friends about the accident, the shaky feeling was starting to wear off, and she was beginning to feel anger toward the driver of the car that had run the red light. Although Mandy was not physically hurt, her mind and body were experiencing a strong emotional reaction to a dangerous situation.

What Are Emotions?

Emotions, often called feelings, include experiences such as love, hate, anger, trust, joy, panic, fear, and grief. Emotions are related to, but different from, mood. Emotions are specific reactions to a particular event that are usually of fairly short duration. Mood is a more general feeling such as happiness, sadness, frustration, contentment, or anxiety that lasts for a longer time.

Although everyone experiences emotions, scientists do not all agree on what emotions are or how they should be measured or studied. Emotions are complex and have both physical and mental components. Generally researchers agree that emotions have the following parts: subjective feelings, physiological (body) responses, and expressive behavior.

The component of emotions that scientists call subjective feelings refers to the way each individual person experiences feelings, and this component is the most difficult to describe or measure. Subjective feelings cannot be observed; instead, the person experiencing the emotion must describe it to others, and each person's description and interpretation of a feeling may be slightly different. For example, two people falling in love will not experience or describe their feeling in exactly the same ways.

Physiological responses are the easiest part of emotion to measure because scientists have developed special tools to measure them. A pounding heart, sweating, blood rushing to the face, or the release of adrenaline* in response to a situation that creates intense emotion can all be measured with scientific accuracy. People have very similar internal responses to the same emotion. For example, regardless of age, race, or gender, when people are under stress, their bodies release adrenaline; this hormone helps prepare the body to either run away or fight, which is called the "fight or flight" reaction. Although the psychological part of emotions may be different for each feeling, several different emotions can produce the same physical reaction.

Expressive behavior is the outward sign that an emotion is being experienced. Outward signs of emotions can include fainting, a flushed face, muscle tensing, facial expressions, tone of voice, rapid breathing, restlessness, or other body language. The outward expression of an emotion gives other people clues to what someone is experiencing and helps to regulate social interactions.

What Are The Sources of Emotions?

Scientists have developed several theories about how emotions are generated based on subjective feelings, physiological responses, and expressive behavior.

* **adrenaline** (a-DREN-a-lin), also called epinephrine, (ep-e-NEF-rin), is a hormone, or chemical messenger, that is released in response to fear, anger, panic, and other emotions. It readies the body to respond to threat by increasing heart rate, breathing rate, and blood flow to the arms and legs. These and other effects prepare the body to run away or fight.

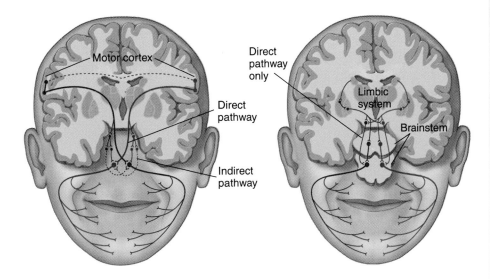

Voluntary Smile Circuit   Spontaneous Smile Circuit

◀

The facial muscles involved in emotional expression are governed by nerves following a complex system of direct and indirect pathways to and from the motor cortex (voluntary smile circuit under conscious control) and the limbic system and brain stem (spontaneous smile circuit not under conscious control). This may explain why people's faces can express emotions like happiness, fear, and disgust without their being aware of it.

The James-Lange theory

American scientist William James (1842–1910) and Danish scientist Carl Lange (1834–1900) both studied the relationship between emotion and physical changes in the body. In about 1885, they independently proposed that feeling an emotion is dependent on two factors: the physical changes that occur in the body and the person's understanding of the body's changes after the emotional event. James and Lange believed that physical changes occur first, and then interpretation of those physical changes occurs. Together, they create the emotion.

According to the this theory, when Mandy experienced a threatening situation (almost being hit by a car), her body first sent out chemical messengers, like adrenaline, that caused physical changes such as increased breathing and a faster heart rate. Her brain then sensed these physical changes and interpreted them as the emotion fear.

One of the problems with the James-Lange theory is that emotions seem to happen too quickly to be accounted for by the release of chemical messengers and the changes they cause. Another problem is that different emotions (for example fear and anger) have been shown to cause the same physical responses.

The Cannon-Bard theory

In 1927, about 40 years after the James-Lange theory was developed, Harvard physiologist Walter Cannon (1871–1945) and his colleague Philip Bard (1898–1977) developed a new theory that related the workings of the nervous system to the expression of emotions. Cannon and Bard found that people could experience emotion without getting physical feedback from chemical messengers. They proposed that upon experiencing a stimulating event, information about the event is collected by the body's senses and is sent through the nervous system to the brain.

*cortex is the part of the brain that controls conscious thought; it is where people experience "thinking and feeling."

In the brain, the message is sent two places at the same time. The message is sent to the cortex*, which creates emotions; in Mandy's case it created fear. At the same time, the message also goes to the hypothalamus (hy-po-THAL-ah-mus). The hypothalamus is the part of the brain that controls automatic body responses. It tells the body to send out chemical messengers that cause the body to respond. Some of these responses are experienced as behaviors such as shaking, rapid breathing, and crying.

The Schacter-Singer model

In 1962, American scientists Stanley Schacter (1922–1997) and Jerome Singer (still teaching at Yale University in 2000) took elements of both the James-Lange and the Cannon-Bard theories and modified them to try to better explain the relationship between physical responses and emotional experience.

According to the Schacter-Singer model, both physical changes and conscious mental processing are needed to fully experience any emotion. In this model, in response to her near-accident, Mandy's body sent out

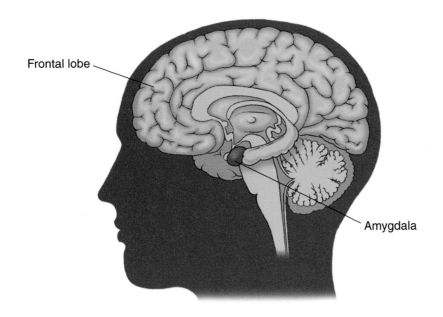

Frontal lobe

Amygdala

Researchers believe that the frontal lobes and the amygdala are among the most important brain structures affecting emotions. Feelings of happiness and pleasure are linked to the prefrontal cortex. Anger, fear, sadness, and other negative emotions are linked to the amygdala.

messages to create physical changes such as an increased heart rate. Mandy's brain sensed these changes and then analyzed them and put a label on them. The emotional label selected for the feelings was fear, and it depended in part on Mandy's experience with large fast cars; in other words, she knew from experience in her past that cars are dangerous. This model explains why the same physical responses can produce different emotions. The brain decides, for example, whether fear or anger or surprise is the appropriate emotion based on mental processing of physical information. Thus, interpretation of information from the environment, body feelings, and experience figure more prominently in the Schacter-Singer model.

Research continues on the relationship between the body, the brain, and the perception of emotions. One current area of research is focused on whether certain areas of the cortex are dedicated to specific emotions and whether a person can feel an emotion when a particular part of the cortex is stimulated directly by an electric impulse.

Why Do We Have Emotions?

Emotions appear to serve several physical and psychological purposes. Some scientists believe that emotions are one of the fundamental traits associated with being human. Emotions color people's lives and give them depth and differentiation. For many people, strong emotions are linked to creativity and expression. Great art, music, and literature deal on a fundamental level with arousing emotions and creating an emotional connection between the artist and the public. Some scientists also believe that emotions serve as motivation to behave in specific ways.

The French neurologist Guillaume Duchenne (1806–1875) studied the body's neuromuscular system. In this experiment (c. 1855), he used an electrical stimulation device to activate the involuntary facial muscles involved in smiling and laughter. *Getty Source/Liaison* ▶

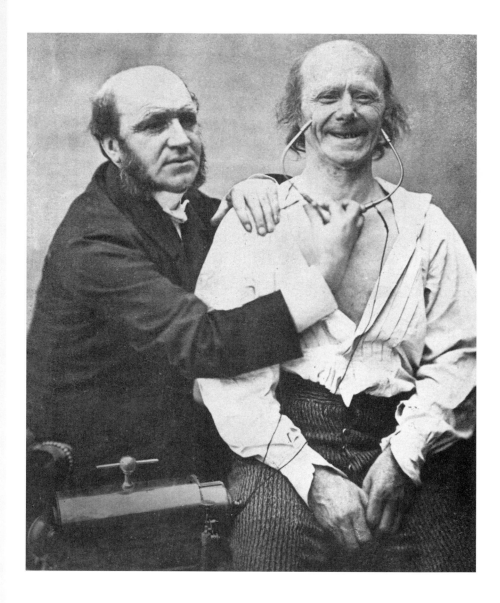

Physiologically, emotions aid in survival. For example, sudden fear often causes a person to freeze like a deer caught by a car's headlights. Because animals usually attack in response to motion, at its simplest level, fear reduces the chances of attack. When Mandy froze in response to a car racing by her, this was an example of a physical response to an emotion that improved her chances of survival.

Emotions also help people monitor their social behavior and regulate their interactions with others. Every person unconsciously learns to "read" the outward expressions of other people and apply past experience to determine what these outward signs indicate about what the other person is feeling. If a person sees a man approaching who is walking very aggressively, holding his body stiffly and frowning, the person might correctly assume that the man is angry. Using this information, the person can decide whether to leave or to stay or what tone of voice and body language to use when approaching the man.

WHAT IS EMOTIONAL INTELLIGENCE?

Emotional intelligence refers to people's ability to monitor their own and other people's emotional states and to use this information to act wisely in relationships. Emotional intelligence has five parts:

1. Self-awareness: recognizing internal feelings

2. Managing emotions: finding ways to handle emotions that are appropriate to the situation

3. Motivation: using self-control to channel emotions toward a goal

4. Empathy: understanding the emotional perspective of other people

5. Handling relationships: using personal information and information about others to handle social relationships and to develop interpersonal skills

Researchers are beginning to develop tests that can measure emotional intelligence. Scientists who study emotions generally believe that people with high emotional intelligence usually work well in cooperative situations and are good at motivating and managing others. People with low emotional intelligence often misinterpret emotional signals and have difficulty with relationships. Although emotional intelligence probably has an inherited component, many psychologists believe that people can be guided into making better use of the emotional intelligence that they possess.

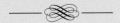

Some outward expressions of emotions (body language) mean different things in different cultures. For example, if a young person avoids looking directly at a person in authority, it is taken as a sign of respect in some cultures. In other cultures, this expression suggests guilt or a lack of trustworthiness.

Resources

Books

Goleman, Daniel. *Emotional Intelligence.* New York: Bantam Books, 1997. This book introduced the idea of emotional intelligence to the public.

▶ See also
Anxiety and Anxiety Disorders
Bipolar Disorder
Stress

LeDoux, Joseph *The Emotional Brain: The Mysterious Underpinnings of Emotional Life*. New York: Simon and Schuster, 1998. This book examines the connection between physical responses and emotions.

Mackler, Carolyn. *Love and Other Four-Letter Words*. New York: Bantam Doubleday Dell, 2000. Young adult fiction that addresses trying to make sense of the strong emotions that occur during adolescence.

Encopresis *See* Soiling

Enuresis *See* Bedwetting

Epilepsy *See* Brain Chemistry (Neurochemistry)

Eye Movement Desensitization Reprocessing (EMDR)
See Therapy

F

Families

A family is a group of people living together, often related by marriage, birth, or other strong bonds.

KEYWORDS
*for searching the Internet
and other reference sources*

Divorce

Stepfamily

Throughout history, people have found that their lives are better, easier, and more rewarding if they live within a group. This group, or family, is a basic unit of almost every society. Which people make up the family, the ways in which they are related, and the nature of their obligations to each other vary greatly through history, across different cultures, and even within a particular culture.

Why Families Matter

Early humans faced many dangers. They banded together in groups of people who were almost always biologically related to each other. These families often were led by one strong, skilled person (usually a man but, in some cultures, a woman). This social structure increased the chances of survival for each individual in the group. Within the family, the young, old, and disabled were protected. Older, more skilled family members taught younger ones. Family life allowed people to pool their labor and resources and develop specialized skills. It gave family members a feeling of security and belonging. Families developed in every culture, because they helped people meet their physical and emotional needs.

In return for receiving the benefits of belonging to a family, each member had certain obligations. These responsibilities usually centered on performing work, respecting the decisions of the head of the family, sharing, and behaving in ways that benefited the family more than the individual. The idea of giving and receiving support, help, knowledge, and protection within a group of trusted people is still the basis of the modern family.

The American Family

The idea of family is ever changing. As immigrants arrived in America from many different cultures, they brought with them their own ideas of family. Technological changes, such as the development of the automobile and the airplane, also have changed the idea of family. Once it was usual for several generations of people to live together in the same house and for brothers and sisters to settle down in the same town. Today, fewer

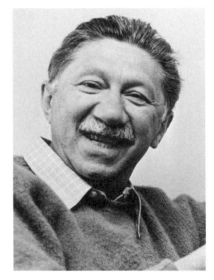

▲

Psychologist Abraham Maslow (1908–1970) believed that all people had needs, which he grouped into a hierarchy of importance. Families meet the needs that Maslow's hierarchy classifies as most basic: food and shelter; safety and security; love, affection, and feelings of belonging; and self-esteem. According to Maslow's theory, people cannot work to satisfy their higher-order needs for knowledge, art, and personal growth until their families have met their most basic needs. *Bettmann/Corbis*

169

families follow this pattern. As children reach adulthood, they are likely to leave their parents' homes and move into separate homes of their own, sometimes at great distances from other members of their family. Today Americans call the people they live with their "immediate family," and groups of other people they are related to either biologically or by marriage are included in their "extended family."

During the mid-twentieth century, the traditional American family usually was defined as consisting of a mother and a father who were married to each other, and their children. This is sometimes called the "nuclear family," meaning that this group is at the center (also called the "nucleus") of family relationships. Although books and television programs often presented this arrangement as the normal American family structure, many families did not fit into this formula even in the 1950s. The second half of the twentieth century brought an easing of divorce laws, more and more immigration from non-European countries, and increasing acceptance of unmarried people living together. As a result, the number of families that do not fit the nuclear family pattern has risen dramatically. Some of this change can be seen in the following United States government statistics:

- The percentage of children living with only one parent increased from 20 percent in 1980 to 27 percent in 1999.

- Although most children living with a single parent live with their mothers, in 1999, 4 percent of children lived in single-parent households headed by their father.

- In 1999 about one in every three babies was born to an unmarried woman. In 1960 only one of every 20 babies was born to an unmarried woman.

- In the late 1990s, about half of unmarried women who gave birth to children lived with, but were not married to, the fathers of their children.

- About half of marriages in the late 1990s are expected to dissolve through divorce.

- About 60 percent of all second marriages end in divorce.

- A significant increase in the number of gay and lesbian couples living together openly has resulted in an increase in the number of children living with adult partners of the same gender. It is estimated that between 8 percent and 20 percent of same-gender couples living in California and between 18 percent and 22 percent of these couples living in South Carolina had minor children living with them in 1999.

- In 2000, Vermont became the first state to put the legal rights of same-gender couples who participate in a civil union on an equal footing with the rights of traditional opposite-gender married couples.

Building Families

In traditional families, marriage between a man and a woman marks the beginning of a new family. In time, the married couple may have children of their own, forming a new nuclear family. Children live from infancy with their parents and siblings, allowing relationships to grow slowly over a period of time.

Sometimes, however, families are created instantly through adoption, remarriage due to the death of a parent or due to divorce, or transfer of responsibility from the parent to another caregiver, such as a grandmother. The majority of these "instant" families come about through the marriage of a parent who already has a child. The Stepfamily Foundation estimates that in 1999 half of the 60 million children in the United States under age 13 were living with one biological parent and that parent's partner.

Although all families experience problems such as sibling rivalry or the adjustment of family relationships when a new baby is born, relationship adjustment difficulties and stresses in so-called instant families are often magnified. When a new family is created that incorporates children past infancy, people may lack the time or skill needed to form close emotional bonds. Older children sometimes feel resentful of the new adult "parent" in their lives. Adults who have not been parents before may be unprepared for the demands of a ready-made family. Adults and children both may be jealous or feel that their security is threatened as a result of issues centering on favoritism.

Families need time to develop new rituals, share experiences, and build emotional bonds of love and trust among family members. Professional counseling or self-help groups often help both children and adults get through the difficult initial stages of forming new family bonds.

Teenagers and Families

Being a teenager and a member of a family normally involves certain types of conflict. As young people move toward adulthood, they need to become more independent of their families. They must develop a sense of self that allows them to establish mature relationships with their peers that will eventually lead to the formation of a new family. At this point in their lives, adolescents sometimes feel that being part of a family prevents them from experiencing the freedom they want. To get away from these restrictions and establish a stronger sense of independence, adolescents may spend a lot of time away from home, sometimes more time with their friends than with family members. The desire for independence often conflicts with family expectations. Parents or heads of households may feel that their teen is ignoring responsibilities to the family or behaving in ways that seem disloyal, put the family at risk, or distress the adults who love them.

Family members may feel uncomfortable with the teenager's changing role in the family. Sometimes parents may try to enforce rules that limit the teens' contact with friends or may become so tired of conflict that they simply give up their role as parents. This can have the unfortunate effect of removing the safety net that families provide for growing teens. While teens are separating from the family, they still need all of the support a family provides.

Finding a balance between the desire for individuality and responsibility to family is one of the greatest challenges of adolescence. Good communication between all members of the family helps everyone adjust to change. If good communication among family members breaks down, it is helpful for teens to find an adult outside the family who can offer a less emotionally involved perspective on family situations. Teens may pass through a stage where they are in conflict with the adults in their families, only to redevelop strong family ties as they grow older and begin families of their own.

Families and the Law

The body of law that deals with marriage, divorce, cohabitation (living together), child custody, the rights of biological and adoptive parents, and juvenile justice is called family law. Legal conflicts can arise when people live in nontraditional groups that are not recognized in law.

Child welfare, inheritance laws, and medical rights are based mainly on the concept of a nuclear family. This can lead to situations where a grandmother who is raising her grandchild may not be able to authorize medical treatment, enroll her grandchild in school, or take the child to another state or country unless she goes to court and becomes recognized as the legal guardian of the child. In other cases, unmarried adults living together as a couple may be unable to receive health insurance coverage available to married partners.

When parents are married and then divorce, both parents are still part of their child's family, but the mother and father do not consider themselves to be part of each other's family anymore. In disputes arising between divorcing parents, the court often is asked to decide who is to be the main caregiver and to determine the rights and responsibilities of each parent. Starting in the 1990s the courts increasingly were asked to address the rights and responsibilities of everyone involved when biological and adoptive parents were in conflict. Courts also began hearing cases involving the rights of homosexual partners who were raising children together.

Generally, the court is charged with making decisions that are in the best interest of a child, but the interpretation of what is in a child's best interest can vary from judge to judge and court to court. Older children may be asked to give their opinion about issues such as custody or visitation, but judges are not required to consider a child's preferences. Young children are rarely consulted in these situations. Often, changes in family law lag behind changes in family structure. More and more families consist of nontraditional groupings of adults and children. Family law is constantly evolving to address the legal challenges that arise from the changing concept of family.

Resources

Books

Jacobs, Thomas A. *What Are My Rights? 95 Questions and Answers About Teens and the Law.* Minneapolis: Free Spirit Publishing, 1997. Written by a lawyer for readers 12 and up, this guide helps teens understand family laws that may affect them.

Packer, Alex J. *Bringing Up Parents: The Teenager's Handbook.* Minneapolis: Free Spirit Publishing, 1993. Written for teens 13 and up, this guide gives advice on how to build trust, take responsibility, earn freedom in their family, and handle common sources of family conflict such as messy rooms and curfews.

Organization

Stepfamily Foundation, Inc., 333 West End Avenue, New York, NY 10023. Provides telephone and in-person counseling from divorce through stepfamily formation.
Telephone 212-877-3244
http://www.stepfamily.org

▶ *See also*
Divorce
Emotions
Homelessness
Love and Intimacy

Family Violence *See* **Abuse**

Fears

Fear is a normal emotion, experienced when a person senses danger. Fear includes physical, mental, and behavioral (bee-HAY-vyor-al) reactions. Certain childhood fears are common and normal.

What Is Fear?

Fear is the emotion that people feel when they sense that they are in danger. It is a protective emotion, which signals danger and helps a person to prepare for and cope with it. Fear includes physical, mental, and behavioral reactions.

KEYWORDS
for searching the Internet and other reference sources

Anxiety disorders

Panic

Phobia

* **nervous system** is a network of specialized tissues made of nerve cells, or neurons, that processes messages to and from different parts of the human body.

* **epinephrine** (e-pe-NE-frin) is a hormone, a chemical that has regulatory effects on different parts of the body. It is produced by the adrenals (a-DREE-nals), a pair of glands found at the top of the kidneys.

The physical reaction to fear is called the "fight or flight" response. "Fight or flight" is an involuntary response, a response that a person cannot control consciously but that is controlled by the body's nervous system*. It is the body's way of preparing to run from danger or to fight. The heart beats faster, and the blood pressure and breathing rate increase. Oxygen-rich blood rushes to the large muscles of the body, which are tensing to prepare to fight. The pupils of the eyes grow larger to help the eyes scan for danger. Epinephrine*, also called adrenaline (a-DREN-al-in), is released to prepare the body for quick action. Sweat is produced to cool the body.

Mentally, fear triggers thoughts about the danger or threat that the person senses. Thoughts may mentally size up the danger, anticipate what might happen, or imagine ways to avoid harm. Behaviorally, the person may startle or jump and then run, freeze, or get ready to fight.

Different Kinds of Fear

Fear, anxiety, and phobia Fear and anxiety (ang-ZY-e-tee) are similar emotions but with an important difference. Fear is the emotion that people feel when a danger is actually present, while anxiety is the fear connected with worrying about danger that might happen. A phobia (FO-bee-a) is an intense fear of specific things, like dogs or spiders or riding in elevators. With a phobia, the fear a person feels is out of proportion to the real danger. The person with a phobia is very worried about the possibility of seeing the feared object or experiencing the feared situation. People with phobias may go to great lengths to avoid any situation that might bring them face to face with the object of their fear. Because of all the worry and avoidance, a phobia can interfere with a person's everyday life.

Childhood fears Certain fears are very common and normal during childhood. In fact, all children have fears at times during their lives. Because so much of the world is new to children, they may fear certain things until they understand them better or are better able to cope. Fear serves a protective purpose, keeping children appropriately cautious while they learn about what is safe and what is dangerous.

Fears of animals, loud noises, or being in water are common in very young children, who are still learning to understand the information their senses are gathering. Babies as young as 8 months old may fear strangers, and this is a sign that the baby is able to recognize his parents and to tell them apart from strangers.

Young children often fear imaginary creatures like monsters, ghosts, and witches. Because imagination is developing at a rapid pace but the young child has not yet developed the ability to tell the difference between what is real and what is make-believe, these imaginary things can seem dangerous. Children tend to outgrow fears of imaginary crea-

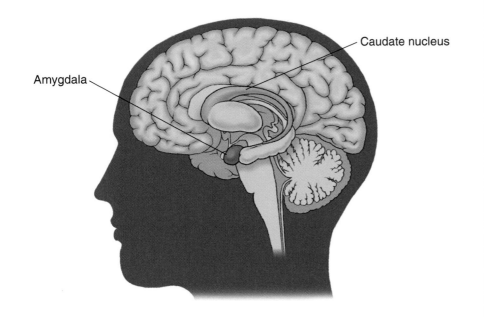

Amygdala

Caudate nucleus

This is a cross-section of a brain showing the amygdala and caudate nucleus—the structures believed to be linked to negative emotions like fear and anger. The amygdala is believed to be fully developed by the time a baby is born. The prefrontal cortex (the front of the brain) where thinking and planning take place, takes longer to mature. This may explain why it takes time for children to learn how to control their fears.

◀

tures as soon as they are able to understand the difference between real and pretend.

Older children are more likely to fear real-life things. Examples might be fear of burglars, fear of getting hurt or lost, or fear of natural disasters like earthquakes or extreme weather like hurricanes. These children may need reassurance and support from parents while they learn to cope with worry and fear and gain confidence in dealing with life's challenges.

Learned fears Fearful parents tend to have fearful children. Without realizing it, parents may teach children to be too fearful or cautious of certain things, not so much by what they say but by how they act. If someone's mother always crosses the street to avoid dogs and gets a little pale when a dog is nearby, chances are the child will learn to be afraid of dogs. Research has found that fears or worries can run in families. It may be that certain fear reactions are inherited, but we do not have to live with them just because they may be inherited.

Fears also can be "unlearned." If the fearful child watches another child calmly approach and pet a dog, she is learning that petting a dog can be safe and pleasant. By watching and then learning to go toward the dog slowly herself, with the right adult support, she can learn to overcome her fear of dogs. When leaving the home, perhaps even to go to school, is too scary or when important activities are avoided because of fearfulness, professional help may be needed to help "unlearn" fears.

What Is So Scary to Children?

Most school-age children report that they have between five and seven fears at any one time. Here are some of the most common childhood fears and the age they usually occur:

- **infants (up to 2 years old):** fear of falling, loud noises, strangers
- **toddlers (2-3 years old):** fear of loud noises, flushing the toilet, dogs and other animals
- **preschoolers (3-5 years old):** fear of monsters, imaginary creatures, getting lost, the dark, insects, thunder and lightning, injury, shots
- **early-school-age children (6-10 years old):** fear of burglars, divorce, tornadoes, hurricanes, injury, being bullied, losing a parent.

175

See also
Anxiety and Anxiety Disorders
Obsessive-Compulsive Disorder
Phobias
Panic
Stress

Fear + Distress or Fear + Excitement?

The feelings and sensations people get when they are afraid or anxious are similar to the excited thrill people feel when they go on a scary ride at an amusement park or see a scary movie. Some people actually like the feeling, while others do not. Research psychologists (sy-KOL-o-jists) have described anxiety as a complex emotion that is made up of fear plus one or more other emotions, such as distress, anger, excitement, shyness, or guilt. Anxiety that is made up of fear plus excitement will be experienced differently from anxiety that is made up of fear plus distress, for example.

▶ *See also*
Anxiety and Anxiety Disorders

Obsessive-Compulsive Disorder

Phobias

Panic

Stress

KEYWORDS
for searching the Internet and other reference sources

Alcohol-related developmental disabilities

Alcohol-related neurodevelopmental disabilities

Are All Fears Outgrown?

Most childhood fears pass with time, learning, and support from caring adults. Childhood fears do not get better by teasing, threatening, or forcing the child to meet the feared object or situation. Such remedies are likely to produce shame and lower self-esteem, and they may even worsen fear. The protective emotion of fear is not outgrown. People feel fear throughout life whenever they sense danger.

When to Get Help for Fears

Sometimes a normal childhood fear can become intense or last well beyond the age when a child usually outgrows it. If this happens, or if fears cause so much distress that they interfere with everyday life, professional help may be needed to help children get over their fears.

Cognitive-behavioral therapy is often helpful. It may involve teaching coping skills, supporting the child's gradual approach to the feared situation, and coaching parents to provide needed reinforcement and support.

Resources

Organizations

Anxiety Disorders Association of America, 11900 Parklawn Drive, Suite 100, Rockville, MD 20852.
http://www.adaa.org

Nemours Center for Children's Health Media, Alfred I. duPont Hospital for Children, 1600 Rockland Road, Wilmington, DE 19803. This organization's KidsHealth website has articles about fear.
http://www.KidsHealth.org

Fetal Alcohol Syndrome

Fetal alcohol syndrome is a group of physical and mental birth defects that can affect the children of mothers who drink alcoholic beverages during pregnancy.

The Leading Known Cause of Mental Retardation

In the United States, the law requires that every bottle or can of beer, wine, or hard liquor that is sold must include the following information on its label: "(1) According to the Surgeon General, women should not drink alcoholic beverages during pregnancy because of the risk of birth defects; (2) Consumption of alcoholic beverages impairs your ability to drive a car or operate machinery and may cause health problems." The first warning refers to the risk of fetal alcohol syndrome (FAS), the leading known cause of mental retardation in the United States. The good news is that this condition is 100 percent preventable as long as a woman does not drink alcohol while she is pregnant.

What Are FAS and FAE?

FAS is a group of physical and mental birth defects that can affect the children of mothers who drink alcohol during pregnancy. Typically, the worst cases are seen in the offspring of mothers who drank heavily. In general, the more the mother drank, the more severe the baby's physical and mental problems are likely to be. The term fetal alcohol effects (FAE) often is used to refer to a less severe form of the syndrome. Since there is no proof that even small amounts of alcohol are safe for unborn children, doctors recommend that women completely avoid alcohol while they are pregnant. Both FAS and FAE have serious long-term consequences for affected children and their families.

According to the American Academy of Pediatrics, there may be as many as 10,000 to 12,000 new cases of FAS each year. In addition, there are probably many more cases of FAE. The exact number is not known, however. Since FAE does not cause the obvious physical defects seen in FAS, it can be difficult to diagnose correctly. To confuse matters further, mothers who drank during pregnancy may hide this fact from their doctors or lie about how much they drank. Experts believe that many children who now are thought to have learning disabilities may actually have undiagnosed FAE.

What Are the Symptoms of FAS and FAE?

Just as alcohol affects the brain of an adult who drinks, it also affects the brain of a developing fetus (FEE-tus), or unborn baby, who is exposed to it before birth. The most serious consequence of a mother's alcohol use during pregnancy is impaired brain development in the fetus, leading to mental retardation. Newborns with FAS often have small brains, indicating poor brain growth while they were inside their mothers, and they typically are small for their age. Other physical defects associated with FAS are narrow eyelids, a flattened midportion of the face, abnormal creases on the palms of the hands, heart defects, hearing and vision problems, and joint abnormalities. These problems are permanent.

Children with FAE may not have these physical defects. However, children with either FAS or FAE are likely to have behavioral and emotional problems. FAS and FAE can cause learning difficulties and slow down a child's development of speech, motor skills, and coordination. Children with these conditions often are impulsive, inattentive, and

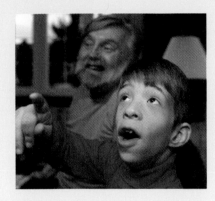

▲

Children with FAS may have attention disorders, mental retardation, and skeletal problems. Many also have distinctive facial characteristics, such as widely spaced eyes, a shortened or flattened nose, and abnormalities in the shape and placement of the ears. *David H. Wells/Corbis*

disorganized. They may have little understanding of the consequences of their behavior. They also may have trouble with following directions, solving problems, listening to people in authority, and socializing with peers. Sometimes these symptoms do not become evident until a child is 3 or 4 years old.

Living With FAS and FAE

Life for children and young people FAS or FAE is often very difficult. Parents, caregivers, teachers, and other adults in authority need to be consistent and firm, setting predictable routines for the young person to follow. Adults may find that they have to repeat instructions again and again, making sure the child knows what is expected. Clear consequences for inappropriate behavior and rewards for appropriate behavior can be used to help the child make better choices. These children also tend to learn best when tasks are broken down into small pieces and new concepts are taught through concrete examples. In addition, medication may be part of the treatment plan.

Many children with FAS or FAE attend special education classes, just like other students who have learning disabilities or mental retardation. This gives them a chance to work with a specially trained teacher that would not be possible in the regular classroom.

Resources

Books

Dorris, Michael. *The Broken Cord.* New York: HarperCollins, 1990. At age 26, writer Michael Dorris adopted a young Native American child with FAS. This book provides compelling insight into what it is like to live with the condition.

Kleinfeld, Judith, and Siobhan Wescott. *Fantastic Antone Succeeds! Experiences in Educating Children with Fetal Alcohol Syndrome.* Fairbanks, AK: University of Alaska Press, 1993. This book features personal stories from children and families affected by FAS and FAE, as well as practical advice for parents and teachers who work with these young people. A sequel, *Fantastic Antone Grows Up: Adolescents and Adults with Fetal Alcohol Syndrome*, was published in 2000.

Organizations

National Organization on Fetal Alcohol Syndrome, 216 G Street Northeast, Washington, DC 20002. This national nonprofit group aims to raise public awareness of FAS.
Telephone 800-666-6327
http://www.nofas.org

U.S. National Center on Birth Defects and Developmental Disabilities, Fetal Alcohol Syndrome section. This section of the U.S. Centers for Disease Control and Prevention website provides the latest information and statistics on FAS.
http://www.cdc.gov/ncbddd/fas

Fugue

Fugue (FYOOG) refers to a psychiatric condition in which people wander or travel and may appear to be functioning normally, but they are unable to remember their identity or details about their past.

Sigmund Freud, one of the fathers of modern psychiatry, believed that the mind has defense mechanisms, or built-in ways of experiencing reality, that prevent it from being overwhelmed by worry or depression*. In fact, Freud believed that people are not even aware of the way their minds take care of them. Dissociation (di-so-see-AY-shun) is a defense mechanism that allows people to separate or "go away from" thoughts, memories, emotions, or events that are highly stressful. This separation helps people successfully cope with situations that would otherwise be intolerable. With dissociation, people can "daydream" themselves away from their troubles or even develop a separate personality to cope with terrible life events.

Fugue, sometimes called dissociative (dis-SO-see-a-tiv) or psychogenic (sy-ko-JEN-ic) fugue, is an uncommon dissociative disorder. Fugue is thought to be caused by the inability to cope with a severe long-lasting stress or conflict. People with dissociative fugue not only mentally "go away from" an intolerable situation through a dissociation defense mechanism, they actually remove themselves physically from the situation by wandering away from home and either partially or completely assuming a new identity. To be diagnosed with fugue, the wandering and memory changes must not be caused by substance abuse, medications, or other psychiatric disorders such as dissociative identity disorder*.

How Do People with Fugue Function?

People diagnosed with fugue unexpectedly travel or wander away from home, work, or familiar places. They may take on new identities, enter new occupations, or develop new interests and hobbies. The degree of fugue can vary from mild to severe and may last anywhere from several hours to years. One study suggests that about half of all fugues last less than 24 hours.

► *See also*
Attention Deficit Hyperactivity Disorder
Mental Retardation

KEYWORDS
for searching the Internet and other reference sources

Dissociative fugue

Psychogenic fugue

* **depression** (de-PRESH-un) is a mental state characterized by feelings of sadness, despair, and discouragement.

* **dissociative identity disorder (DID)**, formerly known as multiple personality disorder (MPD), is a severe psychiatric condition in which a person has two or more distinct sub-personalities that periodically take control of his or her behavior. The sub-personalities are thought to be caused by repeated episodes of an extreme form of dissociation.

* **schizophrenia** (skitz-o-FREE-nee-ah) is a serious mental disorder that causes people to experience hallucinations, delusions, and other confusing thoughts and behaviors, which distort their view of reality.

* **Alzheimer disease** (ALZ-hy-mer) is a condition that leads to a gradually worsening loss of mental abilities, including memory, judgment, and abstract thinking, as well as changes in personality.

* **temporal lobe epilepsy** (EP-i-lep-see), also called complex partial epilepsy, is a form of epilepsy that affects the part of the brain that is located underneath the sides of the head, near the ears. Epilepsy is a condition of the nervous system characterized by recurrent seizures that temporarily affect a person's awareness, movements, or sensations. Seizures occur when powerful, rapid bursts of electrical energy interrupt the normal electrical patterns of the brain.

* **psychotherapy** (sy-ko-THER-a-pea) is the treatment of mental and behavioral disorders by support and insight to encourage healthy behavior patterns and personality growth.

▶ *See also*

Alzheimer Disease

Amnesia

Dissociative Identity Disorder

Schizophrenia

People diagnosed with fugue are often able to perform complex activities and appear to be normal. People with fugue appear to be oriented and to have intact mental functions. However, when questioned, people with fugue are confused about their identity and their past. Some people experience fugue along with other psychiatric disorders such as schizophrenia*, which makes the diagnosis of fugue more difficult.

Do Other Conditions Resemble Fugue?

People with Alzheimer disease* also may wander away from home and lose touch with who they are. This condition, which is believed to be caused by a physical breakdown in the functioning of the brain, is different from dissociative fugue.

Some people who have temporal lobe epilepsy* may have periods of undirected wandering. Neurologists (doctors who study the brain and nervous system) can generally distinguish symptoms that are caused by damage to the brain from those caused by psychological trauma. Drug abuse can also cause fugue-like periods, but these are not considered true dissociative fugue.

Some psychiatrists believe that fugue is a symptom of other psychiatric disorders, rather than a unique, separate disorder. Treatment, as for other dissociative disorders, generally involves psychotherapy* and the treatment of any other psychiatric disorders the person might have.

G

Gender Identity

Gender is the category to which a person is assigned on the basis of sex. Gender is a term used in discussing the different roles, identities, and expectations that our society associates with males and females. Gender identity refers to a person's own sense of being male or female.

KEYWORDS
for searching the Internet and other reference sources

Gender roles

Sexism

There are psychological, cultural, and social characteristics associated with a person's gender identity. The terms feminine or masculine often are used to describe behaviors generally associated with females or males. For example, contact sports have long been considered primarily masculine activities, and taking care of babies has been thought of as a feminine activity. Gender is different from sex. Sex specifically refers to the biological (physical) differences between females and males.

What Do We Know About Ourselves?

In the broadest sense, gender identity refers to each person's own sense of being male or female. We form our gender identities quite naturally. Almost always our gender identities match up to the sexual body parts we have. Most people develop a sense that they are male or female within the first few years of life, and it is generally believed that the majority of children have acquired this sense by the age of 3. It just seems like something that we know automatically! Some people, however, experience confusion over their gender identities. This confusion sometimes leads to a condition known as gender identity disorder. Gender or sex role identity refers to the various attitudes and behaviors that are considered normal and appropriate for people of a particular sex. These attitudes and behaviors vary between cultures and societies and involve a set of expectations about how females and males should think, act, and feel.

What Roles Do Biology and Environment Play in Gender Identity?

Both biological and environmental factors influence the behavior of all individuals as male or female. The most basic biological influence is chromosome* pair 23, the sex chromosomes that mark females and males. These chromosomes influence the development of male or female sex organs in the fetus.

* **chromosome** (KRO-mo-zom) is a threadlike structure inside cells on which the genes are located. Human beings have 46 chromosomes (23 pairs). The X and Y chromosomes determine whether a person is male or female. If you have two X chromosomes, you are female; if you have one X and one Y chromosome, you are male.

The locker room can become a place of fear, shame, and alienation during adolescent years, when teens may be insecure about their bodies and compare themselves to others. Boys may feel pressure to be good at sports and other activities traditionally seen as "masculine." *Photex/Corbis* ▶

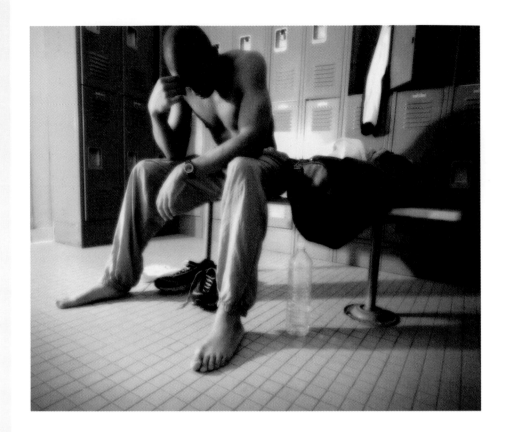

The environmental influences include cultural expectations of males and females. In many countries this begins as early as the child's birth, when boys are clothed in blue and girls in pink. This is followed by differences in hairstyles, clothes, and toys for most children.

Gender identification   One of the strongest influences on the development of gender identity occurs when the child identifies with the same-sex parent. Boys and girls also learn gender roles through imitating the behavior of other adults and watching what adults say and do. Parents, other family members, peers, people at school and in the media, and people from just about every aspect of life with which a child comes into contact exert cultural influences on gender identity.

Media   Considerable attention has been paid to how masculine and feminine roles are portrayed on television, radio, and in the movies. Television and films often show the traditional gender roles for males and females. This reinforces these traditional roles in the viewer's mind. Even language has a gender bias. In English, much of the language children hear is sexist*. Words such as mankind or chairman have been commonly used to refer to everyone, but this is changing. More and more we are seeing the words humankind and chairperson instead.

* **sexist** means promoting stereotypes of social roles based on a person's sex.

Cognition   One's own thought processes or cognitive (intellectual) abilities also contribute to gender identity. As children begin to think about themselves as male or female, the world becomes organized on the basis of gender. For example, most boys know they are boys and want to do things that are associated with boys. This understanding of gender influences each person to behave as a girl or boy as defined by the culture in which he or she lives. As people develop, they adopt a personal version of what is acceptable masculine or feminine behavior.

Nonconformity   Sometimes people do not conform to traditional gender roles. Females may be interested in contact sports, or pursuing a career instead of raising a family. These choices may not conform to the generally accepted notion of being female. Girls interested in more physical activities, like sports, are often called "tomboys." Boys who are interested in such activities as ballet, cooking, or becoming nurses may be called "sissies." These people may have different interests from the norm, whether they think of themselves as male or female. Nonconformity to traditional gender roles does not mean that a person has gender identity disorder.

Changing gender roles   Gender roles are changing in American society as men and women broaden their interests and activities. Today males and females find themselves in many roles that a few decades

BILLY ELLIOT

The movie *Billy Elliot* tells the story of an 11-year-old boy living in the north of England who becomes a dancer. Every week Billy takes boxing lessons at the village hall. Proud of his fancy footwork in the ring, Billy one day happens upon a ballet class being held at the hall. He begins to attend the class on the sly and shows amazing skill, but he must keep his dancing secret. His widowed father and brother work as coal miners, but they are out on strike and are barely able to keep food on the table. When his father finally discovers that Billy has been squandering his boxing money on "unmanly" ballet lessons, he forces Billy to give them up. Later, he chances to see Billy dancing and decides to risk everything to send the boy to London, where Billy can pursue his dream. Billy auditions for the Royal Ballet School. His talent wins him a spot at the school, and he goes on to perform on the London stage.

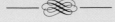

ago would have been the domain of the other sex. Men are staying at home to raise children, and women are captains of the space shuttle. Although gender roles are important because there are differences between men and women, gender roles should not be used to exclude people from following their interests, developing their talents, or using their natural abilities.

Resources

Books

Schwager, Tina, and Michele Schuerger. *Gutsy Girls: Young Women Who Dare.* Minneapolis: Free Spirit Publishing, 1999. True stories of young women who participate in challenging sports and adventure. Inspires girls and boys to achieve their personal best.

Karnes, Frances A., and Suzanne M. Bean. *Girls and Young Women Entrepreneurs: True Stories About Starting and Running a Business Plus How You Can Do It Yourself.* Minneapolis: Free Spirit Publishing, 1997. A resource book for young people who want to start up a business, including first-person advice, step-by-step instructions, and groups for young entrepreneurs to contact.

Karnes, Frances A., and Suzanne M. Bean. *Girls and Young Women Leading the Way.* Minneapolis: Free Spirit Publishing, 1993. First-person stories by girls and young women telling how they became leaders each in her own way.

► See also
Gender Identity Disorder
Sexual Development

KEYWORDS
*for searching the Internet
and other reference sources*

Cross-gender

Transgender

Transsexual

Gender Identity Disorder

Gender identity disorder (GID) is identified by strong and long-lasting gender identification that is opposite to one's biological sex. A person with this condition insists that he or she is of the other sex or desires to be the opposite sex. People with this condition are often referred to as transsexuals.

What Is Gender Identity Disorder?

To understand this disorder, a few terms must be defined:

- **Gender:** is the category (male or female) a person is assigned to on the basis of sex. The term is used in discussing the different roles, identities, and expectations that our society associates with males and females.

- **Gender identity:** This term refers to a person's own perception of their maleness or femaleness.
- **Feminine and masculine:** These terms often are used to describe behaviors generally associated with females or males. For example, contact sports have long been considered primarily masculine activities, and taking care of babies has been considered a feminine activity.
- **Sex:** This term usually refers to the biological (physical) differences between females and males. Specifically, these characteristics are the sex chromosomes* and certain anatomical features, for example, the penis or the vulva*.

Some people identify with, or conform to, traditional roles and expectations the culture sets for males and females. Others do not. For example, someone who is biologically female may like to play football, and someone who is biologically male may like to ballet dance. Still, under most circumstances, this does not interfere with people's sense that that they are female or male, and does not mean that they have gender identity disorder.

What Is Cross-Gender Identification?

GID goes beyond a failure or reluctance to identify with traditional roles or expectations about being female or male. A person with GID who is biologically female has the sense of being male. Likewise, a person with GID who is biologically male has a strong inner sense of being a female. When cross-gender identification causes much distress or impairs a person's functioning in life, that person is said to have GID.

Distress   GID distress may result in a person's refusal to attend school or social events where feminine or masculine clothing or behavior is expected, because they fear teasing or rejection by their peers. This may result in isolation from other children because of the person's insistence on behaving and acting like a member of the opposite sex. Children with this disorder often express wishes to be the other sex or beliefs that they will "grow up to be" the opposite sex. Young children with this condition may be unhappy about their assigned sex. Older children may fail to develop age-appropriate same-sex relationships with their peers. For adolescents, GID can be very difficult, because the person may struggle with feelings of uncertainty about the cross-gender identification or be concerned about being unacceptable to his or her own family or peers.

Intersex conditions   GID is not the same as physical intersex conditions. Intersex conditions may be marked, for example, by genitals* that are not completely male or female. Or the person with this condition may be genetically* male but physically female (or the reverse). For

* **chromosomes** (KRO-mo-some) are threadlike chemical structures inside cells on which the genes are located. There are 46 chromosomes (23 pairs) in normal human cells. Genes on the X and Y chromosomes (known as the sex chromosomes) determine whether a person is male or female. Females have two X chromosomes; males have one X and one Y chromosome.

* **vulva** is the name for the external sex organs of the female.

Stigma

Boys with GID seem to suffer more than girls, probably because of culturally influenced rejection by their peers. In some studies, five times as many boys as girls saw a doctor for GID. Among adults, two or three times as many men as women sought help for GID. This difference probably is due to the greater social difficulties experienced by males who show cross-gender behavior.

* **genitals** (JE-ni-tals) are all the organs of the human reproductive system.

* **genetically** (je-NE-ti-klee) means due to heredity and stemming from genes, the material on the chromosome in cells of the human body that helps determine physical and mental characteristics, such as hair and eye color. The X and Y chromosomes contain gonetic information that determines sex.

example, a male with an intersex condition would have the XY sex chromosomes of males, even though his genitals might appear female. GID should not be confused with nonconformity to traditional or typical gender roles, as may be seen in the case of "tomboyism" or "stay-at-home dads." People who do not conform with all aspects of traditional gender roles seldom have any desire to be the opposite sex.

Cross-dressing There also is a difference between GID and transvestitism. A person who is a transvestite becomes sexually excited by dressing in the clothes of the opposite sex, that is, cross-dressing. This behavior, engaged in for the sole purpose of sexual excitement, most often occurs among heterosexual* or bisexual* men. Transsexuals (people with GID) cross-dress to gain a sense of physical and emotional completeness rather than sexual excitement.

Sexual Reassignment

The causes of GID are uncertain. Some researchers think that biological factors play a role, and others think that environmental factors, such as social learning, are involved. No one can really say why GID occurs. The more important question may be how to resolve the problems that GID may create.

The distress GID causes is real, and, for some adults with this condition, the only effective relief for this distress is a sex-reassignment procedure, which usually involves sex-change operations. These procedures are the subject of a great deal of controversy, and the scientific community continues to debate the possible benefits of sex-change surgery. These procedures can take several years to complete.

Screening These sex-change procedures begin with lengthy and detailed screening interviews. These interviews determine the existence and severity of GID. The person then is instructed about adopting a lifestyle that agrees with his or her gender identity. If people successfully adjust to this lifestyle change over a period of several months to a year, they begin hormone therapy to develop more of the physical traits of the desired sex. This step also can last one year or longer.

Surgery and other treatment If the person continues to adjust successfully to these activities, the final stage is hormone* therapy and sex-change surgery. For males wishing to become females, hormone treatments may produce enough breast development, although some people choose later to have breast enlargement surgeries. In male to female reassignment, body and facial hair growth is reduced by the hormone treatments and hair may also be removed by electrolysis*. People who undergo sex-change surgery to become females are able to have sexual intercourse.

* **heterosexual** (he-te-ro-SEK-shoo-al) refers to a tendency to be sexually attracted to the opposite sex.

* **bisexual** (bi-SEK-shoo-al) means being sexually attracted to both sexes.

* **hormones** are chemicals that are produced by different glands in the body. A hormone is like the body's ambassador. It is created in one place but is sent through the body to have specific effects in different places.

* **electrolysis** (ee-lek-TRAW-li-sis) is a method of destroying hair roots by passing an electric current through them.

Females wishing to become males have surgeries to remove the breasts, the uterus*, and the ovaries* and to seal off the vagina*. The operation to construct a penis is extremely complicated, and the resulting penis is not capable of a natural erection. There are, however, artificial devices available that can help the person successfully engage in sexual intercourse.

Follow-up There have been several worldwide studies conducted to assess the outcomes of sex-change surgery. These studies have shown that 9 of 10 transsexuals who undergo hormonal and surgical sex-reassignment procedures experience a satisfactory result. One of the studies found that 94 percent of the people who underwent the surgery and answered questionnaires stated that if they had it to do over again, they would make the same choice.

Resource

Book

Boenke, Mary. *Trans Forming Families: Real Stories About Transgendered Loved Ones.* Imperial Beach, CA: Walter Trook Publishing, 1999. Includes 31 stories of parents of gender variant children. For older readers.

* **uterus** (YOO-te-rus) is the organ in females for containing and nourishing the fetus during pregnancy. It is also called the womb.

* **ovaries** (O-va-reez) are the sexual glands in females from which eggs are released.

* **vagina** (va-JY-na) is the canal in females that leads from the uterus to the outside of the body.

▶ *See also*
Body Image
Gender Identity
Sexual Development

Genetics and Behavior

Genetics (je-NE-tiks) is the study of how traits are passed from parents to children. Behavior is a person's observable activity. The study of how genetics affects behavior is called behavioral genetics.

Jennifer's Story

At 13 years old, Jennifer is fit and trim. Her mother, however, has been told by her doctor that she is morbidly obese* and must keep to a strict diet and exercise plan to control her weight. Jennifer notices that her aunt and her grandmother are also severely overweight. Jennifer is not sure if her family members are overweight because they do not exercise much and like to eat fatty foods or if there is a problem with the way that their bodies process food.

In school Jennifer has learned that children inherit many traits from their parents. She wonders if she is destined to have a weight problem later in life, since so many of the women in her family do. She decides to ask her doctor if there are diet and exercise programs she can start now to help her avoid having her mother's problem when she gets older.

KEYWORDS
for searching the Internet and other reference sources

Genetic disorder

Human genome

* **morbidly obese** means weighing two or more times a person's ideal body weight.

*__antisocial__ means behaving in ways that purposefully disregard the rights of others and break society's rules or laws.

What Is Behavioral Genetics?

Genetics is the study of how traits are passed from parent to child. The information that children get from their parents is contained in chemical packets of information called genes. These genes make up larger units called chromosomes (KRO-mo-somz). Humans have 46 chromosomes; 23 come from the father, and the other 23 come from the mother. The human genome is the term for all the genetic information contained in humans.

Variations in human behavior are seen every day. Often people are kind and thoughtful. Sometimes people behave in ways that are considered antisocial* or hurtful to themselves. Behavioral genetics is a branch of science that tries to find out what role inherited factors play in how people act and what kinds of genes may lead to different patterns of behavior.

Environmental factors also can influence human behavior. Behavioral geneticists work to discover how much of people's behavior is determined by the genetic information they inherited from their parents and how much is caused by their living conditions, learning choices, and other influences from the world around them.

What Is the Nature Versus Nurture Conflict?

People have long wondered what makes humans act as they do and what produces the differences in human behavior that can be seen every day. Scientists have been especially interested in finding out what causes types of behavior that are considered antisocial or abnormal. For a long time there were two schools of thought. Some scientists believed that everyone is destined to act the way they do because of the genes they inherit from their parents. These scientists believed for the most part that the environment that a person grows up in has little or nothing to do with the way that a person behaves. This idea is called the "nature school of thought," because it was believed that nature has given each person certain genes whose traits cannot be escaped.

Scientists of the "nurture school of thought" believed that humans are not inclined from birth to any certain forms of behavior. They believed that the genes children get from their parents do not matter. The environment that a child grows up in was considered the most important influence on that child's behavior.

Today, however, most scientists agree that both genes and environmental factors are important in forming behavior. There is still debate as to how much nature (genes) and how much nurture (environment) affect behavior. It is generally accepted that for each trait, nature and nurture work together in different proportions. For example, scientists estimate that in deciding how tall a person will be, inherited genes have nine times more influence than the environment a person grows up in (which may influence such factors as a person's nutrition). However, researchers have estimated that in determining whether or not a person will become depressed, genes and the environment are about equally important.

Why Is Behavioral Genetics So Hard to Study?

To study how likely it is that a certain kind of behavior runs in a family, we must be able to separate the genetic factors leading to the behavior from the environmental ones. This is often very difficult. Many times studies on genetics focus on identical twins that are raised in separate homes or on babies of parents with a certain disorder who are adopted into families who do not have the disorder. It is difficult to find cases like these to study, and even when scientists can find them, the results often do not prove anything. Frequently there are many different genetic and environmental factors that could contribute to the disorder, so pinpointing the factors with the most influence can be difficult or impossible.

Some scientists have begun trying to link certain antisocial types of behavior to specific genes. This is also very difficult, but for different reasons. It is estimated that there are more than 50,000 gene pairs in the human genome. Very few have been linked specifically to any particular trait. It is especially hard to link genes to most types of behavior, because most are complex and are determined by more than one gene.

What Are Some Behavioral Disorders That Genes Influence?

Schizophrenia   One of the most serious disorders that causes altered behavior that is linked to a person's genes is schizophrenia (skitz-o-FREE-nee-a). Schizophrenia is a mental disorder in which people have an altered sense of reality. People with the disorder may have hallucinations*, such as hearing voices or seeing things that are not really there, or delusions*, such as believing the FBI is "after them" when they are law abiding. This often causes them to behave in abnormal or odd ways.

Many studies show that there is a strong link between heredity and schizophrenia. If one of a set of identical twins has the disorder, there is a 46 percent chance that the other twin will show symptoms of schizophrenia as well. Children who have two parents with schizophrenia have a 46 percent chance of having the disorder as well. People who come from families where no one has schizophrenia have only a very small chance (1 percent) of developing the disorder.

Genetics is not the only factor that determines whether a person will get schizophrenia. A child whose mother does not have schizophrenia but who is adopted into a family in which one of the adopted parents has the disorder has an 11 percent chance of showing schizophrenic symptoms. This means that the environment also plays a role in the development of schizophrenia.

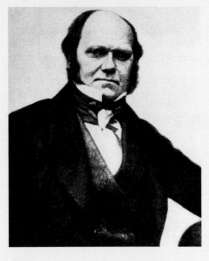

Charles Darwin (1809–1882) was a naturalist, or a scientist who believed that all events could be explained by scientific laws. He was best known for his theory on evolution, which maintained that it was genetic makeup that determined a being's success in its environment. *Bettmann/Corbis*

* **hallucination** (ha-LOO-sin-A-shun) is a sensory perception for which there is no cause in the outside world.

* **delusion** (de-LOO-zhun) is a false belief or judgment that a person continues to hold despite evidence that it is not true.

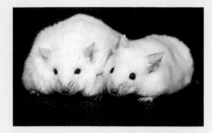

▲

Researchers breed lab mice to study how specific genes affect growth and behavior. The presence, absence, or alteration of even a single gene can make a noticeable difference. *Bettmann/Corbis*

*traumatic** means causing mental or emotional stress or physical injury.

*biochemical** means relating to the chemistry of living organisms.

Alcoholism   For many years scientists have known that people with a family history of alcoholism are more likely to become alcoholics themselves. Using twin and adoption studies, researchers have found that genes probably play a part in determining who will become an alcoholic. As with many behaviors linked to genes, environmental factors are also very important. Researchers are trying to pinpoint genes related to alcoholism, but this is difficult, since it is thought that alcoholism may be caused by many different genes.

Obesity   Obesity is the condition of having much more body fat than is appropriate for a person's age, sex, and height. The chance of becoming obese has been linked to a person's genes. Using the methods of inheritance studies, such as investigating pairs of twins, researchers have concluded that inherited genes contribute about 40 percent and the environment about 60 percent to whether a person becomes obese. Although genes are involved in this disorder, environmental factors, such as income level, social eating habits, cultural values, and exercise also play an important role.

Depression   Depression is present when a person has feelings of sadness, despair, and hopelessness over a long period of time. It is a common condition, and it can be treated. Depression is another disorder that has been linked to the genes that a person inherits, but it is a mental disorder that is also very closely linked to environmental factors, more so than schizophrenia.

It is thought that certain events in life may bring out depression if a person has inherited genes that make it more likely that the condition will develop. People who do not have a family history of depression also can become depressed. Some of the common environmental factors leading to depression include abuse or neglect, poverty, a traumatic* or extremely violent episode in a person's life, and death of a parent or loved one.

What Is the Human Genome Project?

The goal of the Human Genome Project is to identify the approximately 30,000 individual genes that are contained in human DNA. DNA is a double-stranded molecule that contains the genetic code necessary to build a living being. Mapping the human genome is a long and detailed process that uses many complex biochemical* techniques and an enormous amount of computer power. The project was started officially in October 1990, and in January 2000 a very rough draft of the human genome was completed.

Once the gene sequence is worked out for a particular section of chromosome, research can be done to link genes to specific traits. To do this, researchers often use chemicals to remove the gene that they are studying or to make the gene inactive, and then see what kind of changes occur in the animal they are studying.

The Human Genome Project is very important to behavioral genetics. It is hard to determine how much the genetic makeup of a person is responsible for behavioral disorders and how much the environment in which that person grows up is involved. If the genes responsible for certain forms of behavior can be found, researchers can study people who have these genes and try to learn which environmental factors cause the person to act in a particular way. Someday doctors may be able to recommend more ways for people who are genetically inclined to certain behavioral disorders to make lifestyle changes that will lessen the chance that a particular disorder will occur. Doctors may be able to use gene therapy to cure, treat, or even prevent some genetic diseases by replacing or supplementing faulty genes. They might also be able to find out at birth which people have genes that might cause them to get cancer, heart disease, Alzheimer disease, and many other conditions.

Decoding the mysteries of the human genome is a landmark discovery, for other reasons as well. The possibilities for using this information are endless. DNA evidence already has been used to convict criminals and to free innocent people from prison. DNA evidence can also shed light on history. Examining DNA from the bones of people who died near Rome in the fifth century A.D., English scientists have found signs of the disease malaria and have suggested that epidemics of malaria may have led to the fall of the Roman Empire.

There are ethical* considerations that limit how far researchers will be able to take this kind of experiment in humans. How will society use the information learned from the Human Genome Project? At the end of the twentieth century, scientists in Scotland cloned a sheep. Will (and should) scientists make exact replicas of human beings as well?

* **ethical** means having to do with questions of what is right and wrong, or with moral values.

Resources

Organizations

Oak Ridge National Laboratory, P. O. Box 2008, Oak Ridge, TN 37831. This organization sponsors a website on the Human Genome Project that describes its purpose and the progress that has been made in mapping human genes.
http://www.ornl.gov/hgmis

American Society of Human Genetics, 9650 Rockville Pike, Bethesda, MD 20814-3998. This society has a website that provides information about human genetics research. It also has information for anyone interested in pursuing a career in genetics.
Telephone 301-571-1825
http://www.faseb.org/genetics/ashg/ashgmenu.htm

▶ *See also*
Alcoholism
Antisocial Personality Disorder
Bipolar Disorder
Depression
Delusions
Obesity
Schizophrenia

Grief *See* Death and Dying; Emotions

H

Habits and Habit Disorders

A habit is a learned pattern of behavior that is repeated so often that it becomes automatic. Often there is a particular stimulus, or trigger, that activates the automatic behavioral response.

What Is a Habit?

A habit is a learned behavior that a person repeats so often that he or she begins to do it without even thinking about it. Certain habits can be helpful, like the habit of brushing your teeth before going to bed or buckling your seatbelt when you get into a car. These are habits that a person builds on purpose, to achieve a positive objective.

Other habits may seem to serve no particular purpose, like hair twirling. These habits often are built unknowingly. They can include behavior like thumb sucking, nail biting, or chewing on the end of a pencil. Such habits may begin as self-soothing forms of behavior and may help relieve stress. But often, long after the need for that type of soothing is outgrown, the learned habit continues. Some habits are annoying, and some can cause distress or become the focus of teasing. Still others may have harmful effects. For example, thumb sucking, which can go on for years, can cause dental problems.

How Can You Break a Bad Habit?

Most habits can be changed with a bit of effort. When Tenesha wanted to stop biting her nails, she first tried to notice when and where she was biting them. She thought that her habit might have started as a way to relieve the stress she felt while concentrating hard on schoolwork in class. But she had had the habit so long that she bit her nails when she was doing her homework and even when she was sitting and watching TV. Tenesha decided that whenever she noticed her hands going toward her face, she was going to remind herself to stop. Then she was going to squeeze her fingers together for a moment instead of biting her nails. Tenesha tried this every day for a few weeks. Her nails started to grow in, and she rewarded herself with colorful nail polish. Her habit pattern was broken, and her fingers no longer went automatically to her mouth while she was doing schoolwork.

KEYWORDS
for searching the Internet and other reference sources

Behavioral therapy

Habit reversal

Obsessive-compulsive disorder

Tic disorders

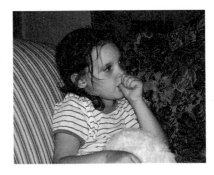

Thumb sucking is a common habit among children that comforts them when they feel tired, sick, or scared. This habit usually disappears on its own by the time the child is about 4 or 5 years old.
Visuals Unlimited

When a Habit Is Not Just a Habit

Most habits can be modified with a bit of effort if people make themselves aware of what they are doing. And the newer the habit (that is, the less practiced the habit), the easier it is to change. But some types of repetitive behavior or movements which may appear to be habits, such as an eye blink or the twitch of one side of a person's mouth, are actually involuntary (that is, they cannot be controlled). For reasons that are not yet clear, such repetitive movements, called tics, can become increasingly frequent and recur in combination with other tics. Stress and fatigue are known to play a role in making tics more frequent.

A condition called Tourette syndrome (also called Tourette disorder) causes a person to have repeated involuntary jerky movements (motor tics), make facial grimaces, and repeat certain sounds or words out loud (vocal tics). These tics can seem surprising and odd to others, who do not understand what is causing them. Another condition called trichotillomania (TRIK-o-til-o-MAY-ni-a) involves the "habit" of pulling out one's own hair, eyebrows, or eyelashes. This is more than a simple habit and stems from powerful urges, produced in the brain, to pull hair. Obsessive-compulsive disorder (OCD) causes people to become trapped in a pattern of repeated unwanted and upsetting thoughts, called obsessions (ob-SESH-unz), and a pattern of repetitive behavior or rituals, called compulsions (kom-PUL-shunz). Rituals (compulsions) are behavioral "habits" that a person with OCD feels the need to repeat over and over again to relieve stressful feelings. While the reward of "relief from anxiety" may play a part in OCD, there is growing evidence that OCD and these other habit-like conditions are the result of involuntary messages sent from nerves in a particular part of the brain. Rituals, compulsive hair pulling, tics, and other repetitive behavior can be very distressing to the person experiencing them. Fortunately, these conditions can be diagnosed and usually treated successfully by mental health professionals.

Behavior therapy techniques are particularly helpful in treating these habit-like disorders. A technique called habit reversal, in which a person learns to substitute a different behavior for the "habit" he or she is trying to control, is effective with trichotillomania. Exposure and ritual prevention is a behavior therapy technique which can effectively manage symptoms of OCD. A person places him or herself in a situation that usually triggers the ritual behaviors. With the help of a therapist, the person learns to apply new methods for coping with the stress caused by the situation, instead of using the ritual to relieve the stress. With supported practice, the stress diminishes and the rituals can be eliminated.

▶ *See also*

**Brain Chemistry
(Neurochemistry)**

**Obsessive-Compulsive
Disorder**

Therapy

Tourette Syndrome

Trichotillomania

Hallucination

A hallucination (ha-LOO-sin-A-shun) is something that a person perceives as real but that is not actually caused by an outside event. It can involve any of the senses: hearing, smell, sight, taste, or touch.

Is It All in Their Heads?

A good magician can make audience members think that they are seeing something they really are not, such as an animal disappearing into thin air or a bouquet appearing from under a handkerchief. These tricks are often referred to as optical illusions. The magician knows how to perform the illusion so that the viewer's eyes and brain are likely to misinterpret what is really happening.

Hallucinations are different from illusions. During a hallucination, the person is not reacting to something real in the outside world. The brain creates its own stimulation instead of relying on input from the five senses. In other words, the entire experience takes place right inside the brain. In her book *Mapping the Mind,* science writer Rita Carter defines hallucinations as "exceptionally intense self-generated sensory experiences."

Dreams are the most common types of hallucinations that people experience on a regular basis. While dreaming, people may think that what they are seeing and hearing is real, but actually it is all in their heads. One frequently occurring "dream hallucination" is the sensation of falling, followed immediately by a jerking reflex that wakes the person up. Hallucinations also commonly occur when a person experiences extremely high fever or when an anesthetic* starts to wear off after surgery.

How can the brain create sights, sounds, feelings, and even tastes and smells that seem so real? For a variety of reasons, the areas of the brain responsible for interpreting sensory input can become activated on their own. When a person dreams, for example, these areas of the brain are still working even though the person is asleep and not processing stimuli from the environment.

Why Does the Brain Hallucinate?

People who have undergone amputation* help researchers understand what may happen in the brain when it hallucinates. Many of these patients report that they feel like the missing body part is still there, even though they know the arm, leg, hand, or other body part is gone. For example, it is not uncommon for people who lose a leg to try to stand up and walk after their surgery. Feeling like an amputated limb is still present is called phantom limb syndrome, and there are two main theories

KEYWORDS
for searching the Internet and other reference sources

Anxiety

Delirium

Mental disorders

Multiple personality disorder

Psychotic disorders

* **anesthetic** (an-es-THET-ik) is a medicine that decreases the sensation of pain.

* **amputation** (am-pyu-TAY-shun) is the removal of a limb or other appendage of the body.

about why it happens. It may be that the nerve cells in the brain area that used to receive signals from that limb go into overdrive and stimulate themselves because that input has disappeared. Another theory is that the brain is programmed for a body where everything is intact and in the right place so that when certain signals are missing, spontaneous nerve cell activity takes over. In either case, the brain is compensating for the lack of sensory input.

That the brain may compensate for a lack of sensory input helps to explain why people who experience vision or hearing loss or who are placed in solitary confinement often experience hallucinations (they start "seeing things" or "hearing things"). Under such circumstances, the different areas of the brain that were used to receiving signals through the senses start to stimulate themselves into action. This also explains why people tend to "see" ghosts at night instead of during the day; the brain is more likely to create the vision of ghosts when other visual stimuli are absent. In other words, people's minds tend to play more tricks on them at twelve midnight than at twelve noon.

Too much stimulation can also result in hallucinations. Excessive anxiety*, intense emotions, certain drugs, and even some mental disorders can essentially flood the brain with too much sensory input. In these cases, the brain's circuits get jammed and it cannot concentrate on making sense of the person's real environment; instead, the brain starts generating its own sensations. For example, people who experience the death of a loved one often report hallucinations in which they see that person or hear his or her voice. Similarly, people who undergo the terrible trauma of abuse sometimes report later visions of their abuser. Hallucinogenic drugs* such as LSD and Ecstasy are artificial sources of overstimulation. They excite the central nervous system* so much that certain areas of the brain produce visions, sounds, and feelings that are not based in reality. Some hallucinogenic drug users continue to experience bizarre visions and sounds even long after they stop using the drug. Researchers have found that subjecting people to constant loud noise and bright lights can also produce hallucinations.

Perhaps the most disturbing hallucinations are those that can accompany psychotic disorders* such as schizophrenia*. People with schizophrenia lose touch with aspects of reality, which affects their thinking and behavior. They often report hearing voices that tell them that they are bad or that they should act in a certain way. Experts who work with these patients have found evidence that these voices actually belong to the patient; patients may be generating "speech" in one part of their brain then experiencing it as sound in another part. People with schizophrenia also tend to see disturbing visions. Medications can help with hallucinations caused by schizophrenia, and in some cases, people can be trained to recognize and even control their hallucinations. This level of improvement usually requires intensive therapy.

* **anxiety** can be experienced as a troubled feeling, a sense of dread, fear of the future, or distress over a possible threat to a person's physical or mental well-being.

* **hallucinogenic drugs** are substances that cause a person to have hallucinations.

* **central nervous system** refers to the brain and the spinal cord, which coordinate the activity of the entire nervous system.

* **psychotic** (sy-KOT-ik) **disorders** are mental disorders, such as schizophrenia, in which the sense of reality is so impaired that a person can not function normally. People with psychotic disorders may experience delusions, hallucinations, incoherent speech, and agitated behavior, but they usually are not aware of their altered mental state.

* **schizophrenia** (skit-so-FREE-nee-ah) is a serious mental disorder that causes people to experience hallucinations, delusions, and other confusing thoughts and behaviors, which distort their view of reality.

Resources

Books

Carter, Rita. *Mapping the Mind.* Berkeley: University of California Press, 2000. See especially Chapter 5, "A World of One's Own."

Siegel, Ronald K. *Fire in the Brain: Clinical Tales of Hallucination.* New York: Penguin, 1993.

Homelessness

Homelessness is the condition of having no fixed, adequate, or secure place to live. In many, though not all cases, homelessness may be a result of mental illness, abuse, or addiction. Even when there is no associated mental health problem, those who are homeless may suffer emotionally because of the lack of the most basic of human needs: safe shelter.

An Eye Opener

Jon and Ryan went for a bike ride one day and were astounded to discover a group of people living in cardboard boxes at the edge of the county park. Before this, it had never occurred to them that at the edges of their suburban community were people who lived on the streets, dependent on social service agencies, charities, friends, and their own ingenuity to find shelter.

The number of people in the United States who are homeless is difficult to estimate because the population of homeless people is constantly changing as some people find housing and others are displaced. One 1999 estimate by the U.S. National Law Center on Homelessness and Poverty indicated that about 700,000 people were homeless on any given night and that over a one year period about 2 million people had experienced a period of homelessness. A study conducted in 1996 by the U.S. Census Bureau for the Department of Housing and Urban Development (HUD) showed that about 70 percent of people who are homeless can be found in cities, about 21 percent in suburbs, and about 9 percent in rural communities.

Who Becomes Homeless?

Homelessness can be either temporary, lasting only a few days or weeks, or semi-permanent, lasting for several years. The number of people who are without shelter is affected by many social factors, including the number of jobs available, the cost of housing, the cost of basic necessities such as food, and the availability of social outreach and assistance programs.

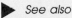

See also

Anxiety and Anxiety Disorders

Delusions

Personality Disorders

Psychosis

Schizophrenia

KEYWORDS
for searching the Internet and other reference sources

Alcoholism

Domestic violence

Drug abuse

Mental illness

Runaway teens

Homeless Teens

Young people can become homeless too. Some teenagers become homeless with their families when financial problems force them from their homes. Other young people become homeless when they run away from home because of abuse, neglect, or indifference on the part of their families.

- The median age of runaway children is between 14 and 16 years.

- About 2.8 million young people living in U.S. households report that they ran away during the previous year.

- Approximately 300,000 people younger than 18 are homeless and on their own each year.

- Young people unaccompanied by parents account for about 3 percent of the homeless in cities.

Of the homeless people in the HUD study, about 15 percent were members of a homeless family and 85 percent were single adults. However, a 1998 study by the U.S. Conference of Mayors found that families made up 38 percent of the people experiencing homelessness, which suggests that the number of families without shelter is increasing. Seventy-seven percent of single adults who were homeless were men, whereas a woman headed the majority of homeless families (84 percent).

In general, people are more likely to be homeless if they are between the ages of 25 and 54, have less than a high school education, belong to a racial minority, have a history of mental illness, and have experienced domestic violence or abuse. Other factors that increase the risk of becoming homeless include having lived in foster care or a group home as a child, childhood physical or sexual abuse, childhood experiences of homelessness, running away from home, and a history of drug or alcohol abuse.

Health Problems Associated with Homelessness

Most people who are homeless have no health insurance and little access to medical care. In the HUD study, almost half of homeless people surveyed had chronic (long-term) health problems such as diabetes*, cancer*, high blood pressure*, or arthritis* for which they were not receiving treatment. Another quarter of the homeless population had an infectious disease such as pneumonia*, tuberculosis*, or AIDS*. In addition, a very high proportion of people who are homeless have problems with drugs, alcohol, and/or mental illness. Almost none of these people receive treatment for their physical or emotional problems. Many people experiencing homelessness also become victims of crime while living on the streets.

What Help Is Available to People Who Are Homeless?

The most common programs available to help people who are homeless provide food (e.g., soup kitchens, food pantries) and emergency shelter. Although many people who are homeless are eligible for government programs such as Medicaid, food stamps, veterans' benefits, or welfare benefits, they often have difficulty claiming these benefits because they have no fixed address or lack the organizational skills necessary to follow through with these programs. Not all people experiencing homelessness are unemployed. In the HUD survey, 44 percent of those interviewed reported that they had done some paid work in the past month. Other sources of cash included gifts from friends and families, money collected panhandling, and money from illegal sources such as drug dealing and prostitution.

Reducing homelessness is the target of many social programs. Studies suggest that the most effective programs not only help people find places to live, but also help people solve the underlying problems that led to their homelessness in the first place.

*diabetes (dy-a-BEE-teez) is an impaired ability to control the levels of sugar in the blood because the body does not produce enough insulin or cannot use the insulin it makes normally.

*cancer is a condition characterized by abnormal overgrowth of certain cells, which may be fatal.

*high blood pressure, or hypertension, is a condition in which the pressure of the blood in the arteries is above normal. Arteries are the blood vessels that carry blood from the heart through the entire body.

*pneumonia (noo-MO-nyah) is an inflammation of the lungs usually caused by a bacterial or viral infection.

*AIDS is short for acquired immunodeficiency (im-yoo-no-de-FISH-un-see) syndrome, the disease caused by the human immunodeficiency virus (HIV). It is characterized by the profound weakening of the body's immune system.

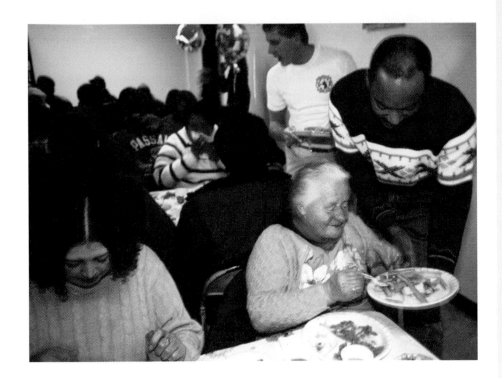

Resources

Books

Eighner, Lars. *Travels with Lizbeth: Three Years on the Road and on the Streets.* New York: St. Martin's Press, 1993. The true story of a homeless person's survival on the streets with his dog, Lizbeth.

Neufeld, John. *Almost a Hero.* New York: Simon and Schuster, 1995. A fictional story about a twelve-year-old's experience with homeless children.

Bolnick, Jamie Pastor, and Tina S. *Living at the Edge of the World: A Teenager's Survival in the Tunnels of Grand Central Station.* New York: St. Martin's Press, 2000. The true story of Tina S., a runaway who survived a year of homelessness in New York and who now helps others who are without shelter.

Organization

National Coalition for the Homeless, 1012 Fourteenth Street, NW, #600, Washington, D.C. 30005-3410. The National Coalition for the Homeless is a national advocacy network for homeless persons and providers of services to end homelessness. Among other services, the organization publishes fact sheets about homelessness and updates about legislation and government policies that affect the homeless.
Telephone 202-737-6444
http://nch.ari.net

▶ *See also*
Abuse
Addiction
Alcoholism
Substance Abuse
Violence

199

Hypnosis

Hypnosis is a passive, relaxed state during which a person's memory and perception are altered and the person is more responsive than usual to suggestion. A hypnotic state typically is caused by the monotonous repetition of words and gestures by the hypnotist.

KEYWORDS
for searching the Internet
and other reference sources

Hypnotherapy

Hypnosis as Entertainment

"Look deep into my eyes," said the hypnotist to his newest subject, 15-year-old Juan. "You are feeling very relaxed," he repeated over and over again in a low, calming voice. It was Spirit Week at Juan's high school, and this assembly was one of the highlights. Much to the delight of his classmates, Juan really did appear to be hypnotized after a couple minutes of listening to the hypnotist's voice. When the hypnotist suggested that Juan recall an event from his childhood, Juan acted as if he were blowing out the candles at his fifth birthday party and then playing with one of his gifts, a fire truck. When asked to think about his favorite kind of music, Juan acted as if he were playing the drums. And when the hypnotist suggested to Juan that he was caught in a snowstorm, he started shivering uncontrollably. Juan's friends roared with laughter as they watched him respond to the hypnotist's suggestions.

Was Juan really hypnotized? Probably not, if we define hypnosis as a state in which a person is unaware of what he or she is doing. More likely, Juan was feeling relaxed and open to suggestions from the hypnotist, and he knew that he was part of the show. So behavior that might have seemed strange in other contexts was perfectly acceptable in this setting. When his friends asked him later if he remembered what had happened, he said that he did.

Hypnosis as a Form of Therapy

Many people think that hypnotism is something done just for fun, but actually it often is used as a way of helping people deal with various behavioral and emotional problems. Experts disagree about how valuable this technique is, and no one has been able to explain exactly how it works. Nevertheless, there is evidence to suggest that hypnosis might be quite helpful in some cases for the treatment of pain, depression, anxiety, stress, sleep disturbances, eating disorders, and many other problems.

Hypnotherapists   Health care professionals who use hypnosis, sometimes called "hypnotherapists," are very different from the "stage hypnotists" who put on entertaining shows at theaters and schools. Typically hypnotherapists are licensed physicians, psychologists (sy-KOL-o-jists), or social workers who have received considerable training in the uses of hypnosis. Unlike entertainers, their goal is not to persuade a person to act strangely or be silly, but instead to produce feelings of relaxation, calmness, and well-being. Usually, they will begin the session by suggesting these states of mind and instructing the person to imagine or think about pleasant experiences. Some people are more easily hypnotized than others, but most people who experience hypnosis report changes in the way they feel, think, or behave. They may feel as if they have entered a different level of consciousness (inner awareness), or they may simply feel more focused, attentive, relaxed, and therefore better able to concentrate on their inner thoughts and feelings without being distracted.

GETTING "MESMERIZED" IN THE EIGHTEENTH AND NINETEENTH CENTURIES

Today we use the term "mesmerize" to mean "fascinate" or "amaze." For example, we might say, "The child was mesmerized by the colorful new toy," or "I am mesmerized by your smile." This modern word is derived from the name of Franz Anton Mesmer, an Austrian physician who introduced the "healing art" of mesmerism in the late 1700s. Mesmer claimed that certain people (including himself) had special powers over the "invisible fluid" he believed was contained within the human body. Mesmer thought that disease was the result of blockages in the flow of this fluid through the body and that he and other special people could use the power of their touch and their gaze to restore healthy flow of this fluid in sick people.

Mesmer used his so-called powers to produce a trancelike state in his patients, who often experienced convulsions (intense shaking) or delirium (confusion and an overly excited state) by the end of the healing session. Many people claimed to have been healed by Mesmer, but the authorities in France, where he was living at the time, soon called his practice into question. In fact, the American statesman Benjamin Franklin was a member of a committee of physicians and scientists appointed by the king of France, Louis XVI, to investigate Mesmer in the 1780s. Nevertheless, mesmerism spread to England, France, and other European countries in the 1800s and became quite popular. While Mesmer's methods may seem questionable to us today, he is credited for his role in the eventual development of hypnotism as a practice that can help some people deal with physical and psychological conditions.

► See also
Consciousness
Relaxation
Therapy

** **heart attack** is an injury to the heart muscle that occurs when blood flow is interrupted, cutting off the supply of oxygen to the heart.*

Suggestion and Choice Contrary to popular belief, people who are hypnotized do not lose control over what they are doing. While they may be more likely to respond to the therapist's suggestions, they can choose whether to follow these instructions. People remain aware of what they are doing and are likely to remember everything after the session is over. Hypnosis is *not* the same as the sleeplike trance that often is portrayed in movies and television shows, and it does not have the magical powers that sometimes are associated with it. Within limits, hypnosis can make a person much more likely to believe in or cooperate with another person (the hypnotist) and do what he or she asks. In other words, it seems that hypnosis is all about the power of suggestion.

Hypochondria

Hypochondria (hy-po-KON-dree-a) is a mental disorder in which people believe or fear that they have a serious disease even though medical examination or tests show no sign of illness.

More Than a Temporary Worry

Everyone has probably worried about their health from time to time. For example, a symptom such as chest pain can have many causes and is usually not serious. But if anyone experiencing this symptom has just read a newspaper article about someone who has had a heart attack*, they might worry that they are about to have one too. This temporary concern is not an example of hypochondria. With true hypochondria the worry is more lasting, and it interferes with one's daily life.

The prevalence of hypochondria among the general public is unknown, but studies have indicated that it accounts for between 4 and 9 percent of visits to doctors. Hypochondria occurs in all age groups and cultures and is about equally prevalent among males and females.

When Medical Reassurance Does Not Help

People with hypochondria may be overly concerned with a variety of symptoms and even with their normal bodily functions. Minor aches and pains, occasional coughing, dizziness, nausea, or small sores can convince people with hypochondria that they are seriously ill. They may also closely monitor normal bodily functions, such as heartbeat, breathing, sweating, and intestinal function, for signs of disease. The health worries of someone with hypochondria may be focused on a particular body organ, such as the heart, or on several parts of the body.

An important characteristic of people with hypochondria is that they are not fully reassured after a medical examination and tests have shown no physical basis for their complaints. Although their fears may be temporarily relieved, the belief that they are ill may still be so strong that they go from one physician to another seeking new tests and treatments.

What Causes Hypochondria?

Why is it that some people are constantly worried about being sick? The cause or causes of hypochondria are not clearly understood, and experts have varying views.

One theory is that people who have hypochondria are excessively sensitive to their bodily sensations and may misinterpret their meaning. In some cases, hypochondria appears to be triggered by the death of a loved one. Researchers have also noted that hypochondria seems to be more common in people who were seriously ill as a child or who have spent a lot of time around sick relatives. Such past experiences may contribute to health worries.

Hypochondria may be one symptom of another mental disorder, such as depression* or anxiety*. For example, in some cases of obsessive-compulsive disorder*, a person may have extreme unfounded health worries and feel compelled to keep seeking reassurance from health professionals.

How Is Hypochondria Diagnosed and Treated?

The first step in diagnosing hypochondria is a thorough physical examination to make sure there is no medical disease or condition causing the patient's complaints. When the patient has been reassured that he or she is not ill, yet the intense health worries continue, the diagnosis of hypochondria may be made. The physician will need to take care not to confuse hypochondria with malingering*, or with such closely related mental conditions as conversion disorder* and Munchausen syndrome*.

Hypochondria can be difficult to treat because the beliefs about illness are usually very strong. Although reassurance that the person is in good health is necessary, it is likely to be helpful only for a short time. Psychotherapy can help a person to make gradual changes in the way they think about their bodily sensations and to cope with health anxiety. When hypochondria is a symptom of depression, anxiety, or obsessive-compulsive disorder, treatment focuses on the underlying disorder.

* **depression** (de-PRESH-un) is a mental state characterized by feelings of sadness, despair, and discouragement.

* **anxiety** can be experienced as a troubled feeling, a sense of dread, fear of the future, or distress over a possible threat to a person's physical or mental well-being.

* **obsessive-compulsive disorder** causes people to feel trapped by distressing thoughts or to feel as if they have to repeat actions, such as washing hands.

* **malingering** (ma-LING-er-ing) means intentionally pretending to be sick or injured to avoid work or responsibility.

* **conversion disorder** is a mental disorder in which psychological symptoms are converted to physical symptoms, such as blindness, paralysis, or seizures. A person with conversion disorder does not intentionally produce symptoms.

* **Munchausen syndrome** (MOON-chow-zen SIN-drome) is a mental disorder in which a person pretends to have symptoms or causes symptoms of a disease in order to be hospitalized or receive tests, medication, or surgery.

▶ *See also*

I

Impulsivity

Impulsivity (IM-pul-SIV-i-tee) is the general term used to describe a tendency to act quickly, often without thinking or caring about the consequences. Impulsivity can be a normal trait. In extreme forms, however, it can be a symptom of certain behavioral disorders.

KEYWORDS
*for searching the Internet
and other reference sources*

Attention deficit hyperactivity disorder

Impulse-control disorders

Acting on Impulse

To understand impulsivity, it is important to understand the word "impulse," which can be used in two different, although related, ways. With regard to behavior, an impulse is a sudden, strong, even irrational urge, desire, or action resulting from a particular feeling or state of mind. Within the central nervous system, a nerve impulse is the electrical and chemical process by which messages are sent along the nerves. People's impulses, or urges to behave, result from nerve impulses, or the sending of messages from one part of the brain to another. As a normal trait, one person may be more impulsive than another.

Babies and very young children consistently act on impulse because they have not yet developed the ability to understand the results of their actions. Babies and young children will obey the impulse to reach for a pot on the stove, draw on the walls, hit another child, or throw a temper tantrum simply because they have not learned how or why to control their impulses. As children mature, though, they develop the skill of impulse control, sometimes simply called self-control. In other words, they learn to think before they act, wait their turn, and consider the consequences of their actions. Good impulse control makes it possible for a child to wait patiently instead of interrupting, to raise his or her hand in class instead of calling out, and to ask for something instead of grabbing it. This skill usually develops as a result of maturity and is shaped by adult guidance and teaching.

What Is Overly Impulsive Behavior?

For some people, overly impulsive behavior lasts into later childhood, the teenage years, and even adulthood. Too much impulsivity, or not enough impulse control, can lead to behavior problems or unsafe actions. For example, children might impulsively run into a busy street without looking, grab a toy from another child, hit others, throw things, or behave in other inappropriate ways. All children may act this way from time to time, but overly impulsive children repeat these behaviors again and again, even after numerous warnings from parents, teachers, and other adults. Teenagers and adults who lack impulse control may blurt out hurtful comments, not finish projects, have trouble listening, interrupt others frequently, or hit others when they're angry. A pattern of such behavior can be a symptom of a behavior disorder. For instance, a greater than normal level of impulsivity is associated with the condition known as attention deficit hyperactivity disorder (ADHD). ADHD is characterized by greater than normal levels of impulsivity, hyperactivity, and distractibility.

What Are Impulse-Control Disorders?

There are several other conditions that are classified in the DSM-IV* as impulse-control disorders. Though they are each quite different from one another, they each involve some form of impulsivity or strong urge for a particular type of problematic behavior. They include:

> ***DSM-IV** is *The Diagnostic and Statistical Manual of Mental Disorders*, 4th revision, published by the American Psychiatric Association. This is the system of classification and diagnosis of mental conditions used in the United States.

- Intermittent explosive disorder: A pattern of behavior in which a person has trouble resisting aggressive impulses, resulting in sudden and severe outbursts of anger, violence, or destruction of property. The person may respond very aggressively to minor sources of stress or frustration. Because people can act aggressively for many different reasons, however, this condition is only diagnosed when the explosive behavior does not stem from another mental disorder, a medical condition, or a drug or medication.

- Kleptomania (KLEP-toe-MAY-nee-a): An abnormal, uncontrollable, and repeated urge to steal. Often, objects are not taken because of their monetary value or because the person needs them, but because the objects have some kind of symbolic meaning for the person.

- Pyromania (PIE-roe-MAY-nee-a): An uncontrollable urge to set fires. The person usually feels tension while setting the fire, followed by pleasure while watching the fire burn.

- Trichotillomania (TRIK-o-TIL-o-MAY-nee-a): An irresistible urge to pull out one's hair, eyelashes, or eyebrows.

Resources

Organizations

Trichotillomania Learning Center, 1215 Mission Street, Suite 2, Santa Cruz, CA 95060. A national nonprofit group devoted to understanding trichotillomania.

Telephone 831-457-1004
http://www.trich.org

CHADD (Children and Adults with Attention-Deficit/Hyperactivity Disorder), 8181 Professional Place, Suite 201, Landover, MD 20785. CHADD is a national organization for education, advocacy and support of people with ADHD.
Telephone 301-306-7070
www.chadd.org

▶ *See also*
Attention Deficit Hyperactivity Disorder
Lying and Stealing
Trichotillomania

Intelligence

Intelligence is the ability to acquire, remember, and use knowledge in order to make judgments, solve problems, and deal with new experiences.

KEYWORDS
for searching the Internet and other reference sources

Giftedness

Intelligence quotient

Mental retardation

Psychometrics

I.Q. Smarts

Not every student will have the experience of taking an I.Q. (intelligence quotient) test. However, almost all students do know what it is like to take a standardized test. Unlike a test taken for a class, which usually is based on specific material already covered in the classroom, standardized tests typically include a wide range of items that ask the test-taker to use words, solve problems, and understand relationships among concepts. The results often show how the student performed compared to others of the same age or grade level. For example, if a student scores at the 80th percentile, that means this person performed better than 8 out of 10 students of the same age or grade who took the test.

I.Q. tests are used to compare an individual's performance to that of others on a sampling of school-related tasks. An individual's performance on all these tasks is averaged and compared to that of other people of the same age. I.Q. varies among people much the way height does. Most people are close to average height, while a small number are much taller or shorter than average. Similarly, the average I.Q. is 100, and most people fall somewhere between 70 and 130. Those who fall below 70 often are diagnosed with mental retardation, while those with an I.Q. higher than 130 often are considered gifted.

What Is I.Q. Testing?

How did the practice of measuring intelligence get started? Back in 1905, public school administrators in Paris asked psychologist Alfred Binet to come up with a test that would identify mentally retarded children who could benefit from special help outside the regular classroom. It was hoped that this would help relieve the problem of overcrowded classes. The Simon-Binet test that resulted set the stage for intelligence testing throughout the 1900s.

Stanford-Binet Intelligence Scale   An American psychologist at Stanford University named Lewis Terman revised the Simon-Binet test in 1916. This revision, known as the Stanford-Binet Intelligence Scale, is still in use today, although it has been revised several more times. The latest version includes sections on abstract/visual reasoning, verbal reasoning (word-related problems), quantitative reasoning (number-related problems), and short-term memory.

Wechsler Intelligence Scales   The Wechsler Intelligence Scales are another well-known set of I.Q. tests. Psychologist David Wechsler developed a number of tests in the 1940s, 50s, and 60s that were tailored to children of different ages as well as to adults. Today, many schools use the Wechsler Intelligence Scale for Children–Third Edition (WISC-III) to evaluate children between the ages of 6 and 16. One of

LEWIS TERMAN AND THE STANFORD STUDY

In the early 1900s, it was widely believed that gifted people were physically inferior, had unusual interests, and found it difficult to relate to others. In the 1920s, psychologist Lewis Terman and his colleagues at Stanford University launched a study of 1,500 children in California who were gifted (I.Q.s over 130). After tracking the children for several years, the researchers found that they actually were healthier, taller, better adjusted, and more popular than the average child. As these gifted children grew into young adults, they were more likely to attend college, achieve academically, pursue advanced degrees, and go on to higher-level professional positions in fields such as science, writing, and business. They also tended to be more satisfied with their lives as adults.

This dispelled the notion that extremely bright people were "eggheads" who were at a disadvantage socially. It also suggested that I.Q. may be a somewhat reliable predictor of later academic and professional success. At the same time, however, the study showed that a high I.Q. is not a guarantee of success, as there were also many individuals who did not achieve at a high level. While many of the "gifted children" were well educated and had good professional jobs, all levels of employment and income were found.

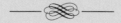

Wechsler's contributions is the notion that intelligence can be broken down into two main types of problem-solving: verbal and nonverbal. A Verbal Scale on the WISC-III measures how well children are able to use words to solve problems of different kinds, including some that involve common sense and others that involve more abstract reasoning. The Performance Scale on the test measures how well children use nonverbal abilities to make sense of visual relationships; for instance, by solving a puzzle or deciphering a code.

What Is Intelligence?

Defining intelligence is not as simple as giving someone an I.Q. test, however. In fact, scientists still are debating what intelligence really is. Harvard psychologist and education expert Howard Gardner has challenged the notion that there is a single human intelligence, or even just verbal and nonverbal intelligences. Instead, Gardner has proposed a theory of multiple intelligences. He argues that human beings have at least seven separate intelligences, each relatively independent of the others:

- linguistic (reading and writing)
- logical-mathematical (using numbers, solving logic problems)

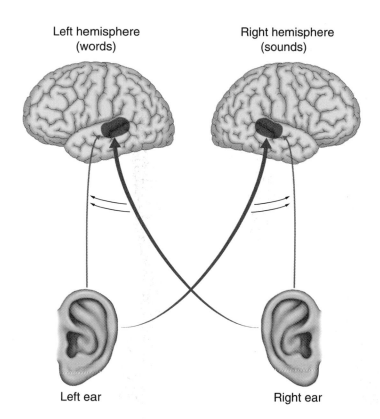

Left hemisphere (words)

Right hemisphere (sounds)

Left ear

Right ear

◀

Intelligence is sometimes classified as left-brained or right-brained, although that is an oversimplification. People can hear words and musical sounds with both ears, but the right ear is believed to have a stronger connection to the left hemisphere of the brain where words and speech are processed. People can hear words spoken into the left ear but they understand them better when assisted by the speech pathway from the right ear. Likewise, the left ear has a stronger connection to the right hemisphere of the brain where musical sounds are processed. People can hear melodies played into the right ear but enjoy them more when assisted by the sound pathway from the left ear.

- spatial (finding one's way around an environment)
- musical (perceiving and creating patterns of pitch and rhythm)
- bodily-kinesthetic (making precise movements, as in performing surgery or dance)
- interpersonal (understanding others)
- intrapersonal (knowing oneself)

Gardner also believes that any definition of intelligence must take into account what the culture values. For example, while we might consider someone intelligent if that person can use words or numbers well, people of another culture might place more value on skills such as hunting, fishing, or understanding nature. Gardner's theory favors observation of people over time, rather than short-answer I.Q. tests, for measuring the different intelligence types.

Other psychologists have suggested still other theories for understanding intelligence. Swiss psychologist Jean Piaget, believed that intelligence should be defined as adaptation to the environment. Piaget looked at how children display intelligence at different stages of life, from infancy through adolescence, and tried to make generalizations about how they are able to cope with their surroundings and meet new challenges. More recently, psychologist Robert Sternberg proposed a three-sided theory of intelligence, arguing that intelligence actually is composed of three parts: the ability to analyze information to solve problems, the creative ability to incorporate insights and new ideas, and the practical ability to size up situations and survive in the real world.

Most likely, all of these theories are at least partly correct and can contribute to our overall understanding of intelligence. However, updated versions of the tests developed by Alfred Binet and David Wechsler still are used to measure I.Q. Many psychologists and educators have strong feelings for or against giving I.Q. tests. Some argue that I.Q. tests are very useful for predicting how well a particular child will do in school and judging whether that child needs extra support or more challenges. However, others fear that children who test poorly may be stereotyped as low achievers and not given the level of attention they otherwise would have received. Still others believe that specific test questions put individuals from certain ethnic groups at a disadvantage. For example, think about how some of the verbal expressions used by African American or Latino students differ from those used by their caucasian classmates. A verbal question that asks about a particular word that is commonly used by people of one ethnic group might be unfamiliar to people from other backgrounds. Finally, some experts are concerned that I.Q. tests may underestimate the abilities of people with speech, movement, and other disabilities.

Resources

Organizations

National Association for Gifted Children, 1707 L Street Northwest, Suite 550, Washington, DC 20036. A national organization for parents and teachers that focuses on the special needs of gifted and talented students.
Telephone 202-785-4268
http://www.nagc.org

U.S. Department of Education, 400 Maryland Avenue Southwest, Washington, DC 20202. The department of the federal government that oversees special education programs for mentally retarded and gifted students.
Telephone 800-872-5327
http://www.ed.gov

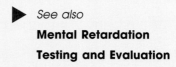

See also

Mental Retardation

Testing and Evaluation

L

Learning Disabilities

Learning disabilities are disorders that affect people's ability to interpret information that they see or hear or to link information processed in different parts of the brain. A person with a learning disability may have specific difficulties with language, visual information, or coordination, which in turn can make it very hard to read, spell, write, or do math.

KEYWORDS
for searching the Internet and other reference sources

Dysgraphia

Dyslexia

Language disorders

Learning disorders

Speech disorders

What Are Learning Disabilities?

Learning disabilities differ from learning problems (which are less severe) and from mental retardation (which refers to more global learning difficulties). Not every learning problem is a true disorder or disability. Some children are just naturally slower than others in developing certain skills, but most children usually catch up and achieve within the normal range for their age and abilities. Children who are mentally retarded, on the other hand, will never be able to learn and function socially like other children their age. Their general intellectual capacity is much lower than average. Children with mental retardation have learning problems but do not truly have learning disabilities.

Children with learning disabilities typically have average or even above-average intelligence, so they have a marked difference between their intellectual capabilities and what they are actually achieving. In a sense, a person with a learning disability is like a radio that is not tuned exactly to a station. There is nothing wrong with the radio itself or with the signal coming from the station, but the music still sounds garbled. Similarly, people with learning disabilities can see and hear as well as others and have normal general learning capacity, but there is a problem with the way their brains process information.

Learning disabilities are generally classified into two main categories: verbal (having to do with the uses of spoken and written words) and non-verbal (having to do with interpreting visual or spatial information).

Verbal learning disabilities Developmental speech disorders are usually diagnosed in very young children who have persistent trouble making certain speech sounds; for example, they may say "wabbit" instead of "rabbit" or "thwim" instead of "swim." Often these speech disabilities improve with age or with the help of a speech therapist.

Developmental language disorders involve the way that children express themselves or how they understand others' speech. Children with this type of disorder may speak in short phrases instead of full sentences, call objects by the wrong names, have disorganized speech, misunderstand words, or have difficulties following directions.

Reading is a very complex task in which a person has to focus attention on the printed marks, control eye movements across the page, recognize sounds associated with letters, understand words and grammar, build images and ideas, compare new ideas to what is already known, and then store the ideas in memory. This process requires a rich, intact network of nerve cells that connect the brain's centers of vision, language, and memory. A problem in any of these areas or the connections among them can lead to difficulties with reading. Dyslexia (dis-LEKS-ee-uh) is the most common and best-known of the reading disorders. It affects 2 to 8 percent of school-age children. Because children with dyslexia have trouble processing the smallest units of language that make up words, they may have trouble with rhyming games or with sounding out individual letters or syllables to form words.

There are other types of reading disorders that affect comprehension (kom-pre-HEN-shun), which is the ability to fully understand and inter-

UNDERSTANDING DYSLEXIA

In the mid-1900s, a doctor named Samuel Orton found that several children he was working with had similar problems with reading. In addition to confusing the letter "b" with "d" and the letter "p" with "q," some could read more easily if they held pages up to a mirror. Orton named this condition strephosymbolia (STREF-oh-sim-BOL-ee-uh), which means "twisted symbols." Now strephosymbolia is called dyslexia, which is derived from the Greek words "dys" (meaning poor or inadequate) and "lexis" (meaning words or language).

Further research has shown that dyslexia involves much more than just seeing letters backwards or reversed. Children with this disorder describe how printed letters and words seem to jump around on the page or that sounds and letters get mixed up or jumbled together. Researchers originally thought that visual and motor problems were at the heart of dyslexia, but they later found that reading disabilities stem from a difficulty with processing the smallest units of language, which are called phonemes (FO-neemz). For example, the "p" of pat and the "f" of fat are two different phonemes, and the word fat has three phonemes linked together. Someone with dyslexia might have trouble telling the difference between these sounds when reading them.

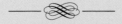

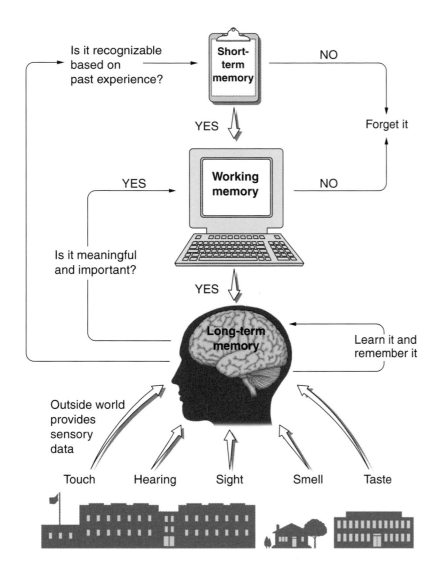

Is it recognizable based on past experience?

Short-term memory

NO

YES

Forget it

YES

Working memory

NO

Is it meaningful and important?

YES

Long-term memory

Learn it and remember it

Outside world provides sensory data

Touch   Hearing   Sight   Smell   Taste

Learning involves a complex series of events. The brain receives new information from the outside world all the time, but in order to learn new information, the brain must recognize the information's importance, interpret it, analyze its meaning, and store it in memory for later use in processing new information. If the brain does not recognize new information as meaningful and important, it will discard it. Learning disorders affect different aspects of this complex process of recognizing, interpreting, understanding, and remembering new information.

◄

pret what one reads. A person with this type of disability can read each word but may find it hard to understand the text, form images, or relate new ideas in the text to those in memory. These reading disabilities usually are discovered at a later age than is dyslexia.

A writing disability can result from problems with any area of the brain that controls grammar, hand movement, vocabulary, and memory. Children who have trouble mastering the motor skill of writing are said to have dysgraphia (dis-GRAF-ee-uh).

Nonverbal learning disorder   Nonverbal learning disorder (also called nonverbal learning disabilities), or NVLD, is not as well understood as verbal learning disabilities. People with NVLD often have problems with visual perception, with recalling visual details, and with spatial relationships. Their eyesight is fine, but they may have trouble processing what they see; for example, a student might find it hard to follow a set of instructions demonstrated by a teacher.

Students with NVLD often find it hard to focus on nonverbal academic material as well, which can make it hard to learn math (a disorder called dyscalculia (dis-KAL-kyoo-lee-uh)) and science. They may have trouble recognizing numbers and symbols, memorizing facts such as the multiplication tables, aligning numbers, and understanding abstract concepts like place value and fractions. In both math and science class, students may have difficulty solving problems, forming complex concepts, and making educated guesses and then testing them out. Reading comprehension may be affected as well. Even though students with NVLD may read words and sentences with ease, they might not understand the underlying organization of the story. Dealing with brand-new material is likely to overwhelm children with NVLD.

Some children with NVLD have trouble in other areas as well. They may have poor motor skills and problems with coordination; for example, learning to ride a bike can be very difficult for a child with NVLD. They also may have trouble socializing with other children because they do not pick up on nonverbal social cues, such as tone of voice and body language, or they tend to say the wrong thing at the wrong time. Children with NVLD tend to be easily frustrated and upset. Any new situation can make them anxious because they may have more difficulty adjusting to it.

Other types of learning disabilities There are many other subtypes of learning disabilities, but verbal and nonverbal learning disabilities are the two main categories. Because many aspects of speaking, listening, reading, writing, and arithmetic overlap and build on the same brain capabilities, it is not unusual for someone to have more than one disorder. For example, most disorders that hinder the ability to understand language will also interfere with learning to read, spell, and write.

Attention Deficit Hyperactivity Disorder*, or ADHD, can also interfere with learning. Children with ADHD often have difficulty focusing on any one task for a period of time. Children with attention problems may have learning problems but attention deficits are not classified as specific learning disabilities. However, more than half of children with ADHD also have learning disabilities.

How Do People Know They Have a Learning Disability?

Parents and teachers are usually the first to notice signs of a possible learning disability. A very young child might not speak or listen as well as other children their age or might have trouble with a game's directions or other activities that other children complete with ease. The classroom teacher may notice persistent difficulties in reading, writing, or math.

*Attention Deficit Hyperactivity Disorder, or ADHD, is a condition that makes it hard for a person to pay attention, sit still, or think before acting.

The first step in diagnosing a learning disability is to rule out any other possible causes, such as vision or hearing problems or some other medical condition. Once a doctor makes sure that other problems are not to blame, the child might be evaluated by a psychologist* who specializes in learning disabilities. Diagnosing a learning disorder often takes time. The psychologist usually takes a careful history of symptoms, interviews the child, and gives certain tests that compare the child's level of ability to what is considered appropriate for a person of that age and intelligence.

Why Do People Have Learning Disabilities?

Why certain children develop learning disabilities and others do not remains a mystery. However, researchers believe that learning disabilities can be traced to differences in early brain development that happen before or after birth. During brain development, a few all-purpose cells must grow into a complex organ made of billions of specialized interconnected nerve cells called neurons [NOR-ons]. Researchers are investigating possible causes for differences or disruptions in brain development that include:

- alcohol, tobacco, or drug use by the mother during pregnancy
- problems during pregnancy or delivery that may cause a decrease in the amount of oxygen that reaches the baby's developing brain
- head injuries
- being exposed to poisonous substances in the environment, such as lead

Also, because some learning disabilities tend to run in families, researchers are looking into how learning differences may be inherited.

Living with a Learning Disability

Because children with learning disabilities typically have normal or above-normal intelligence, they often can find ways to learn in spite of the disorder. They may need special school programs for the learning disabled or to work with a learning specialist several hours each week while attending regular classes.

Special education teachers can help plan out what is called an Individualized Education Program, or IEP, for a learning-disabled child. This plan outlines the specific skills the child needs to develop as well as appropriate learning activities that build on the child's strengths and work around his or her difficulties. For example, a student with dyslexia might be encouraged to listen to a book on tape for English class, while another with a writing disorder might take notes or complete an assignment using a laptop computer.

Children with learning disabilities often need emotional support because they may see themselves as dumb or stupid. They may withdraw

*psychologist (sy-KOL-uh-jist) is a mental health professional who can do psychological testing and provide mental health counseling.

Dyslexia: Separating Myth from Reality

In a 1996 article published in *Scientific American* magazine, one of the country's leading experts on dyslexia tried to correct some of the persistent myths about the disorder, including the following:

MYTH: Mirror writing is a symptom of dyslexia.

REALITY: In fact, backwards writing and reversal of letters are common in the early stages of writing development among children with and without dyslexia. Children with dyslexia have problems in naming letters but not in copying letters.

MYTH: Eye training is an effective treatment for dyslexia.

REALITY: More than two decades of research have shown that dyslexia reflects a linguistic (lin-GWIS-tik; language-related) deficit. There is no evidence that eye training alleviates the disorder.

MYTH: Dyslexia can be outgrown.

REALITY: Yearly monitoring of language processing skills from first through twelfth grade shows that the disability persists into adulthood. Even though most people with dyslexia learn to read accurately, they continue to read slowly and do not read automatically.

MYTH: Smart people cannot be dyslexic.

REALITY: Intelligence is in no way related to language processing skills, and there have been many brilliant and accomplished people with dyslexia, including writers William Butler Yeats and John Irving, scientist Albert Einstein, military leader George Patton, and financial industry leader Charles Schwab.

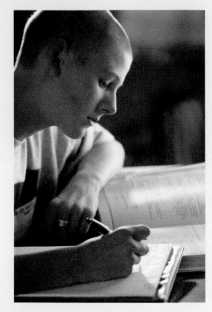

▲

Teens with learning disabilities often find a particular way of learning that works for them. Their methods, along with a regained sense of self-confidence, continue to affect their lives outside the classroom, such as in relationships with others and in their careers. *Photodisc*

▶ *See also*

Attention

Attention Deficit Hyperactivity Disorder

Intelligence

Memory

Mental Retardation

Self-Esteem

Testing and Evaluation

from their classmates at school or even get into trouble because they are frustrated when learning is difficult for them. Children and their families can often benefit by working with a trained counselor or support group.

Resources

Books

Cummings, Rhoda, and Gary Fisher. *The Survival Guide for Teenagers with LD.* Minneapolis: Free Spirit Publishing, 1993.

Lauren, Jill. *Succeeding with LD: 20 True Stories About Real People with LD.* Minneapolis: Free Spirit Publishing, 1997. For ages 11 and up.

Levine, Melvin. *Keeping a Head in School: A Student's Book About Learning Disabilities and Learning Disorders.* Cambridge, MA: Educators Publishing Services, 1996.

Stern, Judith, and Uzi Ben-Ami. *Many Ways to Learn: Young People's Guide to Learning Disabilities.* New York: Magination Press, 1996.

Organizations

The International Dyslexia Association, 8600 LaSalle Road, Chester Building, Suite 382, Baltimore, MD 21286-2044.
Telephone 800-ABCD123
http://www.interdys.org

LD Online is an interactive guide to learning disabilities for parents, teachers, and children. The website includes in-depth information about learning disorders, an interactive chat room and bulletin boards, the latest news and resources, and a KidZone that features artwork and stories by young people.
http://www.ldonline.org

The Learning Disabilities Association of America (LDA), 4156 Library Road, Pittsburgh, PA 15234-1349. LDA is a national non-profit organization that provides education and support for people with learning disabilities and their families.
http://www.ldanatl.org

National Institute of Mental Health (NIMH), National Institutes of Health, 6001 Executive Blvd., Rm. 8184, MSC 9663, Bethesda, MD 20892-9663. The NIMH posts information about learning disabilities at its website.
Telephone 301-443-4513
http://www.nimh.nih.gov/publicat/learndis.htm

NLD on the Web! is a website that provides information about non-verbal learning disabilities.
http://www.nldontheweb.org.

Love and Intimacy

Love is a deep feeling of connection with and affection for another person.

While no one has ever made a scientific count, it is probably true that more songs, books, and poems have been written about love than about any other subject. Most of the world's religions place a high value on the experience and expression of love. Over the centuries, many philosophers have argued that love is the most powerful force in the universe. Without love, people can be lonely, disconnected, sad, or angry. With love, people feel happiness and security.

Kinds of Love

Every time Jason saw Mrs. Smith with her new baby, the infant was crying. Jason could not understand why the endless crying did not annoy Mrs. Smith. "How can she be smiling and cooing at that noisy little thing?" he wondered. The more he thought about it, the more Jason realized that his mother probably had felt the same way about him when he was a crying baby.

The love parents feel for their babies is one of the deepest emotional connections. Parental love grows and changes over time. At first, babies are totally dependent on their parents or other caregivers to take care of them, feed them, and clothe them. Parents are very attached to their children and want to help them feel loved and secure. Children begin to rely less on their parents as they grow up. Yet the more children are loved, the more they later learn to love others as they form relationships and have families of their own. Children's experiences with love can influence their relationships for the rest of their lives. Trusting, close, safe relationships with parents help establish the foundations of good relationships with friends and loved ones. When their relationships with their parents are not loving, children may grow up less able to trust others. They may even have trouble establishing loving or intimate relationships as adults.

Most psychologists (sy-KOL-o-jists) and researchers believe that love is a combination of three things:

- **Intimacy:** a feeling of ease, honesty, and emotional closeness between people
- **Commitment:** devotion or faithfulness
- **Passion:** an excitement and desire to be together.

This is true of all kinds of love, whether it is parental love, friends' affection and loyalty, lovers' romance and attraction, or warm feelings for a pet. Whether they are relationships that involve being "in love" or ones that involve the love of friendship, they bring warmth, connection, and a sense of belonging to people's lives.

KEYWORDS
for searching the Internet and other reference sources

Sexual development

Showing Love

How do people show their love to others? When people are close, or "emotionally intimate," they have feelings of warmth, caring, and familiarity. They might do things together, such as go to the movies or visit each other's houses. Close friends have private experiences, personal conversations, and deep feelings of trust. Helping people, doing them favors, and listening to their troubles are all ways to show love. As people grow older and mature, they have love relationships that involve deepening feelings of caring, tenderness, sacrifice, and an ability to accept the other person's limitations or weaknesses.

Love, however, does not always feel warm and comfortable. Loving someone may mean that a person has to say or do difficult things. For example, a parent who says no to a child's request may seem strict or unfair. But the parent may be acting out of love by protecting the child from something dangerous or hurtful. Sometimes people show their love through physical intimacy. Friends might hug each other or hold hands, a grandchild might snuggle in the arms of a grandparent, or a parent might give a child a backrub. The most mature relationships, such as that between a married couple, are physically and emotionally intimate. The most intense form of physical intimacy is a sexual relationship.

WHY DO WE LOVE MOVIE STARS AND ROCK SINGERS?

The Swiss psychologist Carl G. Jung believed that everyone has an unconscious inner male spirit (which he called the "animus") or an unconscious inner female spirit (the "anima") that remains hidden. According to Jung, a woman has an unconscious male spirit, and a man has an unconscious female spirit. Jung believed that often the people with whom we fall in love are representations of our own inner male or female spirit. Jung thought that people could get in touch with their inner male or female side by studying their dreams.

In 1926, when the popular silent film star Rudolph Valentino died at an early age, Jung observed that thousands of women all over the world wept as if they had lost their own lovers. Jung believed that the women really must have been weeping over the loss of their inner male spirits that seemed to have died. The rock singer Elvis Presley and the actress Marilyn Monroe also captured the hearts of millions of people. When they died, many people felt brokenhearted. Did they symbolize America's inner male and female spirits too?

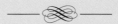

Sexual Attraction

Young children begin to understand the concept of "being in love" when they are 4 or 5 years old, but it is not until the time of puberty, at about the age of 12 or 13, that people begin to have feelings of romantic love. Early on, a young person might have a "crush" on someone or an attraction to someone. This is possible even when people do not know each other well or at all. Girls and boys both have crushes. With a crush, a person might be preoccupied by thoughts of the other person and may even think that he or she is in love.

Young people may develop sexual feelings or desires to be physically close to someone. Usually sexual attraction, a feeling of being drawn or attracted to another person, is accompanied by love, but not always. Most people have sexual feelings and desire for someone of the opposite sex, but some people are attracted romantically and physically to someone of the same sex.

Most adults discourage young people from acting on their feelings of sexual attraction ("making love," or having sex) and encourage them to wait until they are older and more mature, or even until they are married. This is because the most complete kind of love involves deep emotional feelings of caring, responsibility, openness, respect, and affection as well as sexual attraction. For people of all ages, sexual relationships produce complicated feelings and involve a lot of responsibility.

Resource

Book

Harris, Robie H. *It's Perfectly Normal: Changing Bodies, Growing Up, Sex, and Sexual Health.* Cambridge, MA: Candlewick Press, 1994.

▶ *See also*
Emotions
Families
Sexual Development

Lying and Stealing

Lying (purposefully telling an untruth) and stealing (taking what does not belong to you) are dishonest behaviors that break the rules of society. Such misbehaviors in children, adolescents, or adults, especially if they happen often, may be signs of other more significant problems. Sometimes these misbehaviors and others, like cheating, truancy*, destroying property, or hurting others, are called antisocial behaviors, or disruptive behaviors, because they break social rules.

KEYWORDS
for searching the Internet and other reference sources

Antisocial behaviors

Conduct disorder

Disruptive behaviors

* **truancy** means staying out of school or work without permission.

Why Do Children Lie and Take Things That Do Not Belong to Them?

It is normal for very young children to say what is not true or to take what is not theirs. They have not yet learned rules for social behavior. Young children may fib, exaggerate, or tell tall tales because they have not yet learned to tell the difference between what is real and what they can pretend. Very young children may believe that whatever they see or hold belongs to them. They have not yet developed the behavioral controls to resist taking what they want or the understanding of why they shouldn't. Once children learn the difference between truth and untruth, they may lie about their behavior to avoid punishment or because they fear other consequences of telling the truth.

Children who have developmental problems such as mental retardation may be unable to understand or remember societal rules. Other children who have conditions that cause them to be impulsive* may need extra help learning social rules and developing the behavior controls to follow these rules.

*impulsive** means acting quickly before thinking about the effect of a certain action or behavior.

How Do Children Learn to Be Honest?

As children grow, they develop the mental and moral capability to know right from wrong. They learn about the importance of honesty and playing fair through social interactions with adults and with other children. Parents are important role models for children as they learn about honesty, fairness, and positive social behaviors. By being honest, fair, and respectful, parents set a good example for children. Parents who set clear expectations for behavior and follow through with clear consequences for misbehavior help children learn to behave well. Parents who are too harsh or abusive and parents who are too lenient or neglectful may fail to help children develop appropriate social behavior.

As children are learning social rules, they are also developing the behavior controls to follow the rules. This process happens gradually and is made possible by positive coaching, support, and appropriate consequences from parents and teachers. By 8 or 9 years old, most children, as long as they live in an environment where following social rules is encouraged, do not have problems with lying, stealing, or other disruptive behaviors. Most children try to do right and feel rewarded by the praise they receive from adults and the pride they experience when social rules are followed.

When Lying and Stealing Continue

Some children, adolescents, and adults break rules of conduct frequently and on purpose even though they know it is wrong. When lying, stealing, and other antisocial behaviors occur regularly, or beyond the expected age, the person may be said to have a disruptive behavior disorder, such as oppositional defiant disorder, conduct disorder, or antisocial personality disorder.

Oppositional defiant disorder is a disruptive behavior disorder that can be diagnosed in children as young as preschoolers who demonstrate hostile or aggressive behavior and who refuse to follow rules. Conduct disorder is diagnosed in older children and adolescents who have had serious problems with lying, stealing, and aggressive behavior for at least 6 months. Adults who demonstrate a pattern of dishonest, aggressive, or destructive behaviors that violate the rights of others may be diagnosed with antisocial personality disorder.

 See also

Antisocial Personality Disorder

Conduct Disorder

Oppositional Defiant Disorder

M

Malingering

Malingering (ma-LING-er-ing) means intentionally pretending to be sick or injured to avoid work or responsibility. The illnesses faked may be physical, such as the flu, or mental, such as depression*. Similarly, a person may pretend to have severe back pain due to an injury. Sometimes a person may actually have a mild illness or injury and exaggerate the symptoms.

Why Do Some People Malinger?

Although there are rare instances in which malingering may have a positive or useful purpose, such as faking illness as a prisoner of war, it is generally considered to be unacceptable behavior. Why then do people sometimes act this way?

People may fake a disorder for many reasons. They may wish to shirk military service or jury duty or avoid going on trial for some criminal act. Some people feign illness to get extra time off from school or their job. Others may fake or exaggerate an injury or disease to get undeserved money from an insurance company. Some people may malinger to get extra attention, sympathy, or help from family or coworkers.

Telling Malingering from a Real Illness

As long as there have been malingerers, there have likely been others who understood what they were up to. The Greek physician Galen, who lived in the second century A.D., wrote, "People for many reasons may pretend to be ill; it is desirable, then, that the physician should be able to arrive at the truth in such cases." Using their experience with actual diseases, he said, physicians need to distinguish tricks of the malingerer from the "true signs" of disease.

Physicians today face many of the same basic problems with malingering that Galen did. To tell malingering from a real illness, doctors need to perform a thorough physical examination that may include tests to find out whether or not the symptoms a person claims to have are real and are a true sign of disease or injury. Doctors also need to be aware of circumstances in their patients' lives, such as unwanted work or duties, that might cause them to fake a disorder.

Certain mental disorders could be confused with malingering. For example, in hypochondria*, conversion disorder*, and Munchausen*

KEYWORDS
for searching the Internet
and other reference sources

Deception

Factitious disorder

Faking illness

Munchausen syndrome

* **depression** (de-PRESH-un) is a mental state characterized by feelings of sadness, despair, and discouragement.

* **hypochondria** (hy-po-KON-dree-a) is a mental disorder in which people believe that they are sick, but their symptoms are not related to any physical illness.

* **conversion disorder** is a mental disorder in which psychological symptoms are converted to physical symptoms, such as blindness, paralysis, or seizures. A person with conversion disorder does not intentionally produce symptoms.

* **Munchausen syndrome** (MOON-chow-zen SIN-drome) is a mental disorder in which a person pretends to have symptoms or causes symptoms of a disease in order to be hospitalized or receive tests, medication, or surgery.

▶ *See also*

Conversion Disorder

Hypochondria

Munchausen Syndrome

School Avoidance

Somatoform Disorders

syndrome, the patients' symptoms may not arise from actual physical conditions, yet these mental disorders are not the same as malingering. When people miss work or school because of physical symptoms that occur because of stressful changes or emotional upsets in their lives, they are not considered to be malingering. Individuals who are malingering know they are not sick and intentionally pretend to be ill.

Manic Depression   *See* Bipolar Disorder

KEYWORDS
*for searching the Internet
and other reference sources*

Neurotransmitters

Pharmacotherapy

Psychiatry

Psychopharmacology

Medications

Medications for mental, emotional, behavioral, and mood disorders are prescribed by medical doctors called psychiatrists, often as part of a treatment plan that includes psychotherapy (talk therapy).

Psychopharmacology

Psychopharmacology (SY-koe-far-ma-KOL-o-jee) is the study of how medications affect moods, thoughts, and feelings. Psychopharmacology is an exciting new science. When our grandparents were young, there were no medications that helped people with attention deficit hyperactivity disorder concentrate at school or work, no medications that helped people with schizophrenia quiet the voices in their heads, and no medications that helped people with depression find the energy to face a new day. Today there are prescription medications for these disorders and many others.

Psychiatric medications generally are classified into categories that reflect the chemistry of how they work in the body (mechanisms of action) or the symptoms they help relieve. Many medications fall into more than one category. For example, the same medication might improve symptoms of both depression and anxiety. These are some major types of psychiatric medications:

- antidepressant medications, which include tricyclic antidepressants (TCAs), monoamine oxidase inhibitors (MAOIs), and selective serotonin reuptake inhibitors (SSRIs)

- antianxiety medications (tranquilizers), which include barbiturates, benzodiazepines, and the atypical anxiolytic buspirone

- antimanic medications (mood stabilizers)
- anticonvulsant medications
- antipsychotic medications (neuroleptics)
- stimulants.

Examples of well-known psychiatric medications include Prozac and Paxil (antidepressants); Valium, Xanax, and BuSpar (antianxiety medications); lithium (antimanic medication); Tegretol and phenobarbital (anticonvulsants); Thorazine and Haldol (antipsychotics); and Ritalin and Concerta (stimulants).

How Do Psychiatric Medications Work?

Psychiatric medications target the complex chemistry of neurons and neurotransmitters in the brain and central nervous system. Neurotransmitters such as serotonin (ser-o-TONE-in) and dopamine (DOPE-a-meen) are manufactured in neurons (nerve cells) to carry messages from cell to cell, crossing the synaptic gap between the axon (transmitting terminal) of one neuron to the dendrites (receiving terminals) of the next neuron. The chemical structure of each neurotransmitter is designed to fit its neuroreceptor the way a key fits a lock. A change in a neurotransmitter's chemical structure, or an imbalance at any point in this complex process, may affect emotions, moods, thoughts, behaviors, and mental states. Psychiatric medications help restore proper balance. Important neurotransmitters include serotonin, dopamine, epinephrine, norepinephrine (monoamines), acetylcholine, gamma-aminobutyric acid (GABA), glutamic acid, enkephalins, and endorphins.

What Are the Beneficial Effects of Psychiatric Medications?

Psychiatric medications can help improve many of the most distressing symptoms of mental, emotional, and mood disorders. They can reduce the stress of living with chronic diseases and conditions, and they can improve the effectiveness of counseling and psychotherapy. Among their most beneficial effects are:

- decreasing feelings of hopelessness, darkness, and apathy in depression
- preventing relapse of depression
- reducing cravings, anxiety, obsessions, compulsions, and phobias
- preventing panic attacks
- reducing hallucinations, delusions, inappropriate behaviors, and the voices that often accompany schizophrenia
- calming impulsivity, hyperactivity, and mania
- improving concentration, memory, and sleep.

Physicians' Desk Reference (PDR)

Psychiatrists and psychopharmacologists study the research about medications before prescribing them. They attend training sessions, read medical journals, and review descriptions in the *Physicians' Desk Reference* (PDR) medical directory for details about how specific medications work (mechanisms), how they help patients (beneficial effects), whether they cause side effects (adverse effects), and whether they can be used safely with a patient's regular diet and other prescription medications (drug interactions).

The PDR lists medications by generic name (fluoxetine, for example) and also by the trade name given to a particular medication by the company that sells it (Prozac, in this case). Important psychiatric medications include:

Antidepressants

- amoxapine (Asendin)
- bupropion (Wellbutrin)
- clomipramine (Anafranil)
- doxepin (Sinequan or Adapin)
- maprotiline (Ludiomil)
- mirtazapine (Remeron)
- nefazodone (Serzone)
- trazodone (Desyrel)
- venlafaxine (Effexor)

Antidepressants/Tricyclics (TCAs)

- amitriptyline (Elavil)
- desipramine (Norpramin, Pertofrane)
- imipramine (Tofranil)
- nortriptyline (Pamelor, Aventyl)

Antidepressants/Monoamine Oxidase Inhibitors (MAOIs)

- isocarboxazid (Marplan)
- phenelzine (Nardil)
- tranylcypromine (Parnate)

(continued)

Antidepressants/Selective Serotonin Reuptake Inhibitors (SSRIs)

- citalopram (Celexa)
- fluoxetine (Prozac)
- fluvoxamine (Luvox)
- paroxetine (Paxil)
- sertraline (Zoloft)

Antianxiety Medications (Anxiolytics, Minor Tranquilizers)

- alprazolam (Xanax)
- buspirone (BuSpar)
- chlordiazepoxide (Librium, Librax, Libritabs)
- clorazepate (Tranxene, Azene)
- diazepam (Valium)
- halazepam (Paxipam)
- lorazepam (Ativan)
- oxazepam (Serax)
- prazepam (Centrax)

Antimanic Medications (Mood Stabilizers)

- carbamazepine (Tegretol)
- divalproex sodium (Depakote)
- lithium carbonate (Eskalith, Lithane, Lithobid)
- lithium citrate (Cibalith-S)

Anticonvulsants

- carbamazepine (Tegretol)
- clonazepam (Klonopin)
- divalproex sodium (Depakote)
- gabapentin (Neurontin)
- lamotrigine (Lamictil)
- oxcarbazepine (Trileptal)
- topiramate (Topamax)
- valproic acid (Depakene)

Antipsychotic Medications

- chlorpromazine (Thorazine)
- chlorprothixene (Taractan)
- clozapine (Clozaril)
- fluphenazine (Prolixin, Permitil)

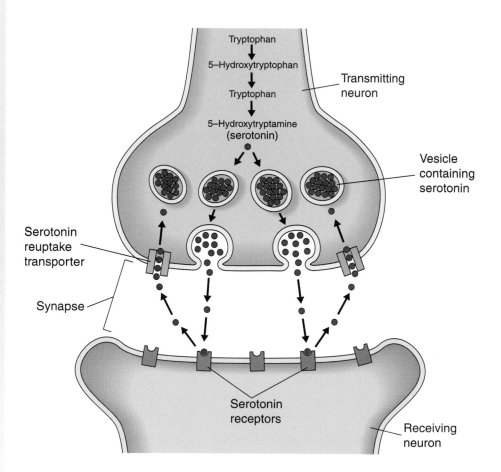

Psychiatric medications can help correct imbalances in the neurotransmitters that affect mood and behavior. Selective serotonin reuptake inhibitors (SSRIs), such as fluoxetine (Prozac), fit into the serotonin neuroreceptors on neuron dendrites. This blocks serotonin from entering the neuron and keeps it active for longer periods of time in the synaptic gaps between transmitting and receiving neurons. Serotonin (5-Hydroxytryptamine) is a calming neurotransmitter that is manufactured in nerve cells from the amino acid tryptophan. Turkey is one good source of tryptophan, which may help explain why people often feel relaxed and sleepy after Thanksgiving dinner.

Selecting the right medication and the right dosage are complicated tasks, requiring that doctors take detailed medical histories from their patients and their patients' families. Doctors must know about other medical conditions the patient may have, about other medications the patient may be taking (including aspirin, alcohol, herbal supplements, and tobacco), and about the patient's diet and daily life. Doctors also must monitor patients who are taking medications to ensure that symptoms improve and to adjust dosages or change prescriptions if side effects occur.

What Are the Adverse Effects of Psychiatric Medications?

Adverse effects are unwanted side effects, and psychiatric medications can have serious adverse effects if not monitored carefully by a doctor. Depending on the medication, adverse effects may include:

- drowsiness or sleepiness at the wrong time of day, making it dangerous to operate machinery or drive a car
- restlessness or wakefulness at night
- headache, dizziness, or blurry vision
- dry mouth or increased thirst
- high blood pressure
- skin rashes
- nausea or vomiting
- unwanted weight loss or unwanted weight gain
- unwanted changes in thoughts or behavior, such as losing interest in dating, losing interest in creativity, or having suicidal thoughts that never occurred before
- seizures, especially if a medication interacts with certain foods or other medications
- muscle spasms, slurred speech, or a movement disorder called tardive dyskinesia.

The complex chemistry of psychiatric medications and the central nervous system also can affect other body organs and systems, such as the blood, bone marrow, thyroid gland, liver, and kidneys. MAOIs can interact with cheeses, wines, or cold medications to cause seizures. Some medications can interfere with a child's normal growth and development. Others can pose serious risks to pregnant women, nursing mothers, and their babies. Older adults who are taking multiple prescriptions are at particular risk for harmful drug interactions. Some psychiatric medications also can lead to addiction, withdrawal symptoms if the medication is stopped, and accidental overdoses. People who use psychiatric medications must see their doctors regularly and report side effects as soon as they notice them.

What Is Next in Psychopharmacology?

The science of psychopharmacology is less than 50 years old, and discoveries are still being made at a rapid pace. Researchers are developing new medications that target more than one neurotransmitter at the same time, which means that they can improve symptoms in multiple categories at once. Also in development and clinical trials are newer medications with fewer adverse effects, reduced risk of addiction and withdrawal symptoms, and less chance for tardive dyskinesia.

- haloperidol (Haldol)
- loxapine (Loxitane, Daxolin)
- mesoridazine (Serentil)
- molindone (Moban, Lidone)
- olanzapine (Zyprexa)
- perphenazine (Trilafon)
- pimozide (Orap)
- quetiapine (Seroquel)
- risperidone (Risperdal)
- thioridazine (Mellaril)
- thiothixene (Navane)
- trifluoperazine (Stelazine)
- triflupromazine (Vesprin)
- ziprasidone (Geodone)

Stimulants

- dextroamphetamine (Adderall, Dexedrine)
- methylphenidate (Concerta, Ritalin)
- pemoline (Cylert)
- mixed amphetamine salts (Adderall)

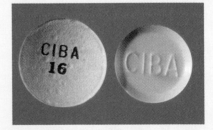

Methylphenidate (Concerta, Ritalin) is a stimulant. It often is prescribed to treat the symptoms of attention deficit hyperactivity disorder (ADHD). When misused, however, methylphenidate can harm the body in the same manner as other forms of amphetamine abuse. *Photo Researchers, Inc.*

Tardive Dyskinesia

Tardive dyskinesia (TAR-div DIS-kuh-NEE-zhuh) is one of the most distressing adverse effects of antipsychotic medication. It is a disorder of the neuromuscular system that causes muscle spasms and tics, which are involuntary movements affecting the eyes, tongue, face, neck, fingers, arms, toes, or legs. Tardive dyskinesia may disappear if the medication is stopped, but sometimes it becomes a chronic condition. People who develop tardive dyskinesia often continue taking their medication because the beneficial effects outweigh this very serious adverse effect.

▶ *See also*

Anxiety and Anxiety Disorders

Attention Deficit Hyperactivity Disorder

Bipolar Disorder

Brain Chemistry (Neurochemistry)

Depression

Obsessive-Compulsive Disorder

Psychosis

Schizophrenia

Tourette Syndrome

KEYWORDS
for searching the Internet and other reference sources

Amnesia

Alzheimer disease

Psychiatric medications are most effective when the people who take them work with psychiatrists and medical doctors to update their prescriptions as often as necessary.

Resources

Organizations

American Academy of Child and Adolescent Psychiatry, 3615 Wisconsin Avenue Northwest, Washington, DC 20016-3007. This professional organization for psychiatrists provides information about medications for children and teenagers.
Telephone 202-966-7300
http://www.aacap.org

American Psychiatric Association, 1400 K Street Northwest, Washington, DC 20005. The leading professional organization for psychiatrists in the United States offers expert information about medications.
Telephone 888-357-7924
http://www.psych.org

U.S. Food and Drug Administration, 5600 Fishers Lane, Rockville, MD 20857-0001. This government agency provides the latest information on new drugs and sound advice about the proper use of medications.
Telephone 888-463-6332
http://www.fda.gov

U.S. National Institute of Mental Health, 6001 Executive Boulevard, Room 8184, MSC 9663, Bethesda, MD 20892-9663. This government institute publishes an informative booklet for families called Medications (publication 95-3929), which also can be downloaded from its website in PDF format. It also posts many other fact sheets at its website offering safe and reliable information.
Telephone 301-443-4513
http://www.nimh.nih.gov

Memory

Memory is the ability to remember and to recall previous sensations, ideas, experiences, or information that has been consciously learned.

The Strange Case of H.M.

It is hard to imagine what it would be like to live without memory. What if the things that people had just seen, learned, or heard simply passed out of their minds after just a few minutes? So many of the activities of daily life, such as reading a book, watching a movie, doing homework, holding a conversation, making friends, and going to the store, would be totally impossible. People, places, and events would always seem brand-new, even if they had been experienced before. Living without memory would mean always having to exist in the present moment with no awareness of the past.

This may sound like a science fiction movie, but it actually happened. In 1953, a 27-year-old man, now known by the initials "H.M.," underwent brain surgery for his severe epilepsy*, a nervous system disorder that caused him to have daily seizures. The surgeons removed his hippocampi*, which are two parts of the lower brain, and portions of his temporal lobes*, which are the side parts of the cortex*. Doctors believed that these areas were diseased and causing H.M.'s severe symptoms. (Today, most cases of epilepsy can be controlled with medication, although sometimes surgery still is required.)

H.M. was cured, but with tragic results: He could no longer remember anything for more than a few minutes. He could remember events that happened more than 2 years before the operation, but new experiences or facts were quickly forgotten. In the more than 40 years that psychologists worked with H.M., his situation did not improve. He could remember a set of numbers or a new fact for a short while, but he would forget it as soon as he was distracted or new information was added. In fact, researchers had to reintroduce themselves every time they met with H.M., constantly reminding him where he was and why he was there. H.M. once said, "Every day is alone by itself," meaning that he could never make sense of today in terms of yesterday. He experienced time in separate chunks that were quickly erased from his mind.

However, H.M. could still learn parts of new motor skills or routines and repeat them at a later time, even though he did not remember that he had learned them. For example, he gradually learned how to draw an image in a mirror, solve puzzles, and mount cigarette lighters on a cardboard display. H.M.'s remarkable case illustrates the fact that there are different types of memory that involve different parts of the brain.

What Are the Main Types of Memory?

Memory is generally divided into two broad categories: short-term and long-term.

Short-term memory   Short-term memory is what a person uses for an activity such as remembering a new phone number after calling directory assistance. The person may repeat the number silently until dialing it, then promptly forget it. If distracted before dialing, the person may have to call directory assistance again. That is because short-term memory is fairly easily disrupted. Think about how students have to study new material in order to learn it, rather than just see it one time.

*   **epilepsy** (EP-i-lep-see) is a disorder of the nervous system characterized by repeated seizures that temporarily affect a person's awareness, movements, or sensations.

*   **hippocampi** (HIP-o-KAM-pie) are two parts of the lower brain that together look like a small pair of ram's horns.

*   **temporal** (TEM-por-al) **lobes** are the side portions of the cortex. They contain the sensory center for hearing and are centers for language function.

*   **cortex** (KOR-teks) is the top outer layer of the brain. It controls the brain's higher functions, such as thinking, learning, and personality.

Research has linked memory to the amygdala and to the hippocampus, two structures deep inside the brain. When surgeons removed the hippocampus from a patient known by the initials H.M., hoping to treat his epilepsy, they discovered that H.M.'s epilepsy improved but his short-term memory disappeared. H.M. could remember events that happened many years before, but not events of the previous day or the previous hour. H.M.'s doctors had to reintroduce themselves to him every single day. ▶

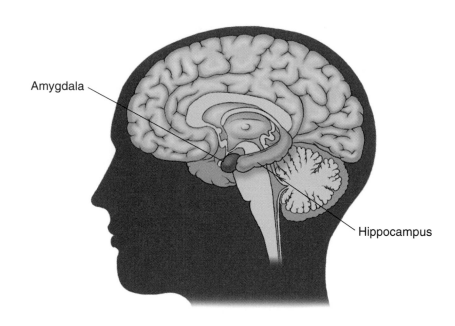

Amygdala

Hippocampus

Basically, they are converting the information from unstable short-term memory into more stable long-term memory by attending to it and rehearsing it.

People who experience severe head injury demonstrate how easily the process of short-term memory can be interrupted. For example, a car accident victim may not recall what happened just before impact or even during the accident itself. Some athletes who are knocked unconscious during an especially physical play may not remember what happened minutes before they were hit. This is because there was not enough time for experiences to be converted from short-term to long-term memory.

Long-term memory   Long-term memory, which is much more permanent and stable, can be further subdivided into two types: implicit and explicit. Implicit memory, or procedural memory, is the ability to repeat automatic tasks or procedures, such as riding a bike, driving a car, typing, or swinging a tennis racket. Of course, these tasks are not automatic at first; just ask any sixteen-year-old who is learning to drive. Over time, though, a person can perform the skill without giving it much thought. Explicit memory is recall for facts or events. This is what comes into play when taking a test, for example, or remembering someone's name. The patient known as H.M. lost the ability to turn new experiences into explicit memory but retained much of his procedural or implicit memory. Implicit memory appears to be controlled not by the hippocampus but by other parts of the brain.

The Anatomy of Explicit Memory

Thanks to H.M. and other patients who have had diseases affecting the hippocampus, scientists who study the brain now know that this structure and the nearby temporal lobes play a crucial role in turning what people hear, see, and experience into long-term memories. A Canadian neurosurgeon named Wilder Penfield also had a key part in identifying the importance of the temporal lobes in long-term memory. In the 1930s, while performing brain surgery on patients with epilepsy, Dr. Penfield used an electrical probe to stimulate different parts of the brain. Because the brain itself does not feel pain, the patients could remain awake during surgery. Dr. Penfield found that some patients experienced vivid events or scenes from their lives when he stimulated the temporal lobes. The memories were so vivid, in fact, that the patients thought they were actually reliving the experiences. Thus, 20 years before H.M. came on the scene, Dr. Penfield concluded that this part of the brain had a critical role in long-term memory.

Today scientists know that other parts of the brain are important to the memory process as well. The thalamus (THAL-a-mus), a structure in the middle of the brain, relays incoming information from our senses to the cortex. These structures together with the hippocampus coordinate facts with their appropriate time and space context to ensure that an event is remembered as a unique happening. In other words, today's breakfast is remembered as distinct from other breakfasts in the past.

What Else Affects Explicit Memory?

A person's emotions affect the process of memory, too. Experiences that make people feel happiness, sadness, or some other strong emotion are more likely to be remembered. For example, most people over the age of 50 can remember exactly where they were and what they were doing when President John F. Kennedy was shot in 1963. Scientists believe that the function of the hippocampus is somehow linked to that of the nearby structures that are involved in controlling a person's emotional responses.

Where do long-term memories go once formed, and how does a person retrieve them? Scientists believe that the entire cortex is involved in long-term memory, but exactly what happens to make or keep these memories is unclear. What is clear is that memories are not exact "videotapes" of an experience. Rather, memories are constructions that are filtered through a person's individual mental abilities and past experiences. Thus, two people seeing the same crime, for example, might remember the events somewhat differently. As a result, when people swear to tell the truth in court, it is only the truth that they have constructed from their memory, not literally "the whole truth and nothing but the truth."

Unable to Forget

Writing things down is an important part of the learning process for most people, whether it is to remember phone numbers and addresses, homework assignments, directions, or the teacher's lecture in class. But what if you had a memory so powerful that, when you encountered new information, you couldn't make yourself *forget* it? Such was the case with S., a man with a memory like a trap: whatever he came across, he could remember for life—and without writing down a thing.

S.'s unusual ability was discovered during his days working as a newspaper reporter, when he never took any notes at news briefings. When his boss became concerned, S recited back to him the briefing, word for word. S went on to work with a psychologist intrigued by his ability, and also became a mnemonist, or a person who demonstrates his extraordinary memory to an audience.

S. had a unique way of remembering that allowed him to experience information through several sensations, such as sound, touch, or taste. He envisioned numbers as forms, for example the number 6 as a man with a swollen foot, and the number 7 as a man with a mustache. Numbers also had textures and colors: the number 2 was a gray-white, and the number 8 a milky blue-green. These personal visualizations are what enabled him to absorb and store data with such extraordinary speed and permanence. After years of memorizing lists, tables, and other tests, S. could always recall anything he had ever learned. It seemed his ability was limitless.

In fact S. tried to invent ways to forget what he learned. It seemed that S. did not really have a short term memory, so he did not experience the usual memory decay. Everything he learned was put into long term memory which is a relatively limitless and permanent storage capacity. Did S. even remember how to forget?

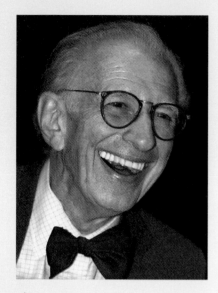

▲

Neuroscientist Eric Kandel received the Nobel Prize for Medicine in 2000. His research showed that learning and memory affect organisms on a cellular level, permanently changing individual neurons. This may help explain why counseling and therapy, even without medication, can help people change mentally, emotionally, and even physically. *AFP/Corbis*

Lessons from a Sea Slug

Many researchers believe that short-term memories are the result of on-going activity by brain cells, while long-term memories actually reflect structural changes in the brain. Basically, long-term memories are thought to be the formation of new connections from cell to cell in the cortex. Eric Kandel, who won the Nobel Prize in Physiology or Medicine in 2000, has found evidence to support this theory in what might seem like the strangest of places: the sea slug.

Because the sea slug has a very simple nervous system, with large nerve cells distributed up and down its body, it is much easier to study than a human. If the slug is touched, it reacts in self-defense by withdrawing its gill. Dr. Kandel found that, if he repeatedly pricked the slug's head or tail for a few days, it would withdraw the gill more quickly and sharply. This heightened reaction would occur even when the slug was touched again at a later date. It was almost as if the slug remembered what had happened to it before and reacted accordingly. Dr. Kandel was able to show that there were actually chemical and structural changes in the synapses (SIN-ap-siz), or connections, between the nerve cells that sense touch and the nerve cells that control motion. More neurotransmitters (noor-o-TRANS-mit-erz), or message-carrying chemicals, were released between these nerve cells, and the connections between them were chemically strengthened.

This is a very simple explanation of just one part of Dr. Kandel's research, but it is enough to show why this work is so important. Now that scientists understand how nerve cells communicate in sea slugs to form memories, they may be able to use this information to better understand how the human brain forms memories.

Resources

Books

Dowling, John E. *Creating Mind: How the Brain Works.* New York: W. W. Norton, 1998. Professor Dowling teaches a popular general education course on the brain at Harvard University.

Greenfield, Susan A. *The Human Brain: A Guided Tour.* New York: Basic Books, 1997. Dr. Greenfield, a professor who lives in Oxford, England, is well-known for her ability to explain scientific concepts in ways that most people can understand.

Kandel, Eric, and Larry Squire. *Memory: From Mind to Molecules.* New York: Scientific American Library, 2000. The authors are two of the scientists at the forefront of memory research. Their book explains some of the most important concepts of how memory works and what can go wrong.

Organizations

Memory Disorders Project at Rutgers University–Newark. This project involves neuroscientists, psychologists, and other researchers at Rutgers University in New Jersey who are studying how the human brain creates and stores memories. The website features easy-to-understand information about memory and memory disorders.
http://www.memory.rutgers.edu

Exploratorium, The Museum of Science, Art, and Perception: Memory Exhibition. From 1998 to 1999, this famous museum in San Francisco, California, hosted an exhibition devoted to the subject of memory. An interactive web version includes games and activities that encourage users to test their memory and even improve it.
http://www.exploratorium.edu/memory

Neuroscience for Kids. This website by a professor at the University of Washington features kid-friendly information about the brain and nervous system, including the functions of learning and memory.
http://faculty.washington.edu/chudler/neurok.html

▶ See also
Alzheimer Disease
Amnesia
Dementia

Mental Retardation

Mental retardation is a condition marked by significantly lower intelligence than the average for individuals of the same age and by delays in developing social skills, communication skills, and the ability to care for oneself and live independently.

What Is Mental Retardation?

The definition of mental retardation changes as researchers study its causes and develop new ways of understanding its effects. Current definitions focus on intelligence levels and on the skills and behaviors for everyday living that people develop as they grow.

Intelligence An intelligence quotient (IQ) is a test score that doctors and schools use to measure thinking, learning, and problem-solving skills. The IQ score for an average person always is set at 100. People who score above 120 are considered gifted. People who score below 80 are considered to have mental retardation. IQ scores define the severity of mental retardation using the following ranges:

- IQ 70–79: borderline
- IQ 55 69: mild
- IQ 40–54: moderate

KEYWORDS
for searching the Internet and other reference sources

Adaptive behaviors

Americans with Disabilities Act

Cognitive disabilities

Developmental disabilities

Individuals with Disabilities Education Act (IDEA)

Intelligence

- About 1 percent of the U.S. population has mental retardation.

- About 85 percent of those people fall into the mild to moderate range, which means that with the proper support they can learn to lead independent lives as adults.

- The other 15 percent fall into the severe to profound range, which means they are likely to need support with activities of daily living for most of their lives.

- Mental retardation affects people of all ethnic, social, and economic backgrounds.

- IQ 25–39: severe
- IQ below 25: profound.

A mentally retarded person is likely to be limited in most or all kinds of intelligence. The lower a person's IQ score, the more impaired his or her learning capacity is apt to be.

Adaptive behaviors   People with mental retardation are more limited than the average person in how well and how quickly they can learn to function in their environment. Limitations often involve language and communication, social skills, self-care, health and safety skills, leisure skills, the ability to live at home and/or in the community, and the ability to perform up to average standards in school or at work. This does not mean all people with mental retardation are unable to take care of themselves, however. Those with borderline mental retardation often are able to lead independent lives as adults if they receive extra support while they catch up to their peers in learning adaptive behaviors.

Mental illness   Mental retardation is not a mental illness. Sometimes people with mental retardation also have depression, anxiety, or other mental illnesses, just as people with average intelligence do. Oftentimes, though, they lead happy and healthy lives.

What Causes Mental Retardation?

Mental retardation sometimes has a genetic cause, resulting from one or more chromosomal abnormalities. Other times, though, mental retardation may be the result of problems during pregnancy that affect development of the fetal brain and central nervous system. Babies may be born with mental retardation if their mothers do not receive proper nutrition and medical care during pregnancy, if their mothers have infections during pregnancy or childbirth, or if their mothers are exposed to alcohol, drugs, or environmental toxins during pregnancy. Many different causes of mental retardation have been identified, but often a specific cause cannot be pinpointed for a specific individual.

Chromosomal abnormalities   Chromosomes are the threadlike structures in body cells that carry genetic information. Most cells in the human body have 23 pairs of chromosomes. Chromosome pair 23 determines whether a person is female (two X chromosomes) or male (one X chromosome and one Y chromosome) as well as other traits. Chromosomes 1 through 22 determine all our other traits and characteristics. Mental retardation may occur when a baby has an extra chromosome, an abnormal or partially missing chromosome, or a mislocated chromosome. The chromosomal abnormalities most often linked to mental retardation are Down syndrome and Fragile X.

DEFINITIONS CHANGE

Just 100 years ago, people with mental retardation were identified as "eternal children," "mentally deficient," "mental defectives," "imbeciles," and the "feeble-minded." Even doctors used those terms, publishing medical texts with titles such as *Mental Defectives: Their History, Treatment and Training* (1904), *Mentally Deficient Children: Their Treatment and Training* (1900), and "On the Permanent Care of the Feeble Minded," published in *The Lancet* medical journal (1903).

Fortunately, times have changed and so have attitudes toward people with mental retardation. We now know that many people with retardation can live meaningful, fulfilling lives, as long as they are in the right environment and get the extra support they need.

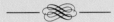

Down syndrome   Down syndrome results from an abnormality on chromosome 21. People with Down syndrome may have three copies of this chromosome throughout the body (trisomy 21), or they may have three copies in some but not all cells (mosaic trisomy 21), or some of the genetic material from chromosome 21 may have become attached to a different chromosome (translocation trisomy 21). The physical differences that may result from chromosome 21 errors include mild to moderate mental retardation, a flat facial profile, an upward slant to the eyes, a short neck, a single deep crease on the palm, and increased risk of hearing loss, vision problems, thyroid disorders, and heart disease. Chromosome 21 errors have been linked to a mother's age. The incidence of Down syndrome in the children of mothers older than age 45 is 1 in 20, while for children of mothers younger than age 30 the incidence is less than 1 in 1,000.

Fragile X   Fragile X results from an abnormality on the X chromosome. It affects girls (XX) about twice as often as boys (XY), but symptoms are more severe in boys, because boys do not have a second X chromosome to help counter the effects of the defective one. The physical differences caused by Fragile X may include severe mental retardation, autism, a large head, protruding ears, a prominent jaw, and large testicles.

Metabolic disorders   Sometimes called "inborn errors of metabolism," these conditions result from abnormalities in the genes that govern how the body produces and handles amino acids, proteins, enzymes, hormones, and nutrients. One metabolic disorder that can cause mental retardation is phenylketonuria (FEN-il-KEE-toe-NOOR-ee-a), which is linked to a lack of the enzyme needed to process the amino acid phenylalanine (FEN-ill-AL-a-neen). Other such disorders include hypothyroidism (HY-poe-THY-royd-iz-um), linked to an underdeveloped, underactive, or damaged thyroid gland, which is needed to produce hormones essential for normal growth and brain development. Many metabolic disorders can be detected at birth by a blood test and treated through special diets, medications, and hormone therapy. If treatment is started early enough, mental retardation often can be prevented.

Brain development disorders   Problems that interfere with fetal development of the brain, spinal cord, and central nervous system may result in mental retardation, making proper prenatal medical care and good nutrition essential for pregnant women. Factors that are linked to brain development disorders include the mother's intake of folic acid (a B vitamin) and her exposure to teratogens (toxins), such as environmental waste, alcohol, tobacco, street drugs, and even some prescription medications. Brain development disorders include anencephaly*, hydrocephalus*, spina bifida*, autism, and fetal alcohol syndrome. Many people with either spina bifida or autism have brain development disorders but are not mentally retarded.

Fetal alcohol syndrome   When a pregnant woman drinks alcohol or takes drugs (legal or illegal), these substances are transmitted directly to the fetus. Mental retardation that is linked to a mother's drinking is known as fetal alcohol syndrome (FAS). In addition to mental retardation, children with FAS may have attention disorders, learning disabilities, skeletal problems, and distinctive facial characteristics, including widely spaced eyes, a shortened or flattened nose, and abnormalities in the shape and placement of the ears.

Infections   Serious infections can harm a baby's developing brain before birth or during early life. Viral infections linked to mental retardation include cytomegalovirus (SIE-toe-MEG-a-lo-VY-rus) and the rubella virus, which causes German measles. Encephalitis (en-SEF-uh-LIE-tis) and meningitis (MEN-in-JY-tis), two infections that involve inflammation of the brain, also can cause mental retardation.

Other causes   Other possible causes of mental retardation include premature or difficult birth, severe head injury, and lead poisoning. In many cases, however, doctors cannot identify specific causes, particularly when the mental retardation is mild. Because mental skills and intelligence are defined statistically by their distribution along a normal (bell) curve and by their variance from an average defined as 100, there always will be some individuals who are classified as intellectually gifted (IQ above 120) and others who are classified as mentally retarded (IQ below 80).

* **anencephaly** (AN-en-SEF-uh-lee) is a condition present at birth in which most of the brain is missing.

* **hydrocephalus** (HY-droe-SEF-uh-lus) is a condition, sometimes present at birth, in which there is an abnormal buildup of fluid within the skull, leading to enlargement of the skull and pressure on the brain.

* **spina bifida** (SPY-nuh BIF-ih-duh) is a condition present at birth in which the spinal column is imperfectly closed, leaving part of the spinal cord exposed and often leading to neurological and other problems.

Diagnosing Mental Retardation

Chromosomal abnormalities and metabolic disorders often are diagnosed by doctors during prenatal testing or at birth. In other cases, however, a parent, caregiver, or teacher may be the first to notice that a baby or young child is not demonstrating new skills at the same pace as his or her peers. For example, the child may not crawl, walk, or talk by the expected age.

Using thorough physical and psychological examinations, doctors try to rule out other possible causes of the child's delays, such as hearing or vision problems, neuromuscular disorders, emotional or behavioral problems, learning or speech disorders, abuse, or a troubled home life. Pediatricians use blood tests, brain scans, genetic testing, and other medical tests to look for underlying physical disorders. Psychologists use developmental tests to help determine whether babies and children actually are behind peers, and they use standardized intelligence tests to compare the abilities of school-aged children to those of average children in the same age group. Psychologists also may observe the child at play, in school, and interacting with family members before making a diagnosis of mental retardation. Because developmental delays are not always linked to mental retardation, and because they may improve with physical treatment or changes in the child's environment, psychologists often schedule repeated evaluations over time to measure delays and assess improvements in intelligence and adaptive behaviors.

Living with Mental Retardation

Families Parents who learn that an infant or child has mental retardation often are shocked, and they may be overwhelmed by feelings of sadness, helplessness, or anger until they adjust to the news. Family counselors and support groups often are needed to help parents learn how to meet the special needs of mentally retarded children and balance those needs with other family responsibilities, particularly to siblings who also must adjust to the situation. To help children with mental retardation, many families work with a team of specialists that includes psychologists, speech and language pathologists, physical and occupational therapists, social workers, and special education teachers.

Children Children with mental retardation face many emotional challenges. They may know that they are "different" from their peers in ways that they may not understand. They may think that their families consider them a burden or an annoyance or a reason for shame, and they may be aware that they are "special needs" students in school. However, children with mental retardation can benefit from treatment and support in learning academic skills and the adaptive behaviors needed for everyday living. They also may get a boost in self-esteem by realizing that they, like other children, are unique and valuable individuals.

IDEA 1990

In 1975, the U.S. Congress passed Public Law 94-142, the Education for All Handicapped Children Act, which was renamed the Individuals with Disabilities Education Act (IDEA) in 1990. IDEA guaranteed all children with disabilities a "free appropriate public education." It said that children with disabilities should be educated alongside their nondisabled peers "to the maximum extent appropriate," a practice known as "mainstreaming." Since then, teachers, principals, parents, civil rights advocates, and even courts of law have debated whether or not students with mental retardation should be educated in the same classrooms as their nondisabled peers. Some argue that this practice places too great a burden on teachers.

In general, current policy favors including students with mental retardation in regular classrooms to whatever extent is possible. Under IDEA, every disabled child has the right to an annual, written individualized education plan (IEP) starting at age 3. Teachers, therapists, and parents work together to develop the best plan for educating the child, which may mean full inclusion in regular classes, partial inclusion supplemented by special education classes, or separate classes full-time. IDEA also ensures that children with special needs get free access to any education-related services they need, including transportation, counseling, and special therapy.

Special Olympics and Best Buddies

Since John Fitzgerald Kennedy became president in 1960, his family often has been in the spotlight. Some members of the Kennedy family have chosen to use their celebrity status to improve the quality of life for people with mental retardation, to honor JFK's sister Rosemary Kennedy, who was born with severe mental retardation in 1918.

Eunice Kennedy Shriver founded the Special Olympics in 1968, when she organized the First International Special Olympics Games in Chicago, Illinois. Since then, the Special Olympics has expanded into an international program of year-round sports training and athletic competition for more than 1 million children and adults with mental retardation. The program is designed to help participants develop physical fitness and motor skills, self-esteem, and a sense of community. In the United States alone, about 25,000 communities now have Special Olympics programs, and 150 countries worldwide also have accredited programs.

Just over a decade ago, Eunice Shriver's son Anthony started his own program to help the mentally retarded. Best Buddies is a mentoring program that pairs people with mental retardation with high school and college students in the community. More than 500 campuses in the United States, Canada, Greece, and Egypt now have a Best Buddies program.

To learn more about these organizations, visit their websites at www.special olympics.org and www.bestbuddies.org.

Adults Adults with severe or profound mental retardation requiring constant supervision often enter nursing homes or other residential facilities that offer intensive 24-hour care. However, the majority of adults with mild to moderate mental retardation can achieve varying degrees of independence. Because they may want or need some support and guidance, many continue to live with family members or in group homes, apartment clusters, or hostels designed especially for people with special needs. Some are able to hold jobs and participate in community events such as the Special Olympics, which can help them develop greater self-esteem. Others are able to get married and start their own families.

Resources

Books

Burke, Chris, and Jo Beth McDaniel. *A Special Kind of Hero: Chris Burke's Own Story.* New York: Doubleday, 1991. This book tells the life story of Chris Burke, a young actor with Down syndrome who starred in the television show *Life Goes On.*

Levitz, Mitchell, and Jason Kingsley. *Count Us In: Growing Up with Down Syndrome.* New York: Harcourt, 1993. Two young men with Down syndrome write about their experiences growing up with the condition and share their viewpoints about education, employment, ambitions, families, and marriage.

Organizations

American Association on Mental Retardation, 444 North Capitol Street Northwest, Suite 846, Washington, DC 20001-1512. Founded in 1876, this is the oldest and largest multidisciplinary organization of professionals and others concerned with mental retardation and related disabilities.
Telephone 800-424-3688
http://www.aamr.org

The Arc of the United States, 1010 Wayne Avenue, Suite 650, Silver Spring, MD, 20910. This is a national organization for people with mental retardation and related developmental disabilities. Its publications include *It's My Future!: Planning for What I Want in My Life,* a spiral-bound planning guide for adults with cognitive and developmental disabilities, and *Different Moms,* a video about parents with developmental disabilities.
Telephone 301-565-3842
http://www.thearc.org

U.S. National Information Center for Children and Youth with Disabilities, P.O. Box 1492, Washington, DC 20013. This national clear-

inghouse offers fact sheets, publications, resources, and referrals in English and Spanish for families and teachers.
Telephone 800-695-0285 (voice/TTY)
http://www.nichcy.org

Mood Disorders   *See* Bipolar Disorder; Depression

Multiple Personality Disorder   *See* Dissociative Identity Disorder

---

Munchausen Syndrome

Munchausen (MUNCH-how-zen) syndrome is a mental disorder in which a person pretends to be physically ill or produces the symptoms of illness in order to take on the role of a patient. In recent years, the condition has been classified as a "factitious* disorder" by the American Psychiatric Association in its Diagnostic and Statistical Manual of Mental Disorders. *Factitious disorders include pretending to be mentally ill.*

How Did Munchausen Syndrome Get Its Name?

The disorder is named for Karl Friedrich Hieronymus, Baron von Münchausen (1720–1797), a German nobleman, soldier, and huntsman who was known for making up exaggerated stories of his exploits and adventures. The disorder itself was not recognized and fully described until the twentieth century, however, when the simpler form of the name, "Munchausen," was applied to it.

What Are the Signs of the Disorder?

There are a great many symptoms that may be faked or produced in Munchausen syndrome. For example, a person may complain of abdominal pain, fever, rashes, bleeding, irregular heartbeat, dizziness, fainting spells, or seizures. These symptoms may appear to be signs of such disorders as appendicitis*, dermatitis*, anemia*, a heart problem, or a brain tumor, even though the person never actually had the symptoms they complained of.

▶ *See also*
Attention Deficit Hyperactivity Disorder
Birth Defects and Brain Development
Disability
Emotions
Fetal Alcohol Syndrome
Genetics and Behavior
Intelligence
Learning Disabilities
Testing and Evaluation

KEYWORDS
for searching the Internet and other reference sources

Hypochondria

Malingering

Somatoform disorders

---

* **factitious** means false. In this case it refers to an impression of illness produced falsely.

* **appendicitis** (a-pen-di-SY-tis) is a painful inflammation of the appendix, a small organ that branches off the large intestine.

* **dermatitis** is a skin condition characterized by a red, itchy rash. It may occur when the skin comes in contact with something to which it is sensitive.

* **anemia** is a blood disorder in which there are too few red blood cells to carry oxygen throughout the body. This condition can make a person weak and dizzy.

People with Munchausen syndrome often are very knowledgeable about medicine and hospitals. They may pretend to have a disease by complaining of a symptom, such as pain, that they do not have. Sometimes they exaggerate or imitate a disorder, such as seizures, that they really do have. Some people may actually injure themselves to create a symptom. For example, they may make themselves bleed to produce anemia. They also may describe an elaborate but false medical history to their physicians and demand medical tests and treatment with drugs or even operations. If the faking of people with Munchausen syndrome is discovered and they are denied treatment, they may start all over again, attempting to fool another doctor at another hospital. In some cases, this process may be repeated throughout a person's life.

What Causes Munchausen Syndrome?

The basic cause for the behavior of people with Munchausen syndrome is believed to be an intense need for care and sympathy. Why people with the disorder have this driving need differs for each person. Often, the disorder begins in early adulthood, after hospitalization for a true medical condition. Other influencing factors may include an important past relationship with a physician, medical employment, or even ill will harbored toward the medical profession.

Diagnosis and Treatment

The two main tasks for a physician diagnosing Munchausen syndrome are to determine that the patient does not really have the illness that the symptoms suggest and that he or she is not malingering. Malingering means that a person is pretending to have an illness because of some life situation, such as wanting to avoid military duty, work, or school.

Munchausen syndrome is treated with psychotherapy. The therapist attempts to help patients understand why they have an excessive need for sympathy, care, and attention. Therapists also help patients find more honest and less destructive ways to satisfy their emotional needs. In the meantime, attempts are made to protect the patient from having unnecessary operations or other medical procedures.

Munchausen Syndrome by Proxy

A variation of Munchausen syndrome, called Munchausen syndrome by proxy, occurs when a caregiver (often the mother) falsely claims that a child is ill. ("By proxy" means acting as a substitute for another.) The caregiver may either pretend that the child is ill or do something to cause a symptom or illness. For example, she may give the child too much of a laxative, causing diarrhea. Sometimes, causing illness may seriously harm the child or even result in death.

It is believed that people with Munchausen syndrome by proxy seek to gain attention as devoted caregivers rather than for being sick patients, as in Munchausen syndrome. They often have troubled marriages or may have suffered some type of abuse as a child. Munchausen syndrome by proxy is considered a form of child abuse, and in most states suspicion of this disorder must be reported to a child protective agency.

Resource

Organization

Selfhelp Magazine. This on-line magazine contains an article on factitious disorder (Munchausen syndrome) that describes a case and discusses treatment.
http://www.shpm.com/articles/chronic/factit.html

▶ *See also*
Abuse
Conversion Disorder
Hypochondria
Malingering
Somatoform Disorders

O

Obesity

Obesity (o-BEE-si-tee) is a significant excess of body fat. Children with obesity are at higher risk for obesity when they grow up. Adults with obesity are at higher risk for high blood pressure, diabetes, and other health problems. In cultures that value being thin, people with obesity also may experience emotional distress as well.

Prevalence rates for obesity are on the rise in the United States and in other parts of the developed world where lifestyles make it easy for people to take in more calories than their bodies use. How do people take in too many calories? Try fast-food burgers and fries, supersize colas, chips, dips, and nachos. How do people use too few calories? Try car rides instead of walking or riding a bike, and television and video games instead of sports. The result? Chubby couch potatoes who are banking extra deposits of adipose (fatty) tissue.

Lifestyle is not the only cause of obesity. Researchers believe that genes and heredity also play a very important role in many cases. People with a history of obesity in one or both parents are at higher risk of becoming obese themselves. People who have inherited "obesity genes" may use calories at a slower rate than others, or they may not have the same appetite "shutoff" control system that helps lean people stop eating when they have taken in enough calories. Also, people who become obese as children may increase the total number of fat cells in their bodies, making it much more likely that they will be obese as adults.

What Happens to People with Obesity?

Children Children who weigh more than 20 percent more than they should for their height and age may be considered overweight, and those who weigh more than 30 percent more may be considered obese. Diets that severely restrict calorie intake often are not a good idea for children because of their need for energy to support normal growth, but doctors may suggest that overweight children be offered fewer calorie-laden foods and find ways to become more physically active after school and on weekends. Certainly they are likelier than normal-weight children to have problems with their peers. They may have trouble keeping up with other kids in sports and other activities, they may tire and get out of breath more quickly, and they may be called cruel names.

KEYWORDS
for searching the Internet
and other reference sources

Adipose

Bariatrics

Binge eating disorder

Body mass index

Diet

Morbid obesity

Nutrition

Weight control

Body Mass Index

Body mass index (BMI) is a mathematical formula that doctors and dietitians use to measure whether people are at a healthy weight relative to their height.[†] It is based on weight measured in kilograms and height measured in meters: $BMI = kg/m^2$. BMI charts classify adult obesity in ranges; for example:

- BMIs 19–21: lean people, such as marathon runners

- BMIs 22–24: people of average weight

- BMIs 25–29: people who are muscular or mildly overweight

- BMIs 30–35: people who are overweight and who are at significantly higher risk for health problems

- BMIs >40: people with severe obesity who are at very high risk for health problems.

[†]Although BMI tends to reflect how much fat a person has, it does not measure body fatness directly. For

(continued)

example, a muscular athlete might have a higher than average weight and BMI measurement despite having a lower than average amount of body fat.

Rx: Weight Loss

The weight-loss industry is a big business, including over-the-counter medications such as Metabolife and organizations such as Weight Watchers. Unfortunately, many media-promoted weight-loss products and programs are based on fads or gimmicks that raise false hopes but have not been shown to produce long-term improvements in weight. Experts stress that weight loss produced by "crash" dieting is almost never sustained unless a person learns to permanently modify eating and exercise habits—and those lifestyle changes are difficult to maintain.

There are also prescription medications for weight loss, presently approved only for treatment of severely obese adults:

- Orlistat (Xenical) reduces the body's ability to absorb fat that has been eaten. However, it also can interfere with the absorption of vitamins, and may cause oily or fatty bowel movements.

- Subutramine (Meridia) is an appetite suppressant that affects the body's brain chemistry. It is not recommended for people with high blood pressure, heart disease, or risk of stroke.

Teens   Teenagers with obesity may have the same problems as obese children, but they also may start having aches and pains as the extra fat in their bodies stresses their joints and overloads their muscles and tendons. Obese teens, as well as some younger children, sometimes may begin to show some of the health problems commonly seen in obese adults such as high blood pressure and diabetes. Also, they may have less active dating and social lives, and they may be at risk for binge eating disorder.

Binge eating disorder   Binge eating disorder also is known as compulsive overeating. Like other eating disorders, it often involves feelings of anxiety, stress, anger, being out of control during a binge, and being remorseful after a binge. It also may involve hiding food and secret eating, behaviors that interfere with social activities. Eventually, it may lead to obesity, still another cause of stress in a culture that seems to believe a person can never be too thin.

Adults   In addition to aches and pains and physical limitations, obese adults face a higher risk of a number of health problems, including high blood pressure, diabetes, heart disease, and stroke. They may face discrimination when they apply for jobs or promotions, and studies have shown that they may be unfairly viewed by others as lazy or less intelligent. Adults with obesity often experience the inconvenience and frustration of needing large-size clothing, large-size movie seats and airplane seats, and large-size seat belts in a world designed by and for medium-size people.

Severe obesity   Severe obesity also is called "morbid" obesity because it is so frequently accompanied by serious health complications. People with severe obesity almost always experience problems with everyday living. They may have trouble walking or exercising, they may have difficulty breathing while they sleep (sleep apnea), and they may be treated with a prescription medication or gastric (stomach) surgery to help bring their weight down to a healthier level.

Is It Possible to Be Fit, Fat, and Happy?

Yes, it is, and there are many media role models showing how, including weightlifter Cheryl Haworth, model Emme, and actress Camryn Manheim. Working with peer support groups and therapists can help people learn ways to resist the stigma attached to being fat in a culture that values thinness. Working with psychotherapists can help people with binge eating disorder learn healthier ways to cope with anxiety and stress. Working with medical doctors can help people with severe obesity get treatment for related health problems, such as high blood pressure or sleep apnea, and it also can help them decide whether prescription medications or surgery are appropriate treatments. Eating a balanced diet can benefit everyone. And getting lots of physical activity can make anyone fitter and happier, no matter how fat or thin the person is.

Resources

Organizations

American Society of Bariatric Physicians, 5600 South Quebec Street, Suite 109A, Englewood, CO 80111. This group is a national professional society for physicians who specialize in the medical treatment of obesity and related conditions.
Telephone 303-779-4833 (for referral to a physician)
http://www.asbp.org

KidsHealth.org. The medical experts at the Nemours Foundation in Wilmington, Delaware, post fact sheets on their website for children, teens, and parents covering obesity, body mass index, eating disorders, activity patterns for children and teens, and other topics.
http://www.KidsHealth.org

Overeaters Anonymous, 6075 Zenith Court Northeast, Rio Rancho, NM 87124. This network of peer support groups helps people find local meetings that use fellowship and a 12-step technique for lifelong control of binge eating disorder.
Telephone 505-891-2664
http://www.overeatersanonymous.org

Weight-Control Information Network (WIN), 1 WIN Way, Bethesda, MD 20892-3665. This division of the U.S. National Institute for Diabetes and Digestive and Kidney Diseases provides information about obesity, weight control, nutrition, weight-loss medications, and gastric surgery.
Telephone 877-946-4627
http://www.niddk.nih.gov/health/nutrit/nutrit.htm

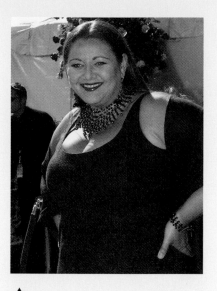

▲

Actress Camryn Manheim won an Emmy award in 1998 for her role in the television series *The Practice*. She has become a role model for people struggling with body-image issues in shattering the stereotype that a beautiful, successful woman must be thin. *AFP/Corbis*

▶ See also
Anorexia
Body Image
Bulimia
Eating Disorders
Genetics and Behavior
Therapy

Obsessive-Compulsive Disorder

Obsessive-compulsive (ob-SES-iv-kom-PUL-siv) disorder (OCD) causes people to become trapped in a pattern of repeated, unwanted thoughts, called obsessions (ob-SESH-unz), and a pattern of repetitive behavior, called compulsions (kom-PUL-shunz). Thoughts that feel impossible to control cause distress and anxiety (ang-ZY-e-tee) that is often neutralized, or offset, by the particular compulsive behavior patterns.

KEYWORDS
for searching the Internet and other reference sources

Anxiety disorders

Brain chemistry (neurochemistry)

Compulsion

Obsession

These PANDAS Are a Bear

PANDAS (Pediatric Autoimmune Neuro-psychiatric Disorders Associated With Streptococcal Infections) is a term for unusual, OCD-like symptoms that arise in a small number of children after strep throat, a common throat infection caused by bacteria. The behavior of the children usually changes quite suddenly. Almost overnight, they develop obsessions, compulsions, or tics; uncontrollable muscle twitches; or verbal outbursts. The cause is still unknown. One theory, though, is that a strep infection in childhood prompts the body to form antibodies (AN-ti-bo-deez), substances in the blood that fight bacteria and other foreign matter. The next time strep develops, the body is ready to fight back. It releases a barrage of antibodies, but some miss their mark and head for the part of the brain that is thought to affect behavior and movement—resulting in OCD symptoms.

*nervous system is a network of specialized tissue made of nerve cells, or neurons, that processes messages to and from different parts of the human body.

*genetic (je-NE-tik) pertains to genes, which are chemicals in the body that help determine a person's characteristics, such as hair or eye color. They are inherited from a person's parents and are contained in the chromosomes, threadlike structures inside the cells of the body.

Many people knock on wood to ward off bad luck. Others may walk around, rather than under, ladders, or they may step over, rather than on, cracks in the sidewalk. These are familiar examples of superstitions. Superstitions are irrational beliefs resulting from false ideas, fear of the unknown, or trust in magic or chance. Superstitions are common in everyday life. However, for people with OCD, rituals go much further than that. People with this disorder may feel driven to wash their hands until they bleed, count objects for hours on end, or go through a complex, 30-minute routine before leaving the house.

What Is Obsessive-Compulsive Disorder?

People with OCD can become trapped in a pattern of repeated, unwanted behaviors and thoughts that are senseless and upsetting but that seem impossible to control. The behaviors and thoughts can take up so much time and energy that people have trouble getting on with their daily lives. The problem often begins with disturbing thoughts, called obsessions. People then go through repeated rituals, called compulsions, in an effort to prevent these thoughts or make the distress caused by the thoughts go away. For example, people may wash their hands, count objects on a shelf, or check a door lock over and over again. For people with OCD, there is no pleasure in doing these things. There is only short-lived relief from the upsetting thoughts (for example, that the house will catch on fire or that a close relative is sick), which all too soon return.

Most people have a few odd habits. For example, they may check an oven to be sure it is off and then recheck it a few seconds later. Such behaviors are signs of OCD only when they take considerable amounts of time each day, cause much distress, and interfere with other activities.

What Causes Obsessive-Compulsive Disorder?

About 2 percent of adults in the United States have OCD in any given year. OCD usually begins during childhood or the teenage years, and it affects men and women equally. In the past, it was believed that OCD was due mainly to family problems or attitudes learned as children. Today, however, researchers stress the link between biological factors and life experiences. Brain imaging studies (special brain "x-rays") have shown that people with OCD have patterns of brain activity that differ from the patterns of people with other mental disorders and of people with no disorders at all.

OCD occurs more often than average in people with certain other conditions that affect the brain and nervous system*. For example, there is an increased risk of OCD in people with Tourette (tu-RET) syndrome, an inherited nervous system disorder that causes repeated, uncontrollable muscle twitches and verbal outbursts. Researchers now are trying to find out if there is a genetic* link between OCD and Tourette syndrome.

What Are Obsessions?

Obsessions are unwanted ideas or wishes that repeatedly well up in the minds of people with OCD. The thoughts create constant worry and fear. People who do not experience OCD believe that the worry is silly or strange. People with OCD also can agree that the worry is needless; however, they cannot stop feeling the worry that comes with the thoughts. Interestingly, thoughts and behaviors may not be related. The thought "I might get sick" could be followed by the behavior of counting to seven. Common obsessions include:

- worries about germs and dirt, for example, worrying about getting germs from shaking hands

- repeated doubts, for example, worrying about leaving a door unlocked

- worries about keeping things in order, for example, becoming very upset when things are out of place

- violent impulses, for example, thinking repetitively about hurting someone

- sexual impulses, for example, thinking repetitively about a sexual act.

What Are Compulsions?

People try to keep these unwanted thoughts in check with repeated actions that they feel driven to perform. Some people have set routines, while others have complex, changing rituals. The actions provide some relief from worry, but only temporarily. Common compulsions include:

- **Washing:** For example, people worried about germs and dirt may spend hours washing their hands.

- **Checking:** For example, people with repeated doubts about leaving a door unlocked may check the lock over and over.

- **Ordering:** For example, people worried about keeping things in order may arrange and rearrange the objects on a shelf.

- **Counting:** For example, people with disturbing violent or sexual thoughts may block them out by counting to 11 again and again.

Teenagers and adults with OCD know that their behavior is pointless, but the distress is so great that they feel unable to stop the behavior. At times, they may even start to believe their own unreasonable fears. People with OCD may be able to keep their behavior under control at school or at work for a while. They often are afraid to tell others, believing that they will be thought of as "weird." Without treatment, though, the problem may get worse over time. For some individuals, the constant worries and time-consuming rituals can take over their lives.

Compelling Reading

The word "compulsive" has more than one meaning in the mental health world. When people talk about obsessive-compulsive disorder, they are using the word in a formal way to refer to a specific kind of repeated ritual. When people talk about compulsive gambling or compulsive internet use, however, they are using the word in a less strict sense to refer to people who have an intense craving that is out of control.

*__serotonin__ (ser-o-TO-nin) is a neurotransmitter, a substance that helps transmit information from one nerve cell to another.

*__debilitating__ (de-BI-li-tay-ting) means making weak or sapping strength.

How Is Obsessive-Compulsive Disorder Treated?

Medications Studies have shown that medicines that affect a brain chemical called serotonin* can reduce the symptoms of OCD. While medicines may help control OCD, the symptoms may return once people stop taking medication. For this reason, doctors often recommend a combination of prescription medication and visits to a behavior therapist. Some individuals whose OCD is not significantly debilitating* might choose behavior therapy alone as the preferred treatment.

Behavioral therapy Behavioral (be-HAY-vyor-al) therapy helps people change specific unwanted behaviors. For OCD, this often means using an approach called exposure and response prevention. In this approach, people purposely are exposed to a feared object or idea, either directly or through imagination. Then they prevent themselves from carrying out the usual response (the compulsion), instead using other methods to manage the anxiety they feel. For example, people with a hand-washing compulsion might be encouraged to touch objects that they believe to be dirty. Then with the therapist's help, they resist the compulsion to wash for several hours. During this time, the anxiety associated with the obsession decreases and so does the compulsion to wash. Research has shown that this approach can be effective for treating OCD. People who remain in therapy may gradually learn to worry less about their obsessive thoughts, and eventually they may learn to go for long periods of time without falling back on their old compulsive actions. With exposure and response prevention, thoughts and compulsions frequently (and sometimes quickly) disappear or become manageable.

Resources

Book

Rapoport, Judith L. *The Boy Who Couldn't Stop Washing.* New York: Plume, reissued 1990. One of the first books to bring obsessive-compulsive disorder to public attention.

Organizations

Anxiety Disorders Association of America, 11900 Parklawn Drive, Suite 100, Rockville, MD 20852. This nonprofit group promotes public awareness of OCD.
Telephone 301-231-9350
http://www.adaa.org

Anxiety Disorders Education Program, U.S. National Institute of Mental Health, 6001 Executive Boulevard, Room 8184, MSC 9663, Bethesda, MD 20892-9663. This government program provides reliable information about OCD.

▶ *See also*
Anxiety and Anxiety Disorders
Brain Chemistry (Neurochemistry)
Habits and Habit Disorders
Medications
Therapy
Tourette Syndrome

Telephone 888-8ANXIETY
http://www.nimh.nih.gov/anxiety

Obsessive-Compulsive Foundation, 337 Notch Hill Road, North
Branford, CT 06471. This organization is for people with OCD and
others with an interest in the disorder.
Telephone 203-315-2190
http://ocfoundation.org

Oppositional Behavior   *See* Conduct Disorders

Oppositional Defiant Disorder

*A child whose behavior is overly hostile, negative, and puposefully dis-
obedient much of the time for a period of more than 6 months may have
oppositional* (op-po-ZI-shun-al) defiant* (dee-FY-ent) disorder.*

What Is Oppositional Defiant Disorder?

Oppositional defiant disorder (ODD) is a type of disruptive behavior
problem in children. Children with ODD often lose their temper, act
stubborn and willful, argue, and refuse to follow rules, and may annoy
others on purpose. Some oppositional behavior is quite common and
normal in children. Examples of oppositional behavior are refusing to
follow rules, directions, or requests given by adults in charge. While all
children may act in these ways occasionally, ODD is diagnosed in those
children who act in these ways frequently and whose oppositional behavior seriously interferes with their ability to get along with others in
school, on the playground, or at home. ODD can start as early as the
preschool years and can be diagnosed in children and adolescents of any
age whose defiant behavior is the cause of problems at home, in school,
or with peers. Children with ODD have at least 5 of the following problem behaviors to a greater degree than expected for their age for at least
6 months:

- become easily annoyed
- lose temper often
- feel and act angry and resentful
- argue with adults
- refuse to do what adults request

KEYWORDS
*for searching the Internet
and other reference sources*

Conduct disorder

Defiant behavior

Disruptive behavior

Oppositional behavior

* **oppositional** (op-po-ZI-shun-al)
is an attitude of going against
something or refusing in a
combative way.

* **defiant** (dee-FY-ent) is an attitude of challenging the rules
in a hostile way or of being dis-
obedient on purpose.

- actively defy the rules of behavior at home or in the classroom
- blame others for mistakes
- deliberately annoy others.

Children with ODD are often set in their ways (inflexible) and stubborn. They may have other problems as well, such as hyperactivity*, anxiety*, or depression. ODD is sometimes an early sign of another behavioral disorder called conduct disorder. Some, but not all, children with ODD go on to show signs of conduct disorder when they are older. While there are some similarities between ODD and conduct disorder, children and adolescents with ODD do not demonstrate the physical aggression or property destruction that is typical of those with conduct disorder.

What Causes Oppositional Defiant Disorder?

There is no single cause of ODD. Some experts believe that certain children may develop oppositional problems because they are less adaptable and overly sensitive by nature. For example, there seem to be some children who find it especially hard to handle frustration and who become easily upset even by minor things. When they are frustrated, such children have extreme difficulty coping and adapting. They may act very stubborn, defiant, and inflexible. Some children are more irritable and touchy by nature. They may be particularly upset by the way certain clothing feels or by tastes or smells, and they may act even more cranky, oppositional, and defiant when they are tired or hungry.

Family environment also can contribute to oppositional defiant disorder. In families where there is much conflict, harsh discipline, aggressive behavior, or inconsistent rules for behavior, children are more likely to develop oppositional defiant disorder because they are learning to relate to others in hostile, argumentative ways.

How Is Oppositional Defiant Disorder Treated?

Children with oppositional defiant disorder may work with a mental health expert. Often children with ODD are referred by their parents or by school personnel because their behavior is so difficult to manage. Treatment involves helping the child learn to handle frustration, develop more cooperative forms of behavior, and acquire more skills for solving problems and adapting to situations. Parents may be coached to make clear and simple rules for the child's behavior, to reward the child's positive behavior patterns, and to enforce consequences for the oppositional ones. When oppositional defiant disorder is treated early, more serious problems with conduct disorder may be prevented.

*__hyperactivity__ (hy-per-ak-TI-vi-tee) is overly active behavior, which makes it hard for a person to sit still.

*__anxiety__ (ang-ZY-i-tee) is a troubling feeling, a sense of dread, fear of the future, or distress over a possible threat to a person's physical or mental well-being.

▶ See also
Conduct Disorder

P

Panic

Panic (PA-nik) is a sudden surge of overwhelming fear that causes both psychological (sy-ko-LAH-je-kal) and physical symptoms. Panic disorder is a condition that leads to repeated attacks of panic that can strike often and without warning.

KEYWORDS
for searching the Internet
and other reference sources

Agoraphobia

Anxiety disorders

Panic attack

Panic disorder

Carla was riding her bicycle to school when a speeding car ran a stop sign. The driver slammed on the brakes, but the car kept skidding toward Carla with a sickening squeal. As Carla watched the car bearing down on her, she felt her heart racing, she broke into a sweat and couldn't catch her breath, and everything seemed to be moving in slow motion. For a moment before the car finally came to a stop, Carla feared she was going to die.

What Are Panic Attacks and Panic Disorder?

Carla was feeling panic, a sudden surge of overwhelming terror that causes both psychological symptoms, such as feeling that things are unreal or fearing that death is approaching, and physical symptoms, such as a racing heart, sweating, trembling, shortness of breath, chest pain, upset stomach, and dizziness. These feelings are the body's natural response to danger or stress. For some people, though, the feelings seem to arise from nowhere. They can occur in seemingly harmless situations, such as while taking a quiet walk or sitting in class. Panic attacks are bursts of intense fear or discomfort that happen, often for no obvious reason. They are part of many anxiety (ang-ZY-e-tee) disorders, in which needless fear becomes so intense and long-lasting that it causes problems at home, in school, at play, or elsewhere.

Panic disorder is a particular type of anxiety disorder in which people have panic attacks that strike often and usually without warning. The attacks are so unpleasant that many people live in constant dread of the next one. People may develop phobias (FO-bee-as), intense, unrealistic fears of certain objects or situations, about things linked to past panic attacks. For example, a boy who has had a panic attack during basketball practice might develop a phobia of the gym. As the problem gets worse, people may start to avoid situations where they believe they might have another panic attack. This avoidance may even turn into agoraphobia (a-gor-a-FO-bee-a), a condition that makes people find it hard

genetics (je-NE-tiks) is the branch of science that deals with heredity (traits inherited from parents), including the ways in which genes control development and behavior.

fraternal twins are born at the same time but develop from two separate fertilized eggs. Unlike identical twins, who develop from only one fertilized egg that splits into two and who look exactly alike, fraternal twins may not look the same at all or be the same gender. Identical twins have the same genes, but fraternal twins are no more likely to share genes than non-twin siblings.

nervous system is a network of specialized tissue made of nerve cells, or neurons, that processes messages to and from different parts of the human body. The brain and spinal cord are part of the nervous system.

to go beyond familiar places or even leave their homes. People with agoraphobia are terrified of having a panic attack in a situation where it would be hard to escape or get help.

How Common Is Panic Disorder?

About 1 in every 63 adults in the United States will have panic disorder at some point in his or her life. The problem usually begins during the late teen or early adult years, but children and older adults can have panic disorder, too. Women are affected twice as often as men. People with panic disorder often have other conditions as well, such as other anxiety disorders or depression.

What Causes Panic Disorder?

Genetics There are probably several causes of panic disorder. Genetics* may play a role in some cases, since panic disorder and other forms of anxiety can run in families. Also, research has shown that twins are more likely both to have panic disorder if they are identical twins rather than fraternal* twins.

Physical factors People with panic disorder may not be able to use the natural substances made by the body to reduce feelings of anxiety. Such people may have flaws in nerve cell structures in the nervous system* that bind to these substances.

THE MYTHOLOGICAL ROOTS OF PANIC

The word "panic" comes from the Greek term "panikos," which means "of Pan." Pan, the son of Hermes, was the Greek god of nature, of shepherds and their flocks (both goats and sheep), and of music. He was not an especially handsome example of a Greek god, having the upper body of a man and the hindquarters and horns of a goat. Nonetheless, within the woods where he made his home, Pan was known for chasing the ladies. The beautiful nymph Syrinx, in an effort to escape him, was changed into a stand of reeds. Pan plucked one of the reeds and made a musical instrument called a panpipe. When lonely travelers wandered through the wild woods at night, it was said that they heard the pipes of Pan in the wind whistling through the trees and were struck with dread and deep fear. This fear of Pan came to be known as panic.

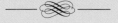

Psychological factors Other research suggests that it takes very little to set off the body's danger alarm in people with panic disorder. These people may have learned to overreact to normal body changes, giving rise to frequent false alarms. Some scientists believe that the faulty learning may be the result of repeated stress. Once people have learned to react this way, a stressful life event may trigger full-blown panic disorder.

What Are the Symptoms of a Panic Attack?

Panic disorder starts with panic attacks that can seem to come out of the blue. People can be struck suddenly by scary and uncomfortable symptoms, often including terror, a sense of unrealness, or a fear of losing control. These symptoms usually last several seconds, but they may go on for several minutes or longer. Confused by the unexpected rush of symptoms, people may worry that they are going crazy or suffering from a disease. Even when the most intense symptoms of panic have stopped, other anxious or nervous feelings may last for a while.

Symptoms of a panic attack may include:

- pounding or racing heart
- sweating
- trembling
- shortness of breath
- a choking feeling
- chest pain
- upset stomach
- dizziness
- faintness
- feeling as if things are unreal
- fear of losing control
- fear of dying
- numbness or tingling.

First panic attacks may occur when people are under great stress, such as when they are trying to do too much or when they have just lost a loved one because of death, divorce, or a move. A panic attack also may follow surgery or a serious accident or illness. In addition, overuse of caffeine or abuse of cocaine and certain other drugs may trigger panic attacks. Whatever the situation, though, first panic attacks usually take people completely by surprise. This is one reason they are so terrifying and most often remembered.

What Are the Symptoms of Panic Disorder?

Some people have a single panic attack or occasional attacks, but they never have a problem serious enough to affect their lives. For others,

Calming Yourself Down

Three things to do if you panic:

- Remind yourself that your feelings and symptoms, though very frightening, are not really dangerous.

- Rate your fear from 0 to 10. Notice how it begins to fall from the highest level after just a few seconds or minutes.

- Distract yourself from your panicky feelings. Count backward from 100 by threes, or snap a rubber band on your wrist. Distracting yourself from the panic will allow the feelings to disappear on their own after a few seconds or minutes, while focusing on the panicky feelings intensifies them.

however, panic attacks can continue and cause much misery. People with panic disorder have attacks so often that they start to live in constant fear of the next one. This "fear of fear" can become so intense and last so long that it greatly interferes with people's lives. Panic disorder tends to get worse over time if it is not properly treated.

How Is Panic Disorder Treated?

Early treatment helps keep panic disorder from reaching the stage where people experience severe problems in everyday life. With proper care, 70 to 90 percent of people with panic disorder can feel much better. Before treatment starts, a medical checkup can determine if there are other possible causes for the person's physical symptoms, such as an overactive thyroid gland*, certain types of epilepsy*, or problems with the rhythm of the heartbeat.

Medications   Certain medications can prevent or lessen the severity of panic attacks. When people find that their panic attacks are less frequent or less severe, they may worry less about future attacks, and they may be able to face situations they have been avoiding. There are several different kinds of medications doctors may use to treat panic disorder, depending on the person's age and condition.

Therapy   A treatment that often works well for panic disorder is cognitive-behavioral (COG-ni-tiv-bee-HAY-vyor-al) therapy, which helps people change specific unwanted behaviors and faulty thinking patterns. People are taught that thoughts such as "I am going to have a panic attack" can be replaced with thoughts like "This is only uneasiness. It will pass." They also may learn to use slow, deep breathing to help ward off the rapid, shallow breathing that many people experience during panic attacks. In another technique, the therapist may have people intentionally bring on some of the sensations of a panic attack. For example, people may exercise to raise the heart rate. Then the therapist can teach them how to cope better with these physical sensations. For example, instead of thinking, "I am having a heart attack," a person may be taught to think, "It is only my heart beating fast. I can handle it."

In this way, cognitive-behavioral therapy focuses on helping people learn to relax when they feel panic. People are taught to understand the thought processes behind their panicky feelings and the way the body physically reacts to stress. Then the therapist can help the person find ways to respond better when they feel the symptoms of a panic attack.

Resource

Organization

Anxiety Disorders Association of America, 11900 Parklawn Drive, Suite 100, Rockville, MD 20852. This nonprofit group promotes

---

*****thyroid** (THY-royd) **gland** is a gland located in the lower part of the front of the neck. The thyroid produces hormones, chemicals that regulate the body's metabolism (me-TA-bo-li-zem), the processes the body uses to convert food to energy. Sometimes problems with the thyroid gland can cause symptoms similar to those of a panic attack.

*****epilepsy** (EP-i-lep-see) is a condition of the nervous system characterized by recurrent seizures that temporarily affect a person's awareness, movements, or sensations. Seizures occur when powerful, rapid bursts of electrical energy interrupt the normal electrical patterns of the brain.

▶ *See also*

Agoraphobia

Anxiety and Anxiety Disorders

Fears

Medications

Phobias

public awareness of panic disorder and other anxiety disorders.
Telephone 301-231-9350
http://www.adaa.org

Paranoia

Paranoia (par-a-NOY-a) refers to either an unreasonable fear of harm by others (delusions* of persecution) or an unrealistic sense of self-importance (delusions of grandeur). While paranoia is often associated with a severe mental illness such as schizophrenia, people without such illnesses can have paranoid feelings, think that people are talking about them, or have difficulties trusting others.

John's Experience

One day John came across a group of his friends huddled together on the soccer field. As he approached, they were all talking and laughing and enjoying themselves. However, when he reached where they were standing, the group suddenly became quiet. John could not help feeling that his friends had been talking about him and that was why they had all stopped talking when he approached. He found himself thinking about this throughout the rest of the day. He even began to believe that his friends had been plotting against him.

The next morning, John saw the same group of guys huddled around his locker. This time when he approached, they shouted "surprise" and presented him with a new CD for his birthday. With embarrassment he realized that they had probably been discussing his birthday surprise the day before on the soccer field. He wondered what had caused him to doubt himself and his friends like that? Was it paranoia or a simple misunderstanding?

What Is Paranoia?

Paranoia is not a particular disorder so much as a way of experiencing (or incorrectly experiencing) reality. For example, John experienced paranoia when he wrongly believed that his friends were out to get him. A person whose phone was once tapped and was thereafter cautious about saying confidential things over the telephone might be considered reasonably concerned rather than paranoid. In contrast, a person who unrealistically feared that his or her phone was tapped even though it never had been before, and who persisted in the belief even when presented with compelling evidence that it was not true, would be considered paranoid. The key issue is not the behavior itself so much as its basis in reality.

KEYWORDS
for searching the Internet and other reference sources

Delusions

Mental illness

Paranoid personality disorder

Schizophrenia

* **delusions** (de-LOO-zhuns) are false beliefs that remain even in the face of proof that they are not true.

Common characteristics of people who tend to be paranoid include:

- poor self-image
- social isolation
- an expectation that others are trying to take advantage of them
- an inability to relax
- an inability to work with others
- a deep mistrust of others
- an inability to let go of insults or to forgive others
- a poor sense of humor

Like many personality traits, paranoia is something that can occur in different degrees of severity. In its milder forms, paranoia may be something that a person feels only occasionally or only in certain situations. John, for example, experienced paranoia one day, but he did not usually feel this way. In its more severe forms, however, paranoia can seriously limit an individual's life. People with significant levels of paranoia may consistently misinterpret reality and experience delusions. Delusions are classified as bizarre or nonbizarre. A person who believes that others are out to get him and are somehow monitoring his actions through the television set is experiencing a bizarre paranoid delusion; this type of delusion is called bizarre because it is completely unbelievable. An example of a nonbizarre paranoid delusion is a person's belief that he or she is under surveillance by the police; while the belief might be false, it is not out of the realm of possibility. Because everyone's experience of reality seems real to them, it is hard to tell individuals with paranoid delusions that they are not in danger. For a person with paranoia, minor hassles or mild insults may be seen as dangerous threats.

Even people with severe paranoia may function normally much of the time if, for instance, they have a paranoid delusion that affects only a part of their life. For example, they might become obsessed with the idea that a particular chain of restaurants is conspiring to poison unsuspecting customers like themselves. They might stop eating in those restaurants and even go so far as to call the health authorities to investigate while they still function normally in other parts of their lives.

What Causes Paranoia?

The cause or causes of paranoia are not precisely known. Many healthy people experience paranoid feelings at some point in their lives, just as John did. Certain situations may make it more likely for someone to experience paranoid feelings. For example, there is evidence to suggest that immigrants are more prone to suspiciousness and paranoia as a result of the language and other cultural barriers they face. People in the majority culture may misunderstand the immigrants' suspiciousness and react with hostility, which creates even more mistrust.

*temporal lobe epilepsy (EP-i-lep-see), also called complex partial epilepsy, is a form of epilepsy that affects the part of the brain that is located underneath the sides of the head, near the ears. Epilepsy is a condition of the nervous system characterized by recurrent seizures that temporarily affect a person's awareness, movements, or sensations. Seizures occur when powerful, rapid bursts of electrical energy interrupt the normal electrical patterns of the brain. Epilepsy is generally treated with medication that helps prevent these "electrical storms" from beginning.

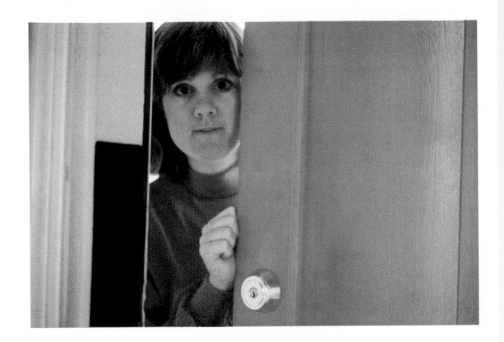

A paranoid person may feel extremely threatened by someone at the door, especially a stranger, and may keep her personal life private and hidden. *Custom Medical Stock Photos*

Paranoia can accompany a number of illnesses. It is associated with certain neurological conditions such as temporal lobe epilepsy* and some forms of dementia* associated with aging, such as Alzheimer disease*. It can be caused by the repeated use of drugs such as cocaine or amphetamines. Paranoia is also known to be associated with mental disorders such as schizophrenia (skit-so-FREE-nee-a) and paranoid personality disorder.

Paranoid schizophrenia Schizophrenia is a serious mental disorder that causes people to experience hallucinations*, delusions, and other confusing thoughts and behaviors that distort their view of reality. Doctors have come to understand that schizophrenia likely is the result of brain differences or chemical imbalances within the brain. However, schizophrenia is a complex and disabling disorder, and there is still much to learn to fully understand it. Schizophrenia is also a disorder that can assume many different forms. These forms (catatonic, disorganized, paranoid, undifferentiated, and residual) are known as subtypes.

Paranoid schizophrenia is characterized by the presence of one or more prominent delusions or auditory hallucinations in a person who seems to have otherwise relatively normal thinking ability and emotions. The delusions are usually organized around a consistent theme relating either to the idea that the person is being persecuted (someone is after him or her) or that he or she has special powers; the hallucinations, when they are present, are typically related to the delusional theme. People with paranoid schizophrenia often act anxious, aloof, angry, and argumentative, and they may also exhibit either a stiff, formal attitude or be quite intense in their interactions with others.

** **dementia** (duh-MEN-shuh) is a decline in mental ability that usually progresses slowly, causing problems with thinking, memory, and judgment. It is most often seen in older individuals and is caused by deterioration in parts of the brain.*

** **Alzheimer** (ALTZ-hy-mer) **disease** is a condition that leads to a gradually worsening loss of mental abilities, including memory, judgment, and abstract thinking, as well as to changes in personality.*

** **hallucinations** (huh-loo-sin-AY-shuns) are sensory perceptions that a person believes are real but that are not actually caused by an outside event. People who experience hallucinations may, for example, hear threatening voices (auditory (AW-dit-or-ee) hallucinations) that are not really there or see things (visual hallucinations) that others cannot see.*

None of the other major characteristics associated with schizophrenia, such as disorganized speech, inappropriate behavior, or inappropriate emotional reactions, are present in people with paranoid schizophrenia, and the age at which this disorder begins tends to be later than it is for the other forms of schizophrenia. People with paranoid schizophrenia are more likely to succeed in holding a job and at living independently when compared to people with other subtypes of schizophrenia.

Paranoid personality disorder   Just as there are several types of schizophrenia, there are also different types of personality disorders (for example, narcissistic, dependent, avoidant, antisocial, and paranoid). All of the personality disorders involve consistent ways of behaving inappropriately across many different situations. Personality disorders lead to problems in social, school, and work settings and to significant internal distress. The personality patterns that later develop into personality disorders typically begin during adolescence or childhood. The long-standing nature of these conditions makes them particularly difficult to treat.

The key characteristic of paranoid personality disorder is a pattern of deep distrust of others. Unlike people with paranoid schizophrenia, whose ideas may be totally bizarre or out of touch with reality, a person with a paranoid personality disorder is not out of touch with reality so much as out of step with it. The belief that other people cannot be trusted colors all of life. As a result, individuals with this disorder have difficulty forming close relationships.

Some common characteristics of people with paranoid personality disorder include:

- suspecting, without justification, that others are trying to harm or trick them
- doubting the loyalty of friends
- avoiding talking about themselves for fear that the information will be used against them
- interpreting casual remarks or events as threats or insults
- carrying grudges and seeking revenge
- overreacting with anger to minor slights
- being overly jealous and suspicious about others (e.g., girlfriend, boyfriend, or spouse) without justification

One of the difficult things about paranoid personality disorder is its self-fulfilling quality; paranoid people's suspicious and combative natures may provoke a hostile response from others, thus confirming their fears that others are hostile and not to be trusted. Rather than seeing their own role in creating the situation, they might instead mistakenly conclude that their suspicions are justified.

Possible signs of paranoid personality disorder that may be seen in childhood or adolescence include difficulties making friends and relating to others, the tendency to be a loner in social situations, and poor performance in school. Paranoid personality disorder is more common in males than in females. Overall, it affects about one percent of the population. The higher likelihood of finding paranoid personality disorder among relatives of individuals with schizophrenia suggests that there may be a genetic link between the two conditions, but further research is needed to confirm this.

Resources

National Institute of Mental Health (NIMH), National Institutes of Health, 6001 Executive Boulevard, Room 8184, MSC 9663, Bethesda, MD 20892-9663. The NIMH posts information about schizophrenia at its website.
Telephone 301-443-4513
http://www.nimh.nih.gov/publicat/schizoph.cfm

The Personality Disorders Foundation has a website that provides information about personality disorders, including paranoid personality disorder.
http://pdf.uchc.edu/

The National Alliance for the Mentally Ill (NAMI) is a nonprofit organization that provides education, support, and advocacy for people with severe mental illnesses and their families. NAMI's website provides information about many mental illnesses.
Telephone 800-950-NAMI
http://www.nami.org

▶ *See also*
Alzheimer Disease
Delusions
Dementia
Hallucination
Personality Disorders
Psychosis
Schizophrenia

Peer Pressure

Peer pressure is the feeling that people get from their friends to conform or behave in a certain way.

A person's friends may dress a certain way, comb their hair in a particular style, and have certain ideas about music and movies. Some teenagers may not share these opinions or adopt these fashions, but they may feel that they should. They may be feeling "peer pressure" and may think that to "fit in" they would have to adopt similar values, beliefs, and goals or participate in the same activities as their friends. Peer pressure can affect people of all ages. A 4-year-old who begs for a toy because her friends all have it is experiencing peer pressure. An adult who buys a luxury car because others in the neighborhood have luxury cars is responding to peer

KEYWORDS
for searching the Internet and other reference sources

Peer group

Social behavior

Social conformity

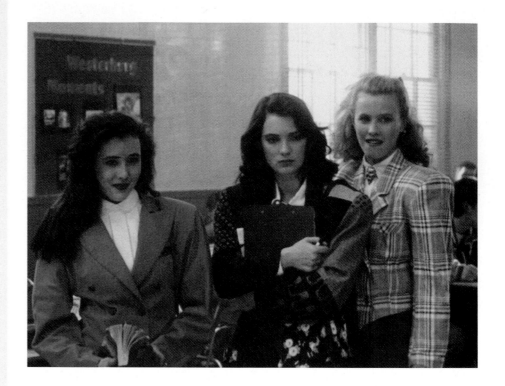

Heathers (1989) portrays a high school in which three girls, all named Heather, use their status as most popular to manipulate and ridicule other students. Veronica (center, played by Winona Ryder) finds herself caught between the Heathers and a rebellious loner at school who seeks revenge on them. *Photofest* ▶

pressure. Peer pressure, in itself, is neither good nor bad. It can encourage a person to study hard and get good grades or to skip school, get drunk, or smoke cigarettes. Peer pressure plays a particularly large role in the lives of teenagers.

In adolescence young people begin to break away from their families and try out different roles and situations to figure out who they are and where they fit into the world. They spend more time with their friends and less time with their families. This is a normal, healthy stage of development, but the growing distance between parents and their children and the increasing importance of friends can be a source of conflict and anger within the family. The desire to feel accepted and to fit in is one of the strongest forces in adolescence. It can lead teens to do things that they know are wrong, dangerous, or risky. On the positive side, pressure to keep up with the peer group can also inspire teens to achieve goals that they might never aim for on their own.

Why Do People Respond to Peer Pressure?

How much a person is influenced by peer pressure depends on many factors. People are less likely to be heavily influenced by their friends and more likely to make their own decisions if they have:

- high self-esteem
- goals and a positive outlook on the future
- good social skills

- the ability to interact with people from many different backgrounds
- strong connections to family and community.

People are more likely to be heavily influenced by their peers and less likely to make decisions for themselves if they:

- have low self-esteem
- are experiencing problems in their family, such as divorce, alcoholism, drug addiction, or unemployment
- come from families where there is little support or communication
- strongly identify with only one ethnic group
- feel distant from school and community activities
- are afraid of not belonging or fitting in.

How Can People Avoid Negative Peer Pressure?

"Just say no" has become a slogan sometimes used to tell youngsters how to respond when they feel pressure to drink or smoke or engage in a harmful activity. Is it a useful strategy to avoid peer pressure? It may be overly simplistic to expect people to reject peer pressure to participate in risky, dangerous, or hurtful behaviors simply by saying no. Different strategies work for different people, but some commonly successful strategies are:

- finding or inventing a reason to leave the scene
- treating the suggestion as if it is not serious or making a joke of it
- getting involved in a new activity with a new group of people
- getting help from a trusted adult (for example, a coach, counselor, or family member).

Social psychologists have studied peer pressure, examining how it can influence people to change their minds to go along with other's opinions. In one study, people consistently changed their answers from what they knew was a correct response to an incorrect response, just because others (who were part of the experiment) gave an incorrect answer. Experiments like these have also shown that people are more likely to stand their ground about what they know is right and stick to their original answers if just one other person joins or agrees with them. Such studies demonstrate that people can more easily resist peer pressure together, and gives new meaning to the conventional wisdom that the friends a person chooses really do matter. The best way for teens, or for that matter people of all ages, to make peer pressure a positive rather than a negative force is to select friends whose values, goals, ambitions, habits, and behaviors they admire and believe are constructive.

Resources

Books

Kaplan, Leslie S. *Coping with Peer Pressure.* New York: Hazelden/Rosen, 1997. A book for young adults that offers suggestions on how to keep peer pressure from controlling your life.

Scott, Sharon. *How to Say No and Keep Your Friends: Peer Pressure Reversal for Teens and Preteens.* Amherst, MA: Human Resource Development Press, 1997.

Spinelli, Jerry. *Wringer.* New York: HarperCollins, 1998. A fictional story about a preteen boy who faces the prospect of having to do something that appalls him just so that he will fit in.

Organization

Nemours Center for Children's Health Media, A. I. duPont Hospital for Children, 1600 Rockland Road, Wilmington, DE 19803. This organization is dedicated to issues of children's health. Their website posts articles for children, teens, and parents on peer pressure, friendships, and related topics. http://www.kidshealth.org

▶ *See also*
Bullying
Emotions
Families
Self-Esteem
Tobacco Addiction

KEYWORDS
for searching the Internet and other reference sources

Personality type

Personality

Personality refers to the collection of traits or characteristics that determine how people usually think and feel about themselves, relate to others, and react to the world around them.

The Neighbors

Dan is a warmhearted, energetic man who knows everyone in the neighborhood. He is always ready to lend a hand or a tool from his well-stocked garage. He loves to organize neighborhood activities. Dan hosts backyard cookouts, plans the yearly spring cleanup and planting of the neighborhood park, and serves mugs of hot chocolate when neighbors shovel snow from the walks in winter. People say that Dan is friendly, outgoing, and enthusiastic.

Pradeep, his next-door neighbor, has a quiet nature and prefers to keep to himself. Pradeep is always on time and very organized. He keeps to a set routine every day—he walks his dog at 6:30 A.M., has coffee and reads the morning paper at 7:00, and then heads off to work at 7:30. At 5:30 every weekday evening, he pulls into his driveway again. Early on Saturdays he shops for groceries for himself and for Mrs. Dunn, a neighbor who cares for her elderly mother. People say that Pradeep is shy, reliable, and thoughtful.

Rudy, who lives at the end of the block, annoys everyone with his grouchy mood and self-centered attitude. He scowls at the neighborhood kids who walk past his house, warning them not to step on his lawn and scolding them to keep the noise down as they get off the school bus on his corner. People say Rudy is selfish and has little patience and a bad temper.

What Is Personality?

The brief descriptions of these three men highlight some of the ways they are different from one another. They capture a few of the main characteristics of each man. These characteristics are what psychologists (sy-KAH-lo-jists) call personality traits.

Personality traits are the ways people usually think and feel about themselves (like insecure, self-centered, or humble), how they relate to others (like suspicious, critical, or friendly), and how they react to events (like easygoing, pessimistic, or short-tempered). Personality is a person's own special blend of these traits. Although each person has a unique personality, there are some groups of personality traits that produce common personality styles.

Some normal and common personality styles have been described with terms like self-confident, dramatic, sensitive, leisurely, adventurous, solitary, and aggressive. Personality style influences how someone will think, feel, and behave in most situations. Well-adjusted people also can adapt to situations that call for a way of thinking or reacting that is different from their usual personality style.

Some individuals have a personality style that causes them to have serious problems in most areas of their lives. Such individuals are set in their ways. They are inflexible and unable to adjust to the demands of a situation that calls for a different way of responding. Such a problematic personality style is called a personality disorder. There are ten different personality disorders that mental health professionals may diagnose. Personality disorder has a harmful effect on most aspects of people's lives, leading to long-term difficulties in relationships with other people.

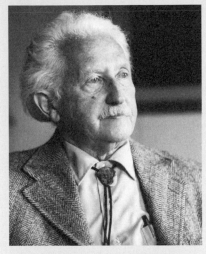

Erik Erikson (1902–1994), a Pulitzer Prize–winning psychoanalyst, was interested in the ways culture influences peoples' personalities. He is known for his term "identity crisis," which he used to describe an event in adolescent personality development. *Ted Streshinsky/Corbis*

▶ *See also*
Antisocial Personality Disorder

Personality Disorders

Self-Esteem

Personality Disorders

A personality disorder may be present when a person's usual way of relating to others, thinking about the world, and reacting to events causes him or her to have problems that interfere with important areas of life, including relationships with other people.

What Are Personality Disorders?

Personality, or personality style, is someone's usual pattern of thinking, feeling, and behaving. Personality style is made up of a number of personality traits or characteristics. A personality disorder is a problematic personality style that negatively affects most areas of a person's life. Personality disorders are diagnosed only in adults, but they reflect difficult personality styles that have been present since adolescence or young adulthood. Personality disorders can cause lifelong psychological problems and difficulty in relating to others.

There are 10 different personality disorders that mental health experts may diagnose. Each has its own set of characteristics, and each causes problems of a certain nature. The 10 personality disorders fall into three groups, called clusters, based on similarities in the personality traits of the disorders in each group.

One cluster includes personality disorders that feature unusual points of view or odd or eccentric behavior of various sorts. In this cluster are the following disorders:

- **Paranoid:** People with paranoid (PAIR-a-noyd) personality disorder distrust other people and may become overly suspicious, believing that other people's actions are always meant to harm them. Someone with paranoid personality disorder may find it difficult to form friendships, and may be very guarded, argumentative, or cold toward others.

- **Schizoid:** A person with schizoid (SKIT-zoyd) personality disorder is typically a loner and does not often show emotion. Such people will not make friends easily and do not even care to spend time with their families. A person with this disorder usually chooses a solitary job and activities and has very little, if any, social life.

- **Schizotypal:** People who have schizotypal (skit-zo-TIE-pal) disorder can be fearful and distrustful of others. They are usually unable to make friends outside their own families. They also can have strange beliefs and superstitions. Often, they will dress oddly or act in a peculiar way that does not seem to "fit in."

Another cluster includes personality disorders that feature personality styles that are overly dramatic, overly emotional, overly reactive, or unpredictable. In this cluster are the following disorders:

- **Antisocial:** A person with antisocial personality disorder is typically in trouble with the law and has no respect for the rights of other people. Such people frequently lie and cheat, and they try to take advantage of others for their own profit or enjoyment. They can be very irritable and often get into fights or even attack others. They also may be quite reckless and put themselves or others in danger, and they frequently do not understand or care that they have done something wrong or hurt another person.

- **Borderline:** A person with borderline personality disorder has difficulty being in relationships. People with this disorder fear that they will be abandoned, and the fear can become so strong that it makes them try to hurt or even kill themselves. Their relationships are often overly intense and they may be very demanding of the time and attention of anyone who is close to them. They may abruptly end relationships and can quickly and drastically change their views about their friends if they think their friends have let them down.

- **Histrionic:** Histrionic (his-tree-AH-nik) personality disorder makes people want to be the center of attention. To draw attention, people with this disorder can be very dramatic, often making up exaggerated stories about themselves. They flirt to attract people, and they may dress and act in a showy or overly sexy way. They may publicly exaggerate their emotions, perhaps through temper tantrums or fits of crying. People with this disorder can be too trusting of other people and too easily influenced by them.

- **Narcissistic:** People who have narcissistic (nar-se-SIS-tik) personality disorder are unusually self-concerned. They often exaggerate their talents and accomplishments. They think of themselves as superior to others, and they tend to imagine themselves as very wealthy or powerful or beautiful or intelligent. Because they feel that they are unique, they also need other people to admire them and to treat them as special. But they usually do not care much about the feelings or needs of other people. In fact, they often take advantage of other people to get what they want.

A third cluster includes difficult personalities that feature anxious, fearful, or extremely cautious behavior. In this cluster are the following disorders

- **Avoidant:** People with avoidant personality disorder fear criticism and disapproval, and for this reason they tend to steer clear of jobs or activities where they must work together with other people. They do not make new friends easily, and they typically are quiet and shy because they fear that other people will embarrass and make fun of them. They often feel out of place in social situations.

- **Dependent:** A person who has dependent personality disorder has a hard time making even small, everyday decisions, for example, what to wear. People with this disorder often rely on others to take care of them and make all their choices in life. When they are alone, they feel helpless, and they typically look around for someone to care for and support them.

- **Obsessive-Compulsive:** People with obsessive-compulsive (ob-SES-iv-kom-PUL-siv) personality disorder have a deep need for order and control. They pay close attention to rules, lists, and schedules, and they can be very hard on themselves when they do not meet their own high standards of perfection. Some may be incredibly neat and orderly, but others may tend to be pack rats, hoarding money or even saving worthless or unnecessary objects just in case they might need them one day. (Obsessive-compulsive personality disorder is not the same as obsessive-compulsive disorder.)

How Are Personality Disorders Diagnosed?

Personality disorders are difficult to diagnose. This is because many, if not all, of these sorts of traits also are found in normal personalities. A personality disorder is diagnosed only when a personality trait, or a set of traits, is present to such an extreme that it causes an individual to have problems almost every day in almost all interactions.

Several of the personality disorders have traits that overlap, making it difficult to tell one from another. Judging personality styles can be subjective, and different people may have different ideas about each personality style. Even experts may not agree about whether a certain trait in an individual is extreme or simply a variation of normal. Also, when some people have problems as a result of trauma or difficult events in their lives, they

▶

The ancient Greek myth of Narcissus tells the story of a beautiful young man who fell in love with his own reflection. So entranced by his image reflected in the water, he threw himself into the pool and drowned. The term "narcissistic," or conceited and self-centered, derives from this myth. *The Bridgeman Art Library International Ltd.*

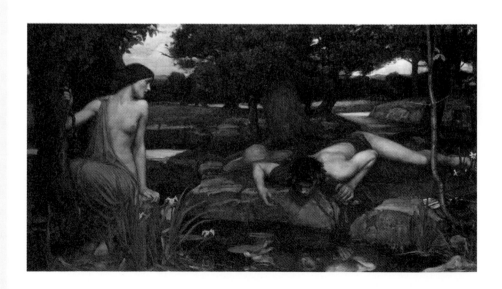

may appear to have problems affecting most parts of their lives. Generally, however, these problems are temporary. Researchers continue to work on finding new ways of classifying and diagnosing personality disorders that will be more reliable and accurate.

What Causes Personality Disorders?

Since each personality disorder is different, there are separate theories about how each one may develop. There is still much to learn about the factors involved in each of these disorders. Most theories focus on a combination of inborn* traits and early experiences that influence and shape how someone begins to think, feel, and act.

*__inborn__ means present from birth, or inherited.

How Are Personality Disorders Treated?

Because personality disorders can be so deeply ingrained and so long-standing, they are among the most difficult conditions to treat. People with personality disorders often resist change. Although some treatment methods can be effective, change may be slow and gradual. Treatment for personality disorders usually involves long-term talk therapy aimed at helping people understand how their particular pattern causes them trouble and then learning new ways to approach and solve specific problems.

▶ *See also*
Antisocial Personality Disorder
Personality
Therapy

Pervasive Developmental Disorders

Pervasive (per-VAY-siv) developmental disorders are a group of conditions in which the brain fails to develop normally, resulting in serious problems with communication, social interaction, and behavioral development.

KEYWORDS
for searching the Internet and other reference sources
Asperger disorder

Rett disorder

Autism

Childhood disintegrative disorder

What are Pervasive Developmental Disorders?

Pervasive developmental disorders are conditions that prevent children from developing normal communication and normal social abilities. Signs of these conditions begin to appear in the very early years of childhood. Some forms of pervasive developmental disorder (PDD) are milder and other forms are more severe. Most children with these conditions have very limited interests and activities, and some engage in unusual behavior, such as rocking, flapping their hands, or even behavior that causes self-injury.

PDDs include autism (AW-tizm), Asperger (AS-per-ger) disorder, Rett disorder, and childhood disintegrative disorder. The term "pervasive developmental disorder" refers to the whole group of conditions, but it sometimes is used to refer to milder forms of autism. The word "pervasive" means affecting all aspects of something. It is used for these conditions because they can affect all aspects of a person's life.

What Are the Types of Pervasive Developmental Disorders?

Autism is a brain disorder that affects children within the first 3 years of life. Sometimes these children may appear to develop normally for a time in early infancy. The word "autism" comes from the Greek word meaning "self." It was chosen for the disorder because of the characteristic self-absorption of people who have it. Indeed, children with autism appear to live in a world of their own, often seeming not even to notice members of their own family around them. They seldom make eye contact with other people or share their interests.

Children with autism are socially isolated. Their social problems are made worse by the fact that their language skills usually do not develop normally. Some children may never learn to talk. Others may talk, but they use language inappropriately, perhaps simply repeating the words of others or reversing the meanings of "I" and "you." They may repeat certain behavior, such as hand-flapping or body-rocking, over and over for no apparent purpose.

Asperger disorder is generally thought to be a milder form of pervasive developmental disorder, and it shares with autism the features of social isolation and lack of responsiveness to other people. The difference between Asperger disorder and what is called "classic" autism is that a child with Asperger disorder has the intellectual function and language skills of a normal child of the same age. In fact, children with this disorder often have excellent vocabularies, but do not use their language skills for appropriate conversation. Socially, they often lack good give-and-take interactions. They may memorize and then recite timetables or lists (for example, facts from almanacs) or have intense and very focused interests (for example, mechanical devices). A child with Asperger disorder may know the names and numbers of every Amtrak engine or be an expert on their town's fire stations. Also, their social interactions often revolve around their overly focused interests ("Which fire station is near your house?" may be a way to say "Hello").

Rett disorder is a severe genetic* developmental condition that affects only girls. At first, the child develops normally, usually for about 1 to 2 years after birth. She may even begin to walk and talk. Then she starts to lose these skills and may show signs of a stiff-legged walk. Losing the ability to use words to communicate, she also may lose interest in making friends. A typical physical sign of Rett disorder is that the child's head stops growing at the normal rate.

Childhood disintegrative disorder has signs that are in many ways similar to those of autism. An important difference is that in childhood disintegrative disorder a child may develop normally for 2 to 10 years. Then the child may begin to lose some combination of social or communicative skills, bowel or bladder control, or motor skills (physical coordination).

* **genetic** (je-NE-tik) pertains to the genes, which are contained in the chromosomes found in the cells of the body. Genes help determine a person's characteristics, such as hair or eye color, and they also are involved in the cause of some medical conditions. They are inherited from a person's parents.

What Causes Pervasive Developmental Disorders?

Rett disorder is now understood to be caused primarily by a faulty gene. The causes of most cases of autism, Asperger disorder, and childhood disintegrative disorder are not yet known. Because autism and Asperger disorder tend to run in families, it is believed that they are at least partly caused by faulty genes. Some authorities believe that childhood disintegrative disorder may be the result of damage to the developing brain, but it is not known how this damage occurs.

How Are Pervasive Developmental Disorders Diagnosed and Treated?

In order to diagnose a developmental disorder, a doctor or psychologist first asks the child's parents questions about the child's early development and then carefully observes the child to identify possible signs of impairment in social activities, behavior, and communication.

There are no cures for pervasive developmental disorders, but many children do improve over time. Early intervention is key to developing social and language skills. Therefore, prompt and proper diagnosis is important, so that well-planned special training and education can begin. Children are taught how to overcome the effects of certain impairments and to build on the skills they have. Medication may be used to treat special problems, such as seizures* or hyperactivity*. One key to treatment is the development of a communication system that can help children with their social skills. One communication system that has proven to be effective uses "picture exchanges." For example, if a child wants a drink, he hands the teacher a picture (symbol) of a drink. Pictures are gradually added together (picture of orange + picture of drink) and paired with words. Often, words then begin to replace the picture exchange system.

Often, children with these disorders can learn to attend to their basic needs such as self-feeding, dressing, and personal care. Many individuals with milder developmental problems learn to use language effectively and learn to relate well enough to gain some degree of independence (have a job; live in a group home) as adults. Some people with autism and Asperger disorder make rapid developmental progress in school and eventually may live by themselves.

Many individuals with PDDs, however, never lean to relate socially, develop a communication system to express their needs, or rid themselves of unusual behaviors such as rocking or hand-flapping.

* **seizures** (SEE-zhurs) are sudden attacks of involuntary (uncontrollable) body movements, changes in behavior, or loss of consciousness that result from bursts of abnormal electrical energy within the brain.

* **hyperactivity** (hy-per-ak-TI-vi-tee) is overly active behavior, which makes it hard for a person to sit still.

Resources

Books

Attwood, Tony. *Asperger's Syndrome: A Guide for Parents and Professionals.* Philadelphia: Jessica Kingsley Publishers, 1997.

Lewis, Jackie, and Debbie Wilson. *Pathways to Learning in Rett Syndrome.* London: David Fulton, 1998. Written for parents.

Seroussi, Karyn. *Unraveling the Mystery of Autism and Pervasive Developmental Disorder: A Mother's Story of Research and Recovery.* New York: Simon and Schuster, 2000. Written for parents.

Organization

Kidshealth.org, A. I. duPont Hospital for Children, 1600 Rockland Road, Wilmington, DE 19803. This organization is dedicated to issues of children's health. Their website has much valuable information for children, teens, and parents. For specific information on autism, go to http://KidsHealth.org.

| **Pharmacotherapy** *See* Medications |

▶ *See also*
Autism
Asperger Disorder
Rett Disorder

Phobias

Phobias (FO-bee-az) are unrealistic, long-lasting, intense fears of certain objects or situations. These fears can be so strong that people go to great lengths to avoid the object of their dread.

Sigmund Freud (1856–1939), one of the greatest psychological thinkers in history, was a psychiatrist and the founder of psychoanalysis (SY-ko-a-NAL-i-sis), a treatment method that focuses on deeply hidden fears and internal conflicts. One of Freud's most famous cases involved Little Hans, a 5-year-old boy who had a great fear of white horses with black mouths. After learning more about Hans and his family, Freud concluded that the horse actually stood for, or represented, the boy's father, a white man with a black mustache. Freud believed the boy was secretly resentful of his father but was too afraid to show his feelings. Instead, he "displaced" these feelings and developed an unreasonable fear of being bitten by a white horse. Freud theorized that phobias were actually displaced fears or conflicts. Modern researchers believe that the tendency for phobias may run in families and that many phobias are learned.

What Are Phobias?

People have long been fascinated by phobias, unreasonable, long-lasting fears of particular objects or situations. These fears can be so serious that

KEYWORDS
for searching the Internet and other reference sources

Anxiety

Fear

Social anxiety disorder

Specific phobias

people will severely limit their lives to avoid the object of their dread. Phobias can affect people of both sexes and all ages, although they are a little more common in women than men. About 8 percent of adults in the United States experience this problem, and many report that their phobias started in childhood. There are three main types of phobias: specific phobias, social phobia (also called social anxiety (ang-ZY-et-tee) disorder), and agoraphobia (a-gore-ra-FO-bee-a), which can be described as a "fear of fear."

Specific phobias People with specific phobias have a deep, unreasonable fear of specific objects or situations. Some common phobias include closed spaces, dogs, heights, escalators, tunnels, water, flying, and blood. The fear is not only extreme but also irrational. For example, a woman who is phobic about walking over a bridge may feel extreme panic in that situation, even though it poses no actual danger. Teenagers and adults with phobias realize that their extreme fears do not make sense, yet they are unable to control how they feel. Children with phobias usually don't realize that their fear is unfounded, and may believe, for example, that thunder is actually dangerous. No matter what someone's age, facing, or even thinking about facing, the feared object or situation brings on severe anxiety, an unpleasant feeling of fear or nervousness. To fend off anxiety, people often avoid what they fear. If the object or situation is a common one, this can limit their activities. To make matters worse, the more people avoid what they fear, the greater the anxiety becomes the next time they are faced with it.

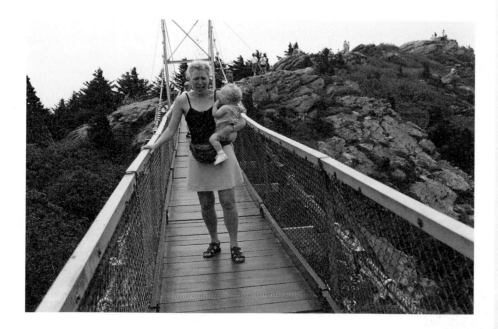

A woman walking over a bridge is seized by intense fear. *Owen Franken/Corbis*

Greek Speak

The word "phobia" comes from the Greek word "phobos," meaning fear. The tongue-twister names for a number of specific phobias have Greek roots as well. For example:

- **Acrophobia (AK-ro-fo-bee-a):** an abnormal fear of heights. The word comes from the Greek "akron," meaning "height."

- **Ailurophobia (ay-LOOR-o-fo-bee-a):** an abnormal fear of cats. The word comes from the Greek "ailouros," meaning "cat."

- **Algophobia (AL-go-fo-bee-a):** an abnormal fear of pain. The word comes from the Greek "algos," meaning "pain."

- **Autophobia (AW-to-fo-bee-a):** an abnormal fear of being alone. The word comes from the Greek "autos," meaning "self."

- **Cynophobia (SY-no-fo-bee-a):** an abnormal fear of dogs. The word comes from the Greek "kyon," meaning "dog."

(continued)

- **Erythrophobia (e-RITH-ro-fo-bee-a):** an abnormal fear of the color red or of blushing. The word comes from the Greek "erythros," meaning "red."

- **Gynephobia (GUY-neh-fo-bee-a):** an abnormal fear of women. The word comes from the Greek "gyne," meaning "woman."

- **Hemophobia (HE-mo-fo-bee-a):** an abnormal fear of blood. The word comes from the Greek "haima," meaning "blood."

- **Mysophobia (MI-so-fo-bee-a):** an abnormal fear of dirt and germs. The word comes from the Greek "mysos," meaning "uncleanness."

- **Nosophobia (NOS-o-fo-bee-a):** an abnormal fear of sickness. The word comes from the Greek "nosos," meaning "disease."

- **Pedophobia (PE-do-fo-bee-a):** an abnormal fear of children. The word comes from the Greek "pais," meaning "child."

- **Xenophobia (ZEN-o-fo-bee-a):** an abnormal fear of strangers. The word comes from the Greek "xenos," meaning "foreign."

*genes are chemicals in the cells of the human body that help determine a person's characteristics, such as hair or eye color. They are inherited from a person's parents.

*amygdala (a-MIG-da-la) is a small almond-shaped structure in the brain that plays a part in processing emotions.

Social phobia or social anxiety disorder People with social phobia (also called social anxiety disorder) have an extreme fear of being judged harshly, being embarrassed, or being criticized by others, which leads them to avoid social situations. Social phobia is much more than normal shyness. For example, people with social phobia may be afraid to eat in a restaurant, go to a party, answer a question in class, or give a speech. Some people have a broad form of the disorder, in which they fear and avoid almost any interaction with other people. This makes it hard for them to go to school or work or to have any friends at all!

Agoraphobia People with agoraphobia are terrified of having a panic attack in a public situation from which it would be hard to escape. For example, they may be frightened of busy streets or crowded stores. If left untreated, the anxiety can become so severe that people refuse to leave their homes. If they do go out, they may be willing to do so only with a family member or friend, and they may still feel great distress.

What Causes Phobias?

Classical conditioning Freud thought that phobias were caused by deeply hidden conflicts in the mind. One of his chief critics was John B. Watson (1878–1958), a psychologist and the founder of behaviorism, a school of psychology that focuses on how behaviors are learned and influenced by the environment. Watson answered Freud's case of Little Hans with his own case of Little Albert, an 11-month-old baby.

Watson wanted to prove that the fear of a particular object could be learned, so he showed the baby a white rat at the same time that he made a loud bang on a metal pipe. Before this, the baby had not been afraid of the white rat and had reached for it playfully when it was presented without the noise. Albert had, however, shown a fear response to the loud noise, as most children his age will do. After seeing the rat and hearing the loud sound together several times, though, Little Albert learned to fear the rat, even without the noise. This is an example of classical conditioning, in which people learn to associate a certain response (fear) with a previously unrelated situation or object (the rat). Given enough pairings of a fear response with a neutral, ordinary object, the object can become feared.

Biological causes Much research has focused on finding biological causes of phobias. A tendency to have phobias seems to run in families, as does the tendency to have anxiety in other forms. Studies have shown that genes* may play a role in some cases. In other cases, anxious family members may unknowingly "teach" others to be fearful or avoidant. Other studies have looked at the part played by the body's fear response, which is rooted in a part of the brain called the amygdala*.

When faced with real or imagined danger, the body sends signals to the amygdala, a part of the brain that connects memory with emotion. The amygdala "remembers" the fear associated with this situation or object and sets in motion the "fight or flight" reaction, physical changes that ready the body to react to a threat. The heart starts to pound and send more blood to the muscles for quick action, while stress hormones* and blood sugar flood the bloodstream to provide extra energy. In people with phobias, a scary experience, even one involving a harmless situation, can create a deeply etched memory of fear. With the help of the amygdala, this memory can trigger an automatic fear response when similar situations come up again, even if the fear is unwarranted.

> * **hormones** are chemicals produced by different glands in the body. A hormone is like the body's ambassador: it is created in one place and sent through the body to have effects in different places.

What Are the Symptoms of Specific Phobias?

Specific phobias cause intense, lasting fear that is excessive or unreasonable. The categories of specific phobias include:

- **Animals:** for example, dogs, snakes, or bugs
- **Natural world:** for example, storms, heights, or water
- **Blood or injuries:** for example, seeing a person who has been hurt in an accident or giving blood at the Red Cross
- **Situations:** for example, traveling through tunnels, crossing bridges, or flying in airplanes
- **Others:** for example, loud noises, choking, or getting a particular illness.

Phobias can start at any age. While it is normal for children to have several fears, occasionally childhood fears become so intense they are considered phobias. Some specific phobias that are common in early childhood (the dark, ghosts) disappear with time. Specific phobias that affect teens and young adults tend to be longer lasting. Only about one in five adult phobias goes away without treatment.

How Are Specific Phobias Treated?

If the phobic object or situation is easy to avoid, people with phobias may not feel the need to seek treatment. When phobias interfere with people's lives, however, treatment can become necessary and often is very helpful. The usual treatment for specific phobias is exposure therapy, in which people are gradually introduced to what frightens them until the fear begins to fade. At least three-fourths of people with phobias improve with exposure therapy. Some may be reluctant to try this at first, since it involves facing fear rather than avoiding it. Relaxation and breathing exercises also can help reduce anxiety, making it easier for people to participate in exposure therapy and face the object or situation they fear. In addition, medications to relieve anxiety sometimes may be prescribed.

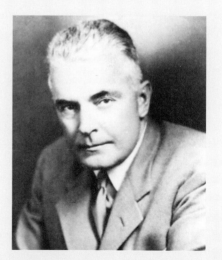

▲

The psychologist John B. Watson (1878–1958) is considered to be the father of behaviorism. He believed that human behavior depends not on the mind or feelings, but instead on our environment and experiences and how we learn to react to them. *Archives of the History of American Psychology, Photograph File—The University of Akron*

Resources

Organizations

Anxiety Disorders Association of America, 11900 Parklawn Drive, Suite 100, Rockville, MD 20852. This group is for people with an interest in phobias and other anxiety disorders.
Telephone 301-231-9350
http://www.adaa.org

Anxiety Disorders Education Program, National Institute of Mental Health, 6001 Executive Boulevard, Room 8184, MSC 9663, Bethesda, MD 20892-9663. This government program provides a wide range of information about phobias and other anxiety disorders.
Telephone 888-8ANXIETY
http://www.nimh.nih.gov/anxiety

www.healthfinder.gov, a resource affiliated with the U.S. Department of Health and Human Services, has an article printed in full called "Fighting Phobias, The Things that go Bump in the Mind" by Lynne L. Hall.
http://www.fda.gov/fdac/features/1997/297_bump.html

▶ *See also*

Agoraphobia

Anxiety and Anxiety Disorders

Medications

Panic

Social Anxiety Disorder

KEYWORDS
for searching the Internet and other reference sources

Abuse

Panic disorder

Traumatic stress

Violence

Post-Traumatic Stress Disorder

Post-traumatic (post-traw-MA-tik) stress disorder is a condition in which a person has long-lasting psychological symptoms after experiencing an extremely stressful event.

Jeff had never belonged to a gang, but a year ago, he was caught in the crossfire of gang violence. As he walked down the street, Jeff was shot in the chest by a boy who mistook him for a member of a rival gang. Luckily, the bullet missed his vital organs, and Jeff recovered without serious damage to his body. His mind did not recover as quickly, however. Several months after the shooting, Jeff began to have terrible nightmares reliving the experience. He felt nervous walking down the street, and would jump at the sound of any loud noise. He also started to have mood swings, shifting from feeling emotionally empty to being filled with rage. Around the first anniversary of the shooting, Jeff sank into a deep despair. At last, his parents took him to a mental health professional, who was able to help him finally deal with the trauma of the shooting and get on with his life.

What Is Post-Traumatic Stress Disorder?

Post-traumatic stress disorder (PTSD) is a condition that occurs in people who have lived through or seen a traumatic, or very stressful, event, such as war, natural disasters, serious accidents, child abuse, or rape. The traumatic event may be any event which involves the threat of death or serious injury, and to which the person responds with fear, helplessness, or horror. People with this disorder often relive the terrifying event again and again through nightmares and strong, disturbing memories. They may have trouble sleeping, and they may feel emotionally numb or cut off from other people. The symptoms can be severe enough and last long enough to cause serious problems in people's lives.

Who Is Affected by PTSD?

It is estimated that about 10 percent of women and 5 percent of men in the United States will have PTSD at some point in their lives, but this is just a small fraction of all those who have experienced a very stressful event. In women, the events most often linked to PTSD are rape, sexual abuse, physical attack, being threatened with a weapon, and childhood abuse. In men, the most common events are rape, war, and childhood neglect and abuse.

Children and teenagers can show signs of PTSD too. Researchers have found that the disorder is extremely common in young people who experience such violence as seeing a parent murdered or raped, witnessing a school shooting, or being the victim of sexual abuse. It is also very common in young people who are exposed to a lot of violence in their community. While it is unclear why PTSD develops in some people but not

Violence Goes to School

- More than three-fourths of students who see a shooting at school may experience PTSD.

- The overall rate of violent crime at school rose slightly during the 1990s.

- One-fourth of students have been victims of a violent act that occurred in or around school.

- One in four high school students say they worry about violence at school.

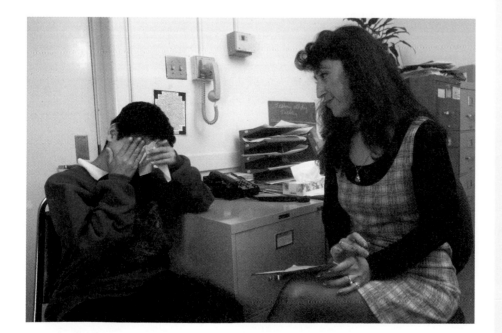

◄

The loss of a friend or loved one, a violent experience, or exposure to a horrifying event may cause a child to develop post-traumatic stress disorder. *PhotoEdit*

*hormones are chemicals produced by different glands in the body. They are created in one place and sent through the body to have effects in different places.

*cortisol (KOR-ti-sol) is a hormone that helps control blood pressure and metabolism, the process of converting food into energy and waste products. It plays a part in the stress response.

*epinephrine (ep-i-NEF-rin) is a hormone that is involved in the body's "fight or flight" stress response. It is also known as adrenaline.

*norepinephrine (NOR-ep-i-NEF-rin) is a hormone and brain chemical that affects blood vessels and plays a part in the regulation of emotion.

*opiates (O-pea-atz) are painkilling chemicals that can cause sleepiness and loss of sensation.

in others, at least one factor, a high degree of family support, lowers the risk of PTSD in young people.

What Causes PTSD?

Researchers are investigating factors that may set apart people who experience PTSD after a very stressful event from those who do not. They have found that people with PTSD tend to have abnormal levels of key hormones* involved in the body's response to stress. In particular, levels of cortisol* are lower than normal, while levels of epinephrine* and norepinephrine* are higher. In addition, when people are in danger, they produce high levels of natural opiates*, body chemicals that temporarily block pain. Scientists have found that people with PTSD keep making higher levels of these substances even after the danger has passed, which may account in part for the emotional numbness often seen in the disorder.

What Are the Symptoms of PTSD?

The symptoms of PTSD may be mild or severe. One person may become slightly cranky, for instance, while another may have violent outbursts. In general, the symptoms seem to be worse if another person caused the event that triggered PTSD. People may have more trouble with their feelings after a rape, for example, than after a flood. Common symptoms of PTSD include:

- reliving the event in nightmares or disturbing memories
- being very distressed by reminders of the event
- avoiding places or situations that bring back the unwanted memories
- trying to avoid thinking or talking about the event
- being unable to recall an important part of the event
- losing interest in things that were once enjoyed
- feeling distant from other people or emotionally numb
- sleep problems
- crankiness or anger
- trouble concentrating
- being easily startled.

Most people who have been through a very frightening event will have a noticeable reaction in the days and weeks just afterward. The diagnosis of PTSD is considered only if the symptoms last more than a month. The course of the disorder varies. Some people with PTSD recover within months, while others have symptoms that last much longer. Occasionally, the onset of symptoms can be delayed and may not show up until years after the stressful event.

What Are Flashbacks?

Among the most disturbing symptoms of PTSD are flashbacks, vivid waking memories in which people relive a terrifying event. Ordinary things that serve as reminders of the event may be the triggers. During flashbacks, people may lose touch with reality and reenact the event for minutes or hours. While having a flashback, people may think they see, hear, or smell things that were part of the original experience. For a while, they can believe that the awful event is happening all over again.

How Are Children Affected?

Young children with PTSD may experience less specific fears, such as being afraid of strangers. They also may start to avoid situations and become preoccupied with words or things that may or may not be linked to the stressful event. They may have sleep problems, and they may lose previously learned skills, such as toilet training. In addition, they may act out parts of the distressing event in their play.

Older children also may reenact part of the event in play or drawings. They may remember things that happened during the event in the wrong order. In addition, they may believe that there were warning signs that predicted the event. As a result, they may think that they can avoid future problems by always staying alert for such signs. Teenagers show symptoms similar to those of adults, but they are more likely to become aggressive or to make poorly thought-out decisions they later regret.

How Is PTSD Treated?

Cognitive behavioral therapy   Cognitive behavioral (COG-ni-tiv bee-HAV-yor-al) therapy helps people change specific, unwanted types of behavior and faulty thinking patterns. In one form of the therapy, people describe and mentally relive a stressful event under safe, controlled conditions. This lets them face and gain control of the fear that was overwhelming during the actual event. In most approaches, gradual exposure to the traumatic event is paired with relaxation in a supportive environment. With systematic desensitization, people start out with less upsetting events and work up to the most severe event, or they confront the stressful event one piece at a time.

Group therapy   In group therapy, several people with similar problems meet as a group with a therapist. This is often an ideal setting for people with PTSD, because it lets them get support and help from others who understand what they are going through. Group therapy may help people feel more confident and able to trust again. In addition, as people share their stories and tips for coping with the fear, rage, grief, and shame caused by their experiences, they may start to focus on the present rather than the past.

Shell-Shocked Veterans

About 30 percent of men and women who have spent time in war zones experience what we now call PTSD. In years past, a number of names were given to the emotional problems some soldiers had after returning from war, including:

- **Civil War:** soldier's heart
- **World War I:** shell shock
- **World War II:** combat fatigue

Play therapy Play therapy may help young children who are not able to talk about their feelings directly. The therapist uses play, games, and art to help children remember and describe the stressful event safely and express their feelings about it.

Medications Medications may help reduce certain symptoms, such as having trouble sleeping and being easily startled. They also may improve conditions that often occur with PTSD, such as depression and panic disorder, in which repeated attacks of overwhelming fear strike often and without warning. Among the medications that may help are antidepressants (an-tee-de-PRES-antz), drugs used for treating depression and anxiety.

How Can PTSD Be Prevented?

Some studies show that counseling people very soon after a disaster may prevent or relieve the symptoms of PTSD. For example, a study of 12,000 children who lived through a hurricane in Hawaii found that those who got counseling early were doing much better 2 years later than those who did not get counseling.

Resources

Organizations

Anxiety Disorders Association of America, 11900 Parklawn Drive, Suite 100, Rockville, MD 20852. This nonprofit group promotes public awareness of PTSD.
Telephone 301-231-9350
http://www.adaa.org

Anxiety Disorders Education Program, National Institute of Mental Health, 6001 Executive Boulevard, Room 8184, MSC 9663, Bethesda, MD 20892-9663. This government program provides reliable information about PTSD.
Telephone 888-8ANXIETY
http://www.nimh.nih.gov/anxiety

Center for the Prevention of School Violence, 313 Chapanoke Road, Suite 140, Raleigh, NC 27603. Based at North Carolina State University, this center works to inform the public about school violence and ways to prevent it.
Telephone 800-299-6054
http://www.ncsu.edu/cpsv

Emergency Services and Disaster Relief Branch, Center for Mental Health Services, Substance Abuse and Mental Health Services Administration, Room 17C-20, 5600 Fishers Lane, Rockville, MD 20857. This

▶ *See also*

Abuse

Amnesia

Anxiety and Anxiety Disorders

Depression

Medications

Panic

Rape

Stress

Therapy

Violence

government agency helps oversee national efforts to provide mental health services to victims of major disasters.
Telephone 301-443-4735
http://www.mentalhealth.org/cmhs/emergencyservices

National Center for PTSD, 215 North Main Street, White River Junction, VT 05009. This center, founded by the U.S. Department of Veterans Affairs, offers a vast amount of excellent information about PTSD in veterans and non-veterans.
Telephone 802-296-5132
http://www.ncptsd.org

Prozac *See* Medications

Psychoanalysis *See* Therapy

Psychological Factors Affecting Physical Condition *See* Somatoform Disorders; Stress

Psychosis

Psychosis (sy-KO-sis) is a broad term covering a range of mental illnesses associated with a loss of connection to reality. Illnesses that involve psychosis may severely impair a person's ability to relate to other people and to perform basic tasks of daily life.

What Is Psychosis?

"Psychosis" is a medical term used to describe serious mental disorders that cause a person to lose touch with reality. People with psychosis may have

KEYWORDS
*for searching the Internet
and other reference sources*

Delusions

Dementia

Hallucinations

Schizophrenia

* **delusions** (duh-LOO-zhunz) are beliefs that are false and have no basis in reality. People may think, for example, that someone is trying to harm them or that they have great importance, power, wealth, intelligence, or ability.

* **hallucinations** (huh-LOO-sin-NAY-shunz) are sensory perceptions without a cause in the outside world. People may hear voices or see things that are not really there.

* **dementia** (duh-MEN-shuh) is a gradually worsening loss of mental abilities, including memory, language, rational thinking, and judgment.

* **chronic** (KRAH-nik) means lasting a long time or recurring frequently.

delusions*, hallucinations*, or dementia*; they may lose the ability to speak coherently or to understand what others say to them; and their thoughts, feelings, and behaviors may be inappropriate and disconnected from the reality around them without their being aware of the disconnection.

Disorders associated with psychotic symptoms In some cases, psychosis lasts only for a few days or weeks (acute or brief psychosis), but sometimes it is a chronic* condition. Some of the disorders associated with psychosis include:

- Schizophrenia (SKIT-zo-free-nee-a) and related conditions, including brief psychotic disorder and schizophreniform (SKIT-zo-fre-ni-form) disorder, which are characterized by hallucinations or delusions and may lead to problems in daily functioning.

- Serious mood disorders, for example major depression or bipolar disorder with psychotic features.

- Alzheimer disease, a progressive disorder that affects the brain, most often in older adults, that usually causes dementia.

- Alcoholism, which causes many physical problems including liver disease and delirium tremens, a temporary condition involving hallucinations, delusions, fears, sweating, and discomfort, which typically occurs in the first few days after people with alcoholism stop drinking completely.

- Wernicke-Korsakoff syndrome (VER-ni-kee KOR-sa-kof SIN-drome), sometimes called Korsakoff's psychosis, which causes confusion, severe memory loss, and inability to control muscle activity, often resulting from advanced alcoholism or thiamine (a B vitamin) deficiency.

- Seizure disorders, which may temporarily disrupt the electrical patterns in the brain and the thought processes controlled by brain cell activity.

- Postpartum psychosis, a disorder that sometimes affects women who recently have given birth.

- Substance abuse, particularly relating to use of opiates, steroids, and hallucinogens like PCP and LSD.

Treatment Psychosis is a sign of serious illness, and people with psychosis must be thoroughly evaluated and should receive appopriate medical treatment. Treatment often involves medication and psychotherapy and sometimes requires that a patient be hospitalized.

Medical treatment for people with psychosis has improved greatly in recent years. Safer and more effective medications have been developed. There also have been many reforms to the laws that safeguard the rights and freedoms of people with mental illnesses, so that they no longer can be hospitalized against their will without a fair hearing and legal representation.

CULTURAL BELIEFS ABOUT MENTAL ILLNESS

The fact that definitions of psychosis and mental illness have changed over the years has led to debate about whether mental illness really exists.

The astronomer Galileo Galilei (1564–1642), for example, was considered to be mentally ill because he believed that the earth revolved around the sun during an era in which everyone else in his culture believed the opposite. Galileo's belief threatened the religious institutions of his day, and he was called before the Inquisition in 1633 and was asked to abandon his belief. When he refused to do so, he was condemned for heresy and held under house arrest for the last nine years of his life. Galileo was not mentally ill. Galileo understood that his culture did not accept his belief, but his personal commitment to scientific reality was more important to him than acceptance by his contemporaries.

British psychiatrist R. D. Laing (1927–1989) believed that mental illness was a form of withdrawal from reality that people chose when they no longer could tolerate situations that other members of their family or society found acceptable. He thought that "mental illness" was a sane response to an insane world. Laing believed that psychiatrists sometimes diagnosed mental illness when the true problems were in fact rebellion and a refusal to live in an unlivable situation. Laing's publications include *Sanity, Madness, and the Family; Self and Others; The Divided Self;* and *The Politics of Experience.*

American psychologist Thomas Szasz (b. 1920) believes that mental illness is a metaphor for thoughts, feelings, and behaviors of which society disapproves. His well-known book *The Myth of Mental Illness* holds that society uses "mental illness" as a label to control people, forcing them to accept unwanted treatment and hospitalization. Dr. Szasz believes that all medical treatment must be voluntary.

While it is certainly true that medical diagnoses sometimes have been misused for social control, most mental health professionals today do not agree with Laing and Szasz that mental illness is a myth, metaphor, or chosen response. To believe this would be to deny a biological basis for many instances of mental illness and to deny the pain, disorientation, and fear that people with mental illnesses experience.

People with psychosis are seriously ill with medical conditions that affect their thoughts, feelings, and ability to understand reality, sometimes even the reality that they need medical treatment. In fact, many patients later thank those who insisted they receive treatment, because when they recover they recognize that their illness had been affecting their thinking.

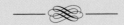

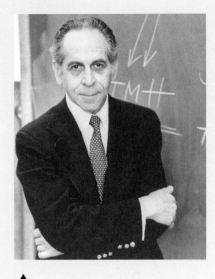

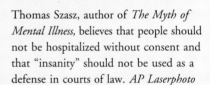

Thomas Szasz, author of *The Myth of Mental Illness,* believes that people should not be hospitalized without consent and that "insanity" should not be used as a defense in courts of law. *AP Laserphoto*

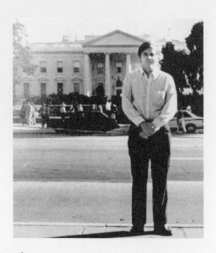

▲

John Hinckley, Jr., tried to assassinate President Ronald Reagan in 1981. In 1982, a Washington, D.C., jury determined that he was "not guilty by reason of insanity." *Ted Streshinsky/Corbis*

Psychosis and the "Insanity Defense"

Our legal system rests on the notion of personal responsibility. To find a person guilty of a crime requires proof that the person committed the crime and that he or she can be found blameworthy. When might a person not be found at fault? One clear case where the law allows for a verdict of innocence, even when a crime has been committed, is when the crime was done in self-defense. The other extreme circumstance that might "excuse" a crime often is called the "insanity defense."

Psychosis is a medical term involving illnesses that cause people to lose touch with reality. *Insanity* is a legal term used to determine whether there are some mental states that limit people's ability to understand their actions so severely that they cannot be held accountable for those actions. Legal tests for determining sanity during court trials using the insanity defense usually focus on whether the people on trial understood what they were doing when they committed crimes, understood the difference between right and wrong, and were able to control their own behavior.

At present, the legal test for insanity varies from location to location. Some states use the British "M'Naghten Rule," named after Daniel M'Naghten, who attempted a political assassination in England in 1843. Other states use the American Law Institute (ALI) Test, also called the Model Penal Code. The ALI test was used during the 1982 trial of John Hinckley, Jr., who attempted to assassinate President Ronald Reagan in 1981. When Hinckley was found "not guilty by reason of insanity," a political backlash occurred, and the U.S. Congress introduced the legal concept of "guilty, but mentally ill."

The American Psychiatric Association (APA), the medical group that publishes standards for classifying mental illnesses and supports research about their treatment, does not use the legal term *insanity*. The APA maintains that psychiatrists may testify in court to help trial participants understand mental illness and psychosis, but that questions of innocence, guilt, and moral responsibility need to be left to judges and juries.

Resources

Organizations

U.S. National Institute of Mental Health, 6001 Executive Boulevard, Room 8184, MSC 9663, Bethesda, MD 20892-9663. This division of the National Institutes of Health oversees research on mental disorders and provides information for professionals and the public. Telephone 301-443-4513 http://www.nimh.nih.gov

American Psychiatric Association, 1400 K Street NW, Washington, DC 20005. An organization of physicians that publishes the *Diagnostic and*

Statistical Manual of Mental Disorders, a guide to the definitions of various disorders. This group also publishes the *Let's Talk Facts* pamphlet series for the public.
Telephone 888-357-7924
http://www.psych.org

American Academy of Psychiatry and the Law, P.O. Box 30, One Regency Drive, Bloomfield, CT, 06002-0030. This organization promotes scientific and educational research in how psychiatry is applied to legal issues (forensic psychiatry).
Telephone 800-331-1389
http://www.aapl.org

National Alliance for the Mentally Ill, Colonial Place Three, 2107 Wilson Blvd., Suite 300, Arlington, VA 22201-3042. An information, advocacy, and support organization for people with serious mental illnesses and their families and friends.
Telephone 800-950-NAMI or 703-524-7600
http://www.nami.org

▶ *See also*
Alcoholism
Alzheimer Disease
Bipolar Disorder
Delusions
Depression
Hallucination
Medications
Schizophrenia
Substance Abuse

Psychotherapy   *See* Therapy

R

Rape

Rape is forced, unwanted sexual intercourse. Rape can happen to males or females, children or adults or elders, healthy people or people with disabilities. Rape is a crime even if the rapist is an acquaintance, a friend, or a member of the family.

What Is Rape?

Rape is forced, unwanted sexual intercourse involving the genitals or any other part of the body. Rape also is called sexual assault. It is an act of violence; it is not a form of consensual sex*, love, or intimacy. Being a rapist does not always mean that a person is mentally ill. Committing a rape is a criminal act. Rape and sexual assault may be committed against females or males; children or elders; wives, dates, or intimate partners. Many rapes are never reported to the police. Rape may be committed by a stranger, but often it is committed by someone known to the person who has been raped. Sometimes physical force is used during a rape. Other times there may be intimidation. Sometimes rape occurs when the victim is drugged, drunk, or otherwise unable to respond.

What Is the Treatment for Rape?

People who have been raped may want to keep the assault secret. They may be upset, confused, and even embarrassed, perhaps mistakenly thinking that they were responsible for the attack. But it is very important that they go to a clinic or hospital emergency room immediately, before showering or changing clothing. Immediate medical examination is necessary to treat injuries, to allow for further medical evaluation, and to gather evidence of the crime. "Rape kit" evidence may include body fluids like saliva or semen* from the rapist or samples of the rapist's hair or clothing. Continuing medical care is necessary to prevent or treat sexually transmitted diseases or pregnancy. Emotional care also is important. Rape crisis workers who understand the trauma that rape can cause often are on hand to provide help, support, and referrals for counseling to aid in emotional recovery from the effects of the rape.

KEYWORDS
for searching the Internet and other reference sources

Acquaintance rape

Child sexual abuse

Date rape

Rape trauma syndrome

Sexual assault

*****consensual sex** is sexual activity in which both people freely agree to participate.

*****semen** is the fluid that carries the sperm produced in the testicles, the male reproductive organs. Sperm are tiny, tadpole-like cells that can unite with a female's egg to result in pregnancy.

Who? Whom? How Often?

The U.S. Centers for Disease Control and Prevention report the following statistics about rape and sexual assault:

- More than 80 percent of people who have been raped do not report the assault to the police.

- Among people who do report the assault to the police, 40 percent are younger than age 18, and 15 percent are younger than age 12.

- Approximately 50 percent of rapes against women are committed by friends or acquaintances, not by strangers

(continued)

- Approximately 25 percent of rapes against women are committed by intimate partners, dates, or husbands.

- More than 25 percent of women in college experience sexual violence that meets the legal definition for rape or attempted rape.

- More than 7 percent of men in college report aggressive sexual behavior that meets the legal definition for rape or attempted rape.

- Women who have been raped experience physical injuries in approximately 40 percent of cases, need to be hospitalized overnight in 3 percent of cases, contract a sexually transmitted disease in 4 percent of cases, and become pregnant in 4 percent of cases.

- Death occurs in approximately 0.1 percent of all rape cases.

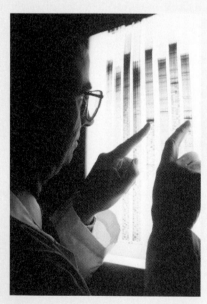

People who have been raped need immediate attention at a clinic or hospital for medical treatment and for the collection of evidence of the crime. Rape kit evidence may include saliva or semen, which can be used to determine the rapist's DNA "fingerprint." *Visuals Unlimited, Inc.*

What Is Rape Trauma Syndrome?

Rape trauma syndrome is a form of post-traumatic stress disorder. In addition to physical distress, people who have been raped may experience psychological symptoms that can include:

- emotional numbness
- alert watchfulness or jumpiness
- sleep disturbances
- nightmares
- disturbing memories (flashbacks) of the sexual assault
- avoidance of healthy sexual activity
- increased levels of alcohol or drug use
- feelings of helplessness, powerlessness, and hopelessness
- depression
- school failure
- suicidal feelings

People who are raped by acquaintances, dates, or family members may experience symptoms that are different from those of people who are raped by strangers. In such cases, in addition to the actual trauma of rape, there is the added trauma of loss of trust. Rape by a stranger may involve a weapon or other types of violence. When people who are raped also fear for their lives, it increases the likelihood of post-traumatic stress disorder. Some symptoms of rape trauma may ease with the passage of time, but often the help of a therapist or support group is necessary for more complete emotional healing to take place.

Prevention of Rape

Important steps toward rape prevention include avoiding alcohol and drugs that can lead to irresponsible or dangerous behavior, always discussing sexual activities with a partner and obtaining agreement about what will happen. It is also important to have friends or family members know details about a date, for example, where the date will take place and the date's name. Speak up or stop a situation whenever abusive sexual behaviors are witnessed. Programs to prevent rape may involve male mentors counseling young men.

Resources

Books

Anderson, Laurie Halse. *Speak.* New York: Puffin Books, 2001.

Draper, Sharon Mills. *Darkness Before Dawn.* New York: Simon and Schuster, 2001.

Organizations

Rape, Abuse, and Incest National Network (RAINN), 635-B Pennsylvania Ave. SE, Washington, DC 20003. This nonprofit organization operates the only national hotline for people who have been raped. It offers free, confidential counseling 24 hours a day.
Telephone 800-656-HOPE
http://www.rainn.org

National Coalition against Sexual Assault, 125 N. Enola Drive, Enola, PA 17025. This organization works to end sexual violence through education and public policy.
Telephone 717-728-9764
http://www.dreamingdesigns.com/other/indexncasa.html

National Center for Injury Prevention and Control, Mailstop K65, 4770 Buford Highway NE, Atlanta, GA 30341-3724. This division of the U. S. Centers for Diseases Control and Prevention posts fact sheets at its website covering rape, dating violence, intimate partner violence, and sexual violence against people with disabilities.
Telephone 770-488-1506
http://www.cdc.gov/ncipc

White Ribbon Campaign, 365 Bloor Street East, Suite 203, Toronto, Ontario, Canada M4W 3L4. This nonprofit organization focuses on men working to end men's violence against women. It publishes a newsletter, fact sheets, and a brochure called *It's Time for Guys to Put an End to This.*
Telephone 416-920-6684 or 800-328-2228
http://www.whiteribbon.ca

KidsHealth, sponsored by the Nemours Foundation and the Alfred I. duPont Hospital for Children, posts articles for teens on rape and related topics.
http://www.KidsHealth.org

Date Rape Drugs

Several medications that are useful when prescribed as sedatives*, muscle relaxants, or sleeping aids also have been used to "force" people to have sex. These drugs have become known as date rape drugs:

- flunitrazepam (sold under the brand name Rohypnol), nicknamed "roofies"
- clonazepam (sold under the brand name Klonopin), also sometimes referred to as "roofies"
- gamma-hydroxybutyrate (GHB), nicknamed "liquid Ecstasy."

When used illegally as club drugs or date rape drugs, these medications can cause euphoria* and loss of consciousness. Sometimes these medications also can cause seizures* or coma. Date rape drugs may be added to drinks as a way of secretly giving them to someone. Caution about accepting drinks from others is one important part of rape prevention.

* **sedatives** are drugs that have a calming effect.

* **euphoria** is an exaggerated feeling of well-being.

* **seizures** occur when the electrical patterns of the brain are interrupted by powerful, rapid bursts of electrical energy, which may cause a person to fall down, make jerky movements, or stare blankly into space.

▶ *See also*
Abuse
Post-Traumatic Stress Disorder
Substance Abuse
Violence

*tai chi (ty chee) is an ancient Chinese system of body movements, practiced as a meditative form of exercise.

*metabolism (me-TA-bo-li-zum) is the chemical processes in the body that convert foods into the energy needed for body functions.

*phobias (FO-bee-as) are intense, unrealistic fears of certain objects or situations.

Relaxation

Relaxation marks a state of ease or rest, often associated with a freedom from routine or work and freedom from stress.

A hot, bubbly bath may ease stress for Shanna, while an on-your-toes racquet ball game releases the day's tensions for Wayne. Maria finds that hot cocoa with a friend is "pure relaxation" and the antidote to stress. Ways to relax are countless. On weekends, city parks teem with children and adults pursuing relaxation as they play chess, practice tai chi*, jog, bicycle, kick soccer balls, shoot baskets, and sit on park benches to read. Still, one person's form of relaxation may be stressful to another.

What Is the Relaxation Response?

The Harvard professor of medicine Herbert Benson reported in the 1970s that the body has the capacity to achieve a special relaxed state, the direct opposite of the state of stress. Benson called this state the "relaxation response" and found that it can easily be achieved through meditation. The relaxation response involves a deep state of rest associated with decreases in heart rate, breathing rate, blood pressure, muscle tension, metabolism*, oxygen consumption, and active thinking. With daily practice of 20 to 30 minutes, the relaxation response reportedly can help keep the body young and the mind alert and might help increase energy, improve concentration, and extend memory.

What Are Other Forms of Relaxation?

There are other ways to achieve a state of deep relaxation. These include abdominal breathing, progressive muscle relaxation, yoga, and creative imagery.

Abdominal breathing   Practicing abdominal breathing (from deep in the stomach) can lead to a state of extreme relaxation. This kind of breathing differs from shallow chest breathing, or panting, which actually can cause an increase in nervousness. Abdominal breathing is the kind of breathing that is practiced in meditation or yoga.

Progressive muscle relaxation   Progressive muscle relaxation was developed in the early twentieth century by Dr. Edmund Jacobson. It is a program of tensing and relaxing muscles in an organized pattern so that that body "learns" how to release muscular tension. This form of relaxation can be paired with the gradual presentation of feared objects or ideas to help reduce phobias* or anxiety. When it is used in this way it is called systematic desensitization.

Yoga Yoga is a system of mental and physical exercise that focuses the mind to eliminate distractions. There are various forms of yoga practice, but stages of the training often involve disciplined behavior, mastery of bodily posture, control of breathing, and meditation. In particular, hatha yoga, which focuses on bodily postures and control of breathing, is believed to improve the overall health of the body.

Creative imagery There are various forms of creative imagery, including guided imagery, in which a therapist or other person describes peaceful scenes or images that create a restful, relaxed state. In some instances, people may form a mental picture of their own place of relaxation. This procedure often is used to lessen the pain and worry of medical procedures. For example, to diminish the pain of needles during injections for kidney disease, 9-year old Luke pictures himself walking on the sands of the beaches of Hawaii, as he did when he was 5 years old, before his illness began. In some instances, self-instruction may be used ("With every breath I take, I relax more deeply") to intensify the relaxation.

Conclusion

The human stress response occurs when people face situations that they perceive as dangerous, difficult, or overwhelming. Anxiety or other psychological symptoms may develop when people believe that inner or outer resources for coping with these stressful aspects of life are lacking or unavailable. The relaxation response is the physiological opposite of stress and can counteract its effects. Effective relaxation restores a person's ability to cope with life's daily hassles and stresses.

Resources

Book

Hipp, Earl. *Fighting Invisible Tigers: A Stress Management Guide for Teens.* Minneapolis: Free Spirit Publishing, 1996. For ages 11 and up.

Organization

www.KidsHealth.org, a website sponsored by the Nemours Foundation and the Alfred I. duPont Hospital for Children, has an article called "Spotlight on Stress" that talks about relaxation. http://kidshealth.org/teen/mind_matters/feelings/stress.html

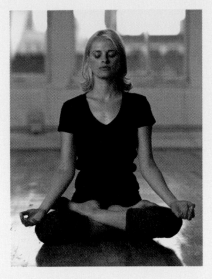

Hatha yoga involves engaging the body in a series of postures designed to connect the body's movement with the breath. This practice increases peoples' awareness of their own bodies and thoughts, which often results in a sense of self-assurance and peace, as well as an ability to calm themselves in stressful situations. *Duomo/Corbis*

▶ *See also*
Hypnosis
Phobias
Resilience
Stress

Resilience

Resilience (re-ZIL-yens) is the ability to overcome difficulty or negative experiences and to rebound or recover quickly from adversity, change, or challenge.

Abraham Lincoln experienced a number of failures that could have left him feeling sorely defeated. He failed in business as a storekeeper. He failed when he farmed. He lost his sweetheart and his first bid for political office. Running for Congress the first time, he lost. He also lost his bid for the United States Senate. He failed to win the vice presidential nomination in 1856. Despite these striking failures, Lincoln became the sixteenth president of the United States, and many people consider him to be the greatest president in history.

What Is Resilience?

Coping skills   While Lincoln may be one of the most famous examples of a resilient person, millions of people regularly demonstrate resilience within their lives. Resilience reflects an individual's coping skills, which are the qualities within an individual that allow him or her to recover from difficulty. While research about resiliency is ongoing, scientists have found that strong coping skills most often develop within individuals during their first ten years of life. Positive parenting during a child's first three years of life contributes to resilience in important ways. However, the need for the ability to bring about change and to find strength for one's life exists at all times.

Setbacks are temporary   A key element of human resilience is an individual's ability to see a difficult situation as temporary and passing. The expression "when life hands you lemons, make lemonade" refers to resilience; a resilient person takes something sour and makes it into something positive. Resilient individuals focus on the future and take steps to bring about changes to improve their situations. They have upbeat beliefs and faith in a brighter future. Such positive beliefs include:

- that negative past events do not necessarily predict or determine the future
- that challenges or tragedies are not a constant part of life
- that setbacks are situations that people can overcome
- that setting goals and planning for the future can help in achieving success
- that something good can come from bad

Resilient individuals manage their stress largely by managing themselves and their beliefs. Viewing difficult circumstances as temporary, they hold the view that humans are capable of rising above adversity.

Finding safety When faced with overwhelming situations, resilient children find a way to stay cool and find a place of safety. Children who are considered resilient seem to bounce back from their difficulties and remain optimistic about the future. However, difficult life events, family stress, illness, and accidents still affect resilient children. No matter how resilient they are, children still need the safety provided by responsible adults.

Education Frequently, resilient individuals place a high value on education. They view achievement in school as a way to rise out of and above difficulties that might hold others back. One study found that the ability to read at grade level by age ten predicted resilience into adulthood. Often resilient people find something they can do well and then practice doing it so they can enjoy ongoing success.

Support networks Another characteristic commonly exhibited by resilient individuals is the ability to enlist support, either from a single individual or from a group. Support prevents a person who is going through tough times from feeling overwhelmingly alone and helps the person understand that difficult circumstances will not last forever. Two important sources of support are religious organizations and therapeutic groups and professionals. Participation in community or religious groups increases resilience by providing connections with others who may have similar beliefs and perspectives for coping with life stresses. A study of 1,500 people in North Carolina over a six-year period found that regular churchgoers had stronger immune systems* than did non-churchgoers. Research also indicates that cognitive-behavioral therapy* and other forms of psychological treatment can help trauma* survivors regain resilience and recover from post-traumatic stress disorder*.

Resources

Book

Desetta, Al, and Sybil Wolin, eds. *The Struggle to be Strong: True Stories by Teens About Overcoming Tough Times.* Minneapolis: Free Spirit Publishing, 2000. Thirty stories by teens tell how they overcame difficult challenges.

Organization

ResilienceNet is a website that provides information for helping children and families overcome adversities.
http://resilnet.uiuc.edu

* **immune system** fights germs and other foreign substances that enter the body.

* **cognitive-behavioral therapy** is counseling that helps people make changes in thinking and behavior that can bring about emotional healing and improve problem solving.

* **trauma** (TRAW-muh), in the broadest sense, refers to a wound or injury, whether psychological or physical. It occurs when a person experiences a sudden or violent injury (physical trauma) or encounters a situation that involves intense fear and loss of control (psychological trauma).

* **post-traumatic stress disorder** is a mental disorder in which people who have survived a terrifying event relive their terror in nightmares, memories, and feelings of fear. It is severe enough to interfere with everyday living and can occur after a natural disaster, military combat, rape, mugging, or other violence.

▶ *See also*
Post-Traumatic Stress Disorder
Relaxation
Stress
Therapy

Rett Disorder

KEYWORDS
for searching the Internet
and other reference sources

Genetic disorders

Rett syndrome

*syndrome is a group or pattern
of symptoms or signs that occur
together.

*Rett disorder is an inherited brain condition that affects only girls. Before
she reaches school age, a girl with the disorder stops developing normally
and begins to lose such skills as walking and talking. Rett disorder is
sometimes called Rett syndrome*. It is rare, occurring in only about 1 in
10,000 girls. Because of the rarity of the disorder and because it has not
been recognized by the medical community for very long, most people
have never heard of it.*

What Are the Signs and Symptoms of Rett Disorder?

A girl with Rett disorder develops and acts normally for some time after she is born. At first she seems to be perfectly healthy. She smiles, sits
up, and may learn how to walk and talk. Then, at some time between
about the ages of 5 months and 2½ years, she begins to lose the use of
her hands to pick up and hold on to things. Instead, she begins to make
certain movements with her hands and arms, which look as if she is
repeatedly wringing or washing her hands. If she can walk, her gait
becomes stiff and poorly coordinated. She also may lose the ability to
say words and to respond to what other people say. She becomes less
interested in playing with other children or in making friends. A typical sign of Rett disorder is that the child's head stops growing at the
rate expected.

A girl who has Rett disorder frequently has other difficulties as well.
She is often, but not always, severely mentally retarded. She may have
seizures* and difficulty breathing at a normal rate, and she also may have
scoliosis (sko-lee-O-sis), or spinal curvature.

*seizures (SEE-zhurs) are sudden
attacks of involuntary (uncontrollable) body movements,
changes in behavior, or loss of
consciousness that result from
bursts of abnormal electrical
energy within the brain.

*genes are chemical sub-
stances in the body that help
determine a person's characteristics, such as hair or eye
color, and also are involved
in determining certain health
conditions. Genes are contained in the chromosomes
found in the cells of the human
body. They are inherited from
parents.

*chromosomes (KRO-mo-somz)
are threadlike chemical structures inside cells on which the
genes are located. There are
46 (23 pairs) of chromosomes
in normal human cells. Genes
on the X and Y chromosomes
(known as the sex chromo-
somes) help determine
whether a person is male or
female. Females have two X
chromosomes; males have one
X and one Y chromosome.

What Causes Rett Disorder?

Rett disorder is an example of a sex-linked genetic (je-NE-tik) disorder.
The disorder is inherited, which means that it is caused by one or more
faulty genes* passed on from a parent. Girls with Rett disorder have one
X-chromosome* that carries the faulty gene and another chromosome
that carries a normal gene. Boys who inherit the disorder, on the other
hand, have one X-chromosome that carries the faulty gene, but they do
not have a matching X-chromosome with a normal gene. If a girl has a
faulty gene for Rett disorder, the normal gene on the other X-chromosome can offset some of the effects of the faulty gene. The girl will live,
but she will show signs of the disorder. It is believed that a boy fetus
with the faulty gene will not survive to the time of birth, because he does
not have a normal copy of the gene. This explains why only girls have
Rett disorder. The faulty gene for Rett disorder was discovered in 1999,
and scientists are still trying to learn more about it and what causes the
disorder.

How Is Rett Syndrome Diagnosed and Treated?

Doctors can diagnose Rett disorder when they see the characteristic signs appear in a girl who had been developing normally. There is no cure for Rett disorder and development is often quite delayed. Treatments such as physical therapy and occupational therapy can lessen motor problems. A speech therapist may join the special education team to help the girl develop specialized ways of communicating, such as with the use of special electronic devices. Girls with the disorder will remain dependent upon others for their care throughout their lives. As they grow to adulthood, some girls become more interested in other people and are able to enjoy family and friends.

Resources

Book

Lewis, Jackie, and Debbie Wilson. *Pathways to Learning in Rett Syndrome.* London: David Fulton, 1998. This book offers special education advice for parents and teachers.

Organizations

International Rett Syndrome Association, 9121 Piscataway Road, Clinton, MD 20735. This organization promotes the study and therapy of Rett disorder and offers information and other types of support to parents and families of children with the disorder.
Telephone 800-818-RETT
http://www.rettsyndrome.org

Rett Syndrome Center of the Baylor College of Medicine and Texas Children's Hospital, 6501 Fannin Street, Houston, TX 77030. This is one of the largest centers in the world engaged in the research of Rett disorder and its treatment.
Telephone 713-798-RETT
http://www.bcm.tmc.edu/neurol/struct/blueb/blueb2.html.

▶ *See also*
Autism
Genetics and Behavior
Mental Retardation
Pervasive Developmental Disorders

Ritalin *See* Medications

S

Schizophrenia

Schizophrenia (SKIT-zo-FREE-ni-a) is a complex, serious, and chronic brain disorder. It results from disruptions in the structure and function of the brain and neurotransmitter pathways of the central nervous system. These disruptions may cause psychotic symptoms, which are frightening distortions in thoughts, feelings, moods, perceptions, and behavior that interfere with daily life. With the correct combination of medication and therapy, the symptoms of schizophrenia often can be managed effectively.

KEYWORDS
for searching the Internet
and other reference sources

Catatonia

Delusions

Hallucinations

Neuroleptics

Neurotransmitters

Psychosis

Information in the form of electrical signals flows down nerve cells in the brain, triggering the release of neurotransmitters. These chemical messengers transmit information from one nerve cell to another. In healthy people, neurotransmitter traffic usually flows smoothly, with occasional hills, valleys, bumps, and potholes that represent the stresses and challenges of growing up and interacting with other people. In people with schizophrenia, however, neurotransmitter traffic runs into major roadblocks, unscheduled stops, and unmapped detours to frightening and unreal places. These traffic disruptions result in periods of psychosis, during which people with schizophrenia lose touch with healthy reality and seem to get trapped in alternate realities. With anti-psychotic medication, people with schizophrenia often find their way back to the healthy realities of everyday life.

What Happens to People with Schizophrenia?

Neurotransmitter disruptions Researchers know that in our chromosomes* are genes that direct the development of all the structures and functions of the brain and central nervous system, including the production and release of neurotransmitters. In schizophrenia, faulty genes may create coding errors affecting several different neurotransmitters. When those miscodings interact with environmental factors during childhood and adolescence, and even before birth, they may affect brain neurotransmitter levels and function, resulting in symptoms that doctors usually classify as positive and negative. Most often, the serious symptoms of schizophrenia do not appear until a person's late teens or early twenties.

*****chromosomes** (KRO-mo-somz) are threadlike chemical structures inside cells on which the genes are located. There are 46 (23 pairs) chromosomes in normal human cells. Genes on the X and Y chromosomes (known as the sex chromosomes) help determine whether a person is male or female. Females have two X chromosomes; males have one X and one Y chromosome.

Positron emission tomography (PET) scans are computer-generated images of brain activity. When compared with PET scans of healthy people, the scans of people with schizophrenia show disruptions in brain activity, changes in brain structures like the ventricles, and decreased function in the frontal cortex. *Photo Researchers, Inc.* ▶

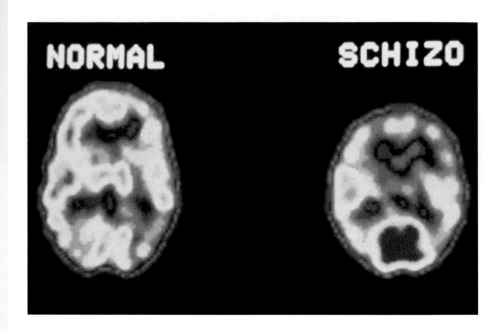

Positive symptoms The positive symptoms of schizophrenia are those that seem to distort and exaggerate sights, sounds, thoughts, perceptions, beliefs, and behaviors. People with schizophrenia usually do not experience positive symptoms until their late teens or early twenties, and doctors usually cannot diagnose schizophrenia before positive symptoms occur. The positive symptoms of schizophrenia may include delusions, hallucinations, and disorganized speech, thoughts, beliefs, movements, and behaviors.

■ **Delusions:** Delusions are false beliefs that a person holds onto even when they are bizarre or could not possibly be true. Delusions may involve fears (paranoid delusions), guilt, jealousy, religion, spirits, one's role in life (delusions of grandeur), one's body, and mind control. People with schizophrenia might believe, for example, that their inner thoughts are being broadcast out loud or that outside people, spirits, or aliens are inserting thoughts into their heads or are touching their bodies.

■ **Hallucinations:** Hallucinations involve seeing, hearing, or feeling things that are not real. People with schizophrenia often "hear voices" in their heads (auditory hallucinations) that other people cannot hear and that are not just their inner thoughts. The voices may tell them what to do, may carry on conversations about them, or may have arguments with each other.

■ **Disorganized speech, thoughts, and beliefs:** People with schizophrenia may lose track of their ideas, meanings, and words ("word salad"). Ideas and images may become jumbled or linked together for illogical reasons, or words and meanings that should be linked instead may become disconnected.

- **Disorganized movements and behaviors:** People with schizophrenia may use exaggerated or repeated gestures, or they may seem to be fidgeting or hyperactive or preoccupied with meaningless physical movements.

Negative symptoms The negative symptoms of schizophrenia usually involve a reduction in a person's normal level of functioning. People with schizophrenia may seem to think, speak, feel, and move less than healthy people do:

- **Alogia (a-LO-jee-a) and poverty of speech:** People with schizophrenia may speak very little, or their speech may have little meaningful content, or they may have long delays between words and sentences, as if the connections between thoughts and speech were interrupted or blocked.

- **Flattening or blunting of affect:** People with schizophrenia may have reduced emotional expression. They may not smile or frown in response to happy or sad events, their voices may not change tone or pitch, and they may not maintain eye contact or other kinds of emotional links with other people.

- **Avolition and anhedonia:** People with schizophrenia may seem to lose interest in and energy for pleasurable activities and achievements.

- **Catatonia and posturing:** People with schizophrenia may seem to freeze into unusual body positions, or they may seem to stop moving entirely.

Remissions and relapses The negative symptoms of schizophrenia sometimes are seen during early childhood, when they may resemble autism and similar developmental disorders. By the late teens or early twenties, the positive symptoms of schizophrenia begin to appear. Mental health activist Ken Steele, for example, reported in *The Day the Voices Stopped: A Memoir of Madness and Hope* that his voices began when he was 14 years old.

Symptoms often occur in cycles, alternating periods of improvement (remissions) with periods of psychosis (relapses). Because schizophrenia is a permanent (chronic) disorder, it often gets worse as a person gets older, as periods of active psychosis interfere with perceptions of reality and activities of daily living. With the correct combination of medication and therapy, however, the positive and negative symptoms of schizophrenia often can be managed and controlled effectively.

How Is Schizophrenia Diagnosed and Treated?

Diagnosis The first step toward diagnosis is a complete medical examination and medical history. This helps the doctor to rule out other

---

The Genetics of Schizophrenia

Scientists know that schizophrenia tends to run in families and that it affects both males and females, but they have not yet located the genetic coding errors that lead to the neurotransmitter disruptions that are seen in schizophrenia.

Studies of inheritance patterns show the following estimates of a person's risk of developing schizophrenia:

- 1%: general population
- 8%: when a sibling has schizophrenia
- 12%: when a parent has schizophrenia
- 14%: when a fraternal twin has schizophrenia
- 25%-35%: when both parents have schizophrenia
- 45%-50%: when an identical twin has schizophrenia.

Identical twins are siblings who develop from the same embryo. They always are the same sex and they share the same genetic material. If schizophrenia were entirely the result of a single genetic coding error, then the risk that identical twins both would inherit schizophrenia would be close to 100%.

Scientists believe that several different genes interacting with environmental factors is the likeliest underlying mechanism for schizophrenia. The U.S. National Institute of Mental Health has launched a Schizophrenia Genetics Initiative to gather data from people and families with schizophrenia. To find out more about it, check their website at www.nimh.nih.gov.

People with schizophrenia experience disruptions in ordinary reality. Through art therapy, they are able to express their energy and subconscious feelings in a creative and uninhibited way. A therapist may be able to interpret the person's experience through this visual, symbolic form of communication.
Paul Almasy/Corbis ▶

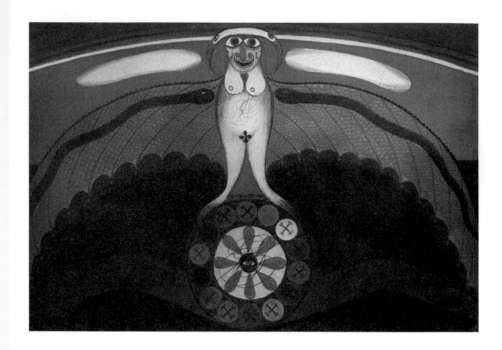

Auditory Hallucinations and "Son of Sam"

During the 1970s, a man who called himself "Son of Sam" killed several people in New York City. When the killer was caught, he was identified as a man named David Berkowitz, who was having auditory hallucinations. In those hallucinations, Berkowitz heard the voice of a neighbor's dog (named "Sam") giving him orders to kill people in parked cars. Berkowitz still is in prison in New York.

possible causes of psychotic symptoms, including substance abuse, bipolar disorder, brain tumors, brain infections, and metabolic disorders that affect the brain and central nervous system. The doctor also may order lab tests or imaging studies. People with schizophrenia often do not have all possible signs and symptoms, but doctors generally will screen patients for delusions, hallucinations, "voices," and disruptions of normal speech, thought, and feeling patterns. Brief psychotic disorder and schizophreniform (SKIT-zo-FREN-ni-form) disorder have symptoms similar to schizophrenia, but these conditions usually last for six months or less. A diagnosis of schizophrenia means that long-term treatment will be necessary.

Medications Schizophrenia is considered a chronic disorder. There is not yet a "cure" for it, but there are medications that can offer relief from psychotic symptoms. These medications, called "antipsychotics," can help quiet the "voices" that interfere with daily activities and can result in dramatic improvements in the quality of life for people with schizophrenia.

Doctors must work very carefully with patients and their families to choose the right medication at the right dosage. When an effective medication is found, it often improves both the positive and negative symptoms of schizophrenia, reducing delusions and hallucinations and increasing social functioning.

Originally introduced during the 1950s, chlorpromazine (Thorazine) was the first medication used to treat schizophrenia. It was considered a "major tranquilizer" and it often produced unpleasant side effects. In the decades since then, researchers have discovered many newer medications that target malfunctioning neurotransmitters more accurately, improve symptoms more effectively, and cause fewer side effects. Newer medications introduced during the 1990s include clozapine (Clozaril), resperidone (Risperdal), olanzapine (Zyprexa), quetiapine (Seroquel), and ziprasidone (Geodon).

Medication dosages often require adjustments over time to maintain effectiveness or to reduce side effects. Sometimes people with schizophrenia stop taking their medication or stop checking in with their doctors, possibly because they feel better or because of unpleasant side effects from the medication. Without medication, however, psychotic symptoms are likely to return or worsen.

Side effects   Antipsychotic medications sometimes result in side effects that can make it difficult or distressing for patients to follow their doctors' recommended treatment plan. The older medications like chlorpromazine (Thorazine) often produced symptoms like sluggishness, emotional numbing, drowsiness, restlessness, muscle spasms or tremors, dry mouth, weight gain, and blurring of vision. A more serious side effect of long-term use of the older medications was a condition called "tardive dyskinesia" (TAR-div dis-ki-NEE-zee-a). People with tardive dyskinesia experienced involuntary movements of the face or arms or legs, movements that sometimes did not disappear when the medication was stopped. Often, people who developed tardive dyskinesia chose to continue taking their medication because the beneficial effects outweighed this serious side effect. It is important to note that each new generation of medications works more effectively than the older ones in relieving psychotic symptoms, reducing the severity of side effects, and reducing the risk of tardive dyskinesia.

Psychotherapy and support networks   As with other chronic diseases, people with schizophrenia need support from doctors, counselors, social workers, family, friends, and other people with the same disorder. Therapy can help people with schizophrenia learn how to accept their diagnosis, manage their symptoms and relapses, and adjust their daily lives to incorporate their medication and treatment plans.

Living with Schizophrenia

Once it was the norm for people with schizophrenia and other psychotic disorders to be hospitalized when they were diagnosed and to remain hospitalized for the rest of their lives. Today it is more common for patients to be hospitalized for only a short period of time, while their psychotic symptoms are being brought under control. As long as they remain on medication under a doctor's supervision, many people with schizophrenia are now able to remain at home with their families or in supervised group homes.

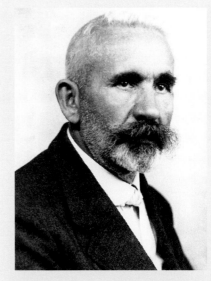

▲

Emil Kraepelin was a German psychiatrist who identified "dementia praecox" as a disorder in which people lost touch with reality. Kraepelin's colleague Eugen Bleuler later renamed the disorder "schizophrenia." *National Library of Medicine*

"Dementia Praecox" and "Schizophrenia": Emil Kraepelin and Eugen Bleuler

Psychosis has been written about since before the time of the ancient Greeks, but the scientific study of mental disorders is still rather new in human history. Previous generations often believed that psychosis was a form of possession by supernatural spirits because people with schizophrenia seemed to "see things" and "hear voices" that were not real. Often people with schizophrenia and other psychotic disorders were put in prisons or in lunatic asylums.

It was not until 1896 that the German psychiatrist Emil Kraepelin (1856–1926) developed a classification system for mental illnesses in which he identified a group of psychotic symptoms that he called "dementia praecox" (de-MEN-sha PRAY-cox), from the Latin term meaning "precocious" or "premature" dementia. Kraepelin took note of many of the distorted thoughts and perceptions that signaled the start of the disorder, the age at which it seemed to occur most often, the periods of remission and relapse, and the fact that the disorder was chronic and usually got worse with the passage of time.

The Swiss psychiatrist Eugen Bleuler (1857–1939) later renamed the disorder "schizophrenia" from the Latin phrase for "splitting of the mind." Bleuler did not mean that people with schizophrenia had dissociative identity disorder ("multiple personality disorder") or "Jekyll and Hyde" personalities. Rather he meant that people with schizophrenia had minds that seemed to become fragmented and disrupted when they needed to coordinate thoughts, emotions, and behavior with the real world. Processes of mind that ran smoothly in healthy people instead seemed to split into fragments in people with schizophrenia.

Current research suggests that Bleuler was on the right track. As researchers identify the specific functions of the neurotransmitters that become disrupted in schizophrenia, the medications designed to target those neurotransmitters become more effective and cause fewer side effects.

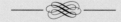

Therapy for people with schizophrenia Psychotherapy often helps people with schizophrenia learn to manage the behaviors that accompany psychotic symptoms and adjust to the rhythms and requirements of chronic illness. Therapy may involve a "token economy" technique that uses rewards for behavioral change. It also may involve rehabilitation and social skills training so that people with schizophrenia can catch up with the everyday skills and opportunities that had to be put on hold during periods of psychosis. Taking care of oneself, talking and listening during ordinary conversations, and interacting with friends, family, coworkers, and community in the real world all are skills that can be learned or relearned.

Family education Family members also must learn how to overcome the confusion, shame, guilt, regret, grief, and stigma often attached to mental illness. Help in understanding the biology of schizophrenia is important, as is acceptance by family members that the signs and symptoms of schizophrenia are real and not just a way to avoid accepting reality and responsibility.

Family members must learn how to cope with specific symptoms like delusions and with alternating cycles of remission and relapse. People with schizophrenia are at a higher risk for depression and suicide, making it essential that family members know when to intervene and summon professional help. During periods of active psychosis, it usually is not helpful for friends and families to challenge delusions. But it is possible for them to communicate openly and honestly that they do not share the psychotic delusions even though they know that they are real for the person with schizophrenia.

Family members also play an important role in helping patients stick to their prescribed treatment plan. Patients with disorganized thinking may forget to take their medications, or their "voices" may tell them they do not need medication at all. At such times, family members who recognize the signs and symptoms of schizophrenia can take action to get immediate treatment, to prevent a relapse, and to keep the person with schizophrenia in touch with the reality of managing his or her disorder.

Resources

Books

Greenberg, Joanne. *I Never Promised You a Rose Garden.* New York: New American Library, 1984. Originally written under the pseudonym "Hannah Green" to protect the author from the stigma of mental illness, Joanne Greenberg's classic novel about a girl with schizophrenia was published in 1964 and has been in print continuously ever since.

Steele, Ken, and Claire Berman. *The Day the Voices Stopped: A Memoir of Madness and Hope.* New York: Basic Books, 2000. This moving autobiography tells the story of mental health activist Ken Steele, whose voices began when he was 14 years old and continued for decades until his doctors found the right medication to control his symptoms.

Organizations

U.S. National Institute of Mental Health, 6001 Executive Boulevard, Room 8184, MSC 9663, Bethesda, MD 20892-9663. This division of the National Institutes of Health oversees research on schizophrenia and other mental illnesses. It publishes the *Schizophrenia Bulletin* for researchers and many helpful fact sheets for the public.
Telephone 301-443-4513
http://www.nimh.nih.gov

American Academy of Child and Adolescent Psychiatry, 3615 Wisconsin Ave. NW, Washington, DC, 20016-3007. The American Academy of Child and Adolescent Psychiatry website posts *Facts for Families* about schizophrenia and other psychiatric disorders.
Telephone 202-966-7300
http://www.aacap.org

National Alliance for Research on Schizophrenia and Depression, 60 Cutter Mill Road, Suite 404, Great Neck, NY 11021. This nonprofit organization supports scientific research on brain and behavior disorders.
Telephone 516-829-0091 or 800-829-8289
http://www.narsad.org

National Alliance for the Mentally Ill (NAMI), Colonial Place Three, 2107 Wilson Blvd., Suite 300, Arlington, VA 22201-3042. This information, advocacy, and support group for people with mental illness and their families and friends sponsors a self-help education program called *Living with Schizophrenia and Other Mental Illnesses (LWS)*. LWS programs currently are active in more than 30 states.
Telephone 800-950-NAMI or 703-524-7600
http://www.nami.org

American Psychiatric Association, 1400 K Street NW, Washington, DC, 20005. An organization of physicians that provides information about schizophrenia.
Telephone 888-357-7924
http://www.psych.org

National Mental Health Association, 1021 Prince Street, Alexandria, VA 22314-2971. A nonprofit organization that addresses all aspects of mental illness and health and supports education and research to improve mental health.
Telephone 800-969-6642 or 703-684-7722
http://www.nmha.org

National Mental Health Consumers' Self-Help Clearinghouse, 1211 Chestnut Street, Suite 1207, Philadelphia, PA 19107. This organization makes information available to consumers about various mental health issues, including mental health services and resources.

Telephone 800-553-4539 or 215-751-1810
http://www.mhselfhelp.org

School Avoidance

School avoidance occurs when children and teens repeatedly stay home from school, or are repeatedly sent home from school, because of emotional problems or because of aches and pains that are caused by emotions or stress and not by medical illness.

KEYWORDS
*for searching the Internet
and other reference sources*

Anxiety disorders

Separation anxiety

Stress

Ben's Story

Ben missed a lot of school because of his stomachaches. His stomach felt especially bad on Monday mornings. Often, while he was getting dressed for school, he felt as if he might throw up. His mother didn't want him to go to school if he was sick. On days he stayed home, Ben got back into bed, and by lunchtime he felt much better. But by the next morning, he felt miserable all over again. He managed to get himself to school sometimes, but it was getting harder and harder. He would be embarrassed if he threw up on the bus. Ben's doctor had examined him and found him to be in excellent health despite his stomach pains. Still his stomachaches continued, and Ben's mother had started to worry about how many school days he was missing.

What Is School Avoidance?

Ben has school avoidance, a common condition among schoolchildren and adolescents. Sometimes called school "phobia"* (FO-bee-a) or school refusal, school avoidance is a pattern of missing school for symptoms that are caused by emotions or stress, rather than physical illness. School avoidance is different from truancy (TROO-an-see), which is a pattern of repeated unexcused absences from school. The student who is truant, or skips school, is neither at home nor at school. In school avoidance, the student stays home.

* **phobia** is an intense, persistent, unreasonable fear of (and avoidance of) a particular thing or situation.

What Causes School Avoidance?

There are two main reasons someone has school avoidance. One reason is that the student feels anxiety (ang-ZY-eh-tee), fear, or worry about some aspect of going to school or about leaving home. The other reason is that there is some benefit, or a secondary gain, to staying home from school.

Anxiety-related school avoidance Most children have some anxiety about attending school for the first time. This is known as "separation anxiety." It is not surprising when separation anxiety occurs when a child is about to enter kindergarten or first grade. For many children this is the first time they are away from home or separated from their parents. But some children have separation anxiety that lasts beyond the expected age. Children who have recently been through other difficult separations, such as divorce, or the death of a parent, or the illness of a family member, may have an especially difficult time leaving home to go to school.

Children with school avoidance may have headaches, stomachaches, chest pain, or other symptoms brought on by the stress of separation. These pains are real, but they are caused by the body's response to stress and not by an illness. Usually, a checkup by the doctor finds the child or teen to be in good physical health. Students with anxiety-related school avoidance are often good students and like school, but because of their stress-related symptoms, they feel that they need to stay home.

Some students with school avoidance may have anxiety about school itself. They may worry about grades, about being bullied, about being called on by the teacher in class, or about having to undress for gym. Some schools have rules about when students may use the bathroom, and this may be a worry to children who may need to go more often. Dirty school bathrooms without enough privacy or issues about safety may be real concerns for some children.

In many cases, anxiety-related school avoidance begins with an upsetting event that happens at school, for example, being teased or experiencing something disturbing in class. Students who are shy and sensitive by nature and those who have an overprotective parent may be more likely to have anxiety-related school avoidance.

Secondary-gain school avoidance Not all children and teens with school avoidance are anxious or shy. Some may simply find that it is more comfortable staying home than attending school. This is called secondary-gain school avoidance. "Secondary gain" is a term that refers to the bonus or positive side of something unpleasant. For example, though it is unpleasant to be sick, it may be pleasant to watch television during the day and to have meals in bed. Another secondary gain of being sick might be not to have to do homework or having the personal attention and care of a parent at home.

Secondary-gain school avoidance often starts with an illness that lasts for a few days and causes the student to miss school. The student may get behind in homework and begin to think about how hard it will be to catch up. To avoid the hard work ahead, the student may stretch out the illness a bit longer. Receiving the secondary gains of sympathy, the care and attention of parents, and the fun of watching daytime TV can contribute to school avoidance. Lenient parents or parents who do not view school as important can contribute to secondary-gain school avoidance. Sometimes students exaggerate symptoms or claim to have symptoms they really do not have (like sore throat or leg pain) just to avoid school.

How Is School Avoidance Diagnosed?

School avoidance is diagnosed when a student has repeatedly missed school due to aches and pains or other symptoms, and a careful checkup by the doctor has found the student to be in good health. The doctor will check for school avoidance by evaluating the pattern of symptoms and asking about stresses. The doctor may explain how stress can cause certain physical symptoms and may have the student keep track of symptoms by writing them down.

Ben's doctor asked him about some of the worries that were on his mind lately. Ben mentioned that since his parents had divorced last year and his dad had moved across town, he had started to worry about his mom being lonely. He had seen her cry a lot this year, and it made him sad. He said he missed his dad and wished they could be a family again, but without the arguing. Although he looked forward to the weekends he spent with his dad, he was sad that his mom had to spend weekends alone. Ben's doctor explained how people could get stomachaches from stress and sadness. She asked Ben to keep track of his stomachaches in a diary, and she told him to go to school anyway. She gave Ben and his mom the name of a therapist who would help him talk about his feelings and about how to adjust to all the changes in his family.

How Is School Avoidance Treated?

The first step in treating school avoidance is to help the student get back to school right away. The longer a student avoids school, the harder it is to return. Students with anxiety usually need reassurance that they are in good health. Students and their parents are helped by taking a "yes but" approach. The symptoms are real, but are not cause to miss school. Parents are guided about what symptoms are grounds to stay home, and find ways to help a student attend school despite discomfort caused by aches and pains. The treatment often includes a plan for what to do when the student begins to feel ill at school. The plan may be for the student to go to the nurse's office to lie down for 5 to 10 minutes and then return to class, but not to go home. Medications to treat anxiety may be helpful in some cases.

Another important part of treatment may involve working with school personnel to solve problems that are causing anxiety, such as bullying or lack of privacy in bathrooms. Students who have separation anxiety or generalized worry may benefit from counseling to learn to cope with painful feelings or loss. The usual treatment for students with secondary-gain school avoidance also is to return to school right away. Clear limits, appropriate expectations, and support for regular school attendance are critical factors for successfully addressing the problem.

▶ *See also*

Anxiety and Anxiety Disorders

Bullying

Malingering

School Failure

Stress

School Failure

School failure is a person's inability to meet the minimum academic standards of an educational institution.

School failure is a process where a student slips farther and farther behind his peers and gradually disconnects from the educational system. The end result of school failure is dropping out before graduation. Many cases of school failure happen among students who have the ability and intelligence to succeed but who are unable or unwilling to apply these abilities in the school setting.

Students can begin the slide into failing patterns at any time during their school career, but school failure is more likely to occur at transitional stages, such as when graduating from elementary to middle school or after a family move to a new school system. Failing grades typically are symptoms of emotional, behavioral, or learning problems.

Why Do People Fail in School?

People who fail in school may feel "stupid," but emotional or mental health problems and "hidden" learning disorders, not low intelligence, often are the root causes of their inability to meet the standards of a school. There are several factors that can lead to school failure, among them depression, anxiety, problems in the family, and learning disabilities.

Depression Depression is one of the most common causes of school difficulties. It is a condition that can make people feel sad for long periods of time, have low energy, and lose interest in activities that normally give them pleasure. People with depression have continuing negative thoughts about themselves and the future, and they may experience changes in eating and sleeping patterns and in their ability to concentrate and make decisions. They may feel hopeless and may even think about suicide. Depression has been shown to be a leading cause of school failure in young people with learning disabilities. Depression can also cause school failure in students without learning disabilities.

Anxiety Anxiety is a feeling of excessive worry about a possible danger or an uncomfortable situation that is intense enough to interfere with a person's ability to concentrate and focus. Students can have genuine reasons to be anxious. People who have been bullied at school may worry that they will be bullied again. Students may legitimately fear personal violence on the way to or from school. They might worry about their families going through a divorce or about a parent who is ill. On the other hand, ordinary adolescent worries about looking right and fitting in can be blown so far out of proportion that a student may try to be

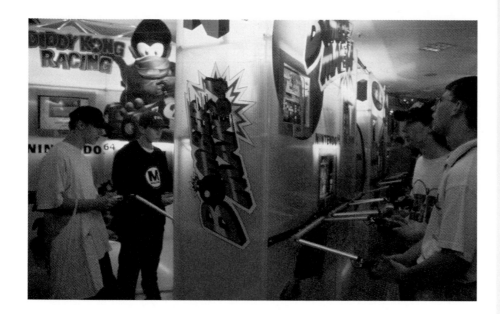

Teens with learning disabilities or who feel anxiety about school may neglect schoolwork for other distracting activities. *Peter Arnold, Inc.*

absent from school just to avoid a possibly embarrassing or uncomfortable situation. This is called "school avoidance." Anxiety in any of its forms can interfere with a student's performance in school.

Problems in the family   Students also may bring their problems at home to school with them. If a student's family is experiencing violence, unemployment, alcohol or drug use by a family member, problems with the law, or any other upsetting experience, it can be difficult to concentrate on schoolwork. Many students who are having family problems might have trouble controlling their anger and frustration at school, and they may end up in trouble because of their behavior. Some students who are overburdened at home by circumstances that make it necessary for them to "parent" siblings, hold a job, or care for an ill or impaired parent may find it impossible to keep up. Many times students who face overwhelming family or personal problems keep these problems to themselves. School counselors can help support a student and prevent failure if they are made aware of the problem.

Learning disabilities   Learning disabilities are conditions that interfere with gaining specific academic skills, such as reading or writing. Learning disorders can hinder a person's ability to concentrate or to process or remember information. When these difficulties are recognized early, certain teaching strategies can help a student overcome the learning disability. Unfortunately, many learning problems may go undiagnosed or may be diagnosed incorrectly as behavior problems. The frustration and depression that can result from undetected learning disabilities is a major cause of school failure or dropping out of school.

* **truancy** is staying out of school without permission.

* **chronic** (KRAH-nik) **illness** is an illness with symptoms that last a long time or that recur frequently.

Other causes Many social factors can increase the risk of school failure. These include homelessness, poverty, frequent moves from school to school, and the inability to speak English. Other circumstances such as truancy*, teenage pregnancy, and chronic illness* may also affect a student's ability to do his or her best in school.

Helping People at Risk of School Failure

Students at risk of school failure need to be identified as early as possible in their school careers if they are to receive the help they need. This task usually falls to the teacher, school counselor, or parents, because many failing students are hostile to or disconnected from the educational system and will not or do not know how to ask for help. To bring failing students back to school and foster their success, the reasons for school failure need to be recognized and treated. Parents, teachers, counselors, and mental health professionals are people the student can ask for help.

Parents can help by:

- taking a genuine interest in their child's school life and attending school events
- listening to and understanding their child's concerns about school
- taking seriously sudden changes in behavior, sleeping, or eating
- intervening for the student when unsafe situations are causing anxiety or school avoidance
- setting and enforcing appropriate standards of school behavior
- setting realistic goals for school attendance and academic improvement
- eliminating barriers to homework completion and school attendance
- working as a team with teachers and counselors to get children appropriate help
- helping children identify their strengths and pinpointing career options that involve these strengths
- getting help in recognizing the reasons for school failure.

Teachers can help by:

- developing learning plans that support the student's strengths
- referring the student for evaluations for possible learning disabilities
- providing referrals to programs that offer extra academic help or arranging peer tutoring
- teaching study skills and strategies to support learning

- encouraging students to participate in school activities, such as sports, plays, or clubs, so that they feel they are a part of the school
- arranging a mentor for the student
- promoting a tolerant, violence-free school environment
- communicating concerns or changes in school performance to parents right away.

Mental health professionals can help by:

- screening for emotional problems and offering appropriate treatment
- listening to the student's concerns about family and school difficulties
- performing evaluations for learning disabilities or attention deficit hyperactivity disorder
- working with the school to formulate appropriate learning strategies for the student
- working with teachers and parents to help them eliminate barriers to school failure.

Resources

Books

Heacox, Anne. *Up from Underachievements: How Teachers, Students, and Parents Can Work Together to Promote Student Success.* Minneapolis: Free Spirit Publishing, 1991.

Levine, Melvin. *Keeping a Head in School: A Student's Book About Learning Abilities and Learning Disorders.* Cambridge, MA: Educators Publishing Service, Inc., 1996.

Shumm, Jeanne Shay. *School Power: Strategies for Succeeding in School.* Minneapolis: Free Spirit Publishing, 2001.

▶ *See also*
Attention Deficit Hyperactivity Disorder
Depression
Learning Disabilities
School Avoidance
Self-Esteem

| **School Violence** *See* Violence |

Seasonal Affective Disorder

KEYWORDS
for searching the Internet
and other reference sources

Depression

Disthymia

Seasonal affective disorder (SAD) is a form of depression that occurs at the same time each year (usually with the onset of winter) and disappears at the same time each year (typically at the start of spring). SAD is linked to the availability of daylight and is found most often in the Northern Hemisphere.

More Than the Winter Blahs

Many people get the winter blahs or cabin fever as the days get shorter and colder, but for about 10 million Americans with SAD, shorter days mean a slide into true depression. SAD is a seasonal pattern of depression. It occurs in about 5 of every 100 people. Four times more women than men experience SAD, and it can also occur in children and teens. The farther away from the equator someone lives, the higher the risk that he or she will experience SAD. One study has estimated the incidence of SAD in the general population as only 1.4 percent in Florida but 9.7 percent in New Hampshire. This comparison suggests that in the southern United States only about 1 person in 100 has this condition, but in the north, the number may be as high as 1 in 10 people.

What Causes Seasonal Affective Disorder?

As autumn arrives, the number of daylight hours declines. The effect is greater the farther north a person travels from the equator. Daylight also can be decreased by cloud cover in specific areas of the United States, such as the Great Lakes region.

*neurotransmitter (NUR-o-tranz-mit-er) is a chemical messenger that lets brain cells communicate with each other and therefore allows the brain to function properly.

It is believed that for some people the decrease in available daylight causes a decline in the neurotransmitter* serotonin (ser-a-TO-nin), in the brain. A decrease in the amount of serotonin in the brain has been linked to depression, because serotonin typically is associated with feelings of well-being. In the autumn, after a few weeks of reduced serotonin levels, a person can start to show signs of depression. If left untreated, the depression may continue throughout the winter and then disappear in the spring as the number of daylight hours increases.

SAD is diagnosed in people if they become depressed in the fall and winter for two or more consecutive years, with periods of normal moods in the spring and summer, and if they have no other problems that might account for seasonal depression. A rare form of SAD, called summer SAD, occurs in reverse of the normal pattern. People with summer SAD become depressed during the summer and feel better in the winter.

What Are the Symptoms of SAD?

Not everyone who has SAD experiences all the same symptoms. Often people with SAD report feeling fatigue and oversleeping and a craving for carbohydrates, along with the tendency to gain a little weight. These

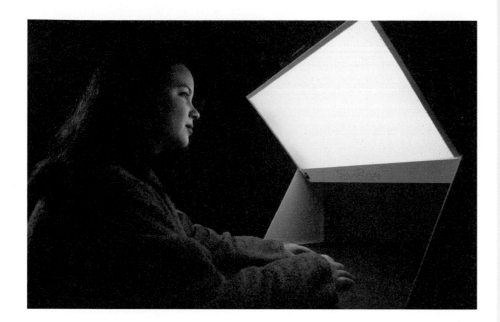

Winter depression is a common type of SAD that is caused by the dramatic decrease in sunlight when the seasons change. Patients who undergo light therapy may sit in a light box for about a half hour a day throughout the fall and winter, until springtime when there is more natural sunshine. *Stock Boston*

symptoms occur along with other common symptoms of depression such as:

- depressed mood
- feelings of helplessness, hopelessness, or guilt
- pessimistic thoughts
- loss of pleasure in previously enjoyable activities
- difficulty concentrating or making decisions.

How Is SAD Treated?

Once it has been diagnosed correctly, seasonal affective disorder can be treated with light therapy. People with SAD sit in front of special bright light boxes or wear light visors for a period of 30 minutes to 2 hours every day, glancing occasionally at the light. To be effective, the light must enter the eyes and not just fall on the skin. Occasionally, people report eyestrain or headaches from the light devices, but usually there are no negative side effects. When natural daylight increases, people with SAD discontinue light treatment.

Resource

Organization

Depression and Related Affective Disorders Association (DRADA), Meyer 3-181, 600 North Wolfe Street, Baltimore, MD 21287-7381. A self-help and educational organization for people with depressive illnesses and their families.
Telephone 410-955-4647
http://www.med.jhu.edu/drada

▶ *See also*
Depression

Seizures *See* The Brain and Nervous System (Introduction); Brain Chemistry (Neurochemistry)

Selective Mutism

Selective mutism (se-LEK-tiv MU-ti-zum) is a condition in which children feel so inhibited and anxious that they do not speak in particular situations, most commonly in school. Children with selective mutism are capable of speaking and communicating normally, and do so in other situations, for example, at home.

When Brandon first started kindergarten, his teacher just thought he was a very quiet boy, that he would come out of his shell in a week or two. As the weeks passed into months, though, Brandon still never spoke a word at school, even when the teacher called on him. Sometimes if he needed something, he would point or gesture, but he would never speak. His teacher was concerned, and when she called his parents, they told her that Brandon spoke easily at home, and that he had always been a little shy around others. It was clear that Brandon's problem was more than normal shyness. Since it was interfering with his ability to participate in class and on the playground, Brandon's parents took him to a mental health professional, who diagnosed his problem as selective mutism.

What Is Selective Mutism?

Selective mutism is a condition in which children feel anxious and inhibited and do not speak in certain situations. Children with selective mutism are capable of speaking normally, and do so in other situations where they feel more comfortable. These children often talk normally at home, but they may completely stop talking around teachers, other children, or other adults. Their behavior gets in the way of making friends and doing well in school.

Selective mutism, once thought to be quite rare, is beginning to be more widely recognized. It used to be called elective mutism, because it was thought that children were purposely choosing not to talk. It was sometimes thought that a child's refusal to speak was a way to rebel against adults, or a sign of anger. It affects at least 1 in 100 school-age children. It usually begins before age 5, but it may not cause problems until children start school. The condition may last for just a few months, but in some cases, if left untreated, selective mutism can last for years. Some experts believe that untreated selective mutism in children leads to social anxiety disorder in their adult years. Experts now believe that selective mutism is an extreme form of social anxiety in a child. Social anxiety is an intense, lasting fear or extreme discomfort in social situations, and usually leads to avoidance of many social situations. With selective mutism, children seem to feel so self-consious or anxious in certain situations that they avoid talking altogether.

What Causes Selective Mutism?

There is no single cause of selective mutism. As with other forms of anxiety, some children may be more likely to have this problem if anxiety or extreme shyness runs in the family, or if they are born with a shy nature. Beyond genetics, in some families where adults are anxious, children may learn to feel socially anxious by watching the way adults react and behave. Upsetting or stressful events such as divorce, the death of a loved one, or frequent moves may trigger selective mutism in a child who is prone to anxiety.

What Are the Symptoms of Selective Mutism?

Many children are shy for a while when they first start kindergarten, but most eventually become comfortable in school, make friends, and talk to the teacher. For those with selective mutism, silence continues and lasts for a month or longer. Some children with selective mutism make gestures, nod, or write notes to communicate. Others use one-syllable words or whispers. Many children with selective mutism are very shy and fearful and may have nervous habits, such as biting their nails. They may cling to their parents and sulk around strangers but might throw temper tantrums and be stubborn and demanding at home. When pushed to speak, they may become stubborn in their refusal. It is sometimes hard for adults to understand that fear, not stubbornness, is at the root of selective mutism, and that children with this condition experience speaking as risky, scary, or dangerous. Understood in this way, it is possible to see a child's stubborn refusal to speak when forced as a strong, but misguided, attempt at self-protection.

How Is Selective Mutism Diagnosed?

Some children with selective mutism will speak to a mental health professional, but others will not. Even if children are silent, though, a skilled professional therapist still can learn a lot by watching how they behave. The therapist also can talk to parents and teachers to find out more about the problem and possible factors that contribute to it. In addition, a number of tests may be needed to exclude other possible causes for failing to speak. These include special medical tests to rule out brain damage, intelligence and academic tests to rule out learning problems, speech and language tests to rule out communication disorders*, and hearing tests to rule out hearing loss.

*communication disorders affect a person's ability to use or understand speech and language.

315

How Is Selective Mutism Treated?

Most children who have selective mutism want to feel comfortable talking. Though they resist efforts to help them talk at first, therapy can be very helpful in treating this problem. The most common treatment for selective mutism is behavioral (bee-HAY-vyor-al) therapy, which helps people gradually change specific, unwanted types of behavior. For example, after the therapist helps the child to feel comfortable, the child might be rewarded for speaking softly and clearly into a tape recorder. Once they have succeeded at this several times, they can move on to being rewarded for speaking to one child at school. Children who are selectively mute may speak to specific children. They then might be invited to participate in a group with the children the selectively mute child speaks to.

Often family therapy is added, which helps identify and change behavior patterns within the family that may play a role in maintaining mutism. When a child has selective mutism, it is common for the family members to speak for the child. While they begin to do this out of love and concern and the desire to be helpful, these patterns must be discontinued to help motivate a reluctant child to begin to speak for herself. Play therapy and drawing are often used to help these children to express their feelings and worries. In addition, some children with selective mutism are prescribed medications used for treating anxiety. These medications help lessen the anxiety that plays an important role in the selectively mute child's behavior, allowing the child to take the risks involved in talking out loud.

Resource

Organization

Selective Mutism Group, 30 South J Street, 3A, Lake Worth, FL 33460. This organization provides online support for the parents of children with selective mutism.
http://www.selectivemutism.org

▶ *See also*

Anxiety and Anxiety Disorders

Social Anxiety Disorder

KEYWORDS
for searching the Internet and other reference sources

Self-confidence

Self-image

Self-Esteem

Self-esteem is the value that people put on the mental image that they have of themselves.

What Is Self-Esteem?

Everyone has a mental picture of his or her strengths, weaknesses, characteristics, and abilities. This mental picture, often called self-image, begins to develop in infancy and continues to grow and change throughout life. People develop their self-image through their interactions with other people and the world. Self-esteem is a person's overall sense of being lovable, acceptable, worthy, and capable.

Self-esteem has three main parts:

- feeling loved and accepted by others
- having feelings of self-acceptance and self-worth
- feeling competent and capable of solving problems and using skills

How Does Self-Esteem Develop?

The first ideas that babies and young children have about themselves are strongly influenced by the things their parents do and say. If a caregiver tells a toddler that she is bad often enough, the child will begin to believe that she is bad. If a parent constantly tells a school-age child that he is dumb, there is a good chance that he will believe that he can never do well in school. As children grow, the judgments of teachers, friends, coaches, and other people in their lives influence the image they have of themselves.

People also have a mental image of what they would like to be. Everyone's mental image of the ideal person is different. Some people admire athletic skills. Others admire academic abilities, courage, compassion, or the ability to get along with others. People whose mental self-image matches fairly well with the qualities they admire generally feel good about themselves and have high self-esteem. People whose self-image does not match well with the things they think are important tend to be unhappy, dissatisfied, negative about themselves, and have low self-esteem. With low self-esteem, people may see themselves as unlovable, unacceptable, unworthy, or incompetent.

Why Does Self-Esteem Matter?

The way people feel about themselves has a big effect on their behavior. People with high self-esteem who feel good about themselves and see themselves as competent, independent problem solvers are more likely to meet challenges at home, school, and work. People who feel lovable and worthy have better relationships and tend to ask for help and support when they need it. Self-acceptance helps people cope with failures and learn from mistakes. High self-esteem allows people to accept their imperfections.

Low self-esteem has been linked to violent and delinquent behavior and to school failure. Teenagers with low self-esteem are more likely to be involved in gangs, drug and alcohol abuse, sexually promiscuous activities, or antisocial behaviors* that lead to confrontations with the law. Low self-esteem is also linked to depression*, poor body image*, and eating disorders*. People with low self-esteem tend to have a harder time coping with failure, mistakes, and their own imperfections.

*__antisocial behaviors__ are behaviors that differ significantly from the norms of society and are considered harmful to society.

*__depression__ (de-PRESH-un) is a mental state characterized by feelings of sadness, despair, and discouragement.

*__body image__ is a person's impressions, thoughts, feelings, and opinions about his or her body.

*__eating disorders__ are conditions in which a person's eating behaviors and food habits are so unbalanced that they cause physical and emotional problems.

Can People Improve Their Self-Esteem?

Unlike a person's height or eye color, self-esteem is not fixed for life. Self-esteem can be nourished and improved. Studies have shown that positive thinking or positive self-talk helps raise self-esteem. For example, people who think, "I'm so dumb, I'll never solve this math problem" reinforce their low self-esteem. They can help raise their self-esteem by mentally correcting themselves and thinking instead, "I might have to work harder than some of my friends to solve this problem, but I am sure I can figure it out."

Parents, teachers, coaches, and friends can help people develop high self-esteem by:

- helping them learn new skills that are suited to their age and interest
- encouraging them to try new things
- offering genuine praise for trying hard, as well as for success
- not comparing people's abilities (especially with siblings or classmates)
- expressing acceptance and caring
- being a good listener and letting the person know that his or her ideas and feelings are important

Resources

Book

Canfield, Jack, Mark Victor Hansen, and Kimberly Kirberger, eds. *Chicken Soup for the Teenage Soul: 101 Stories of Life, Love and Learning.* Deerfield Beech, FL: Health Communications, Inc., 1997.

Organizations

The National Association for Self-Esteem (NASE), 1776 Lincoln Street, Suite 1012, Denver, CO 80203-1027. The National Association for Self-Esteem has a website that provides information on the latest research on self-esteem and its relationship to behavior. http://www.self-esteem-nase.org

Nemours Center for Children's Health Media, Alfred I. duPont Hospital for Chidren, 1600 Rockland Road, Wilmington, DE 19803. This organization's KidsHealth website has articles about self-esteem. http://www.KidsHealth.org

▶ *See also*

Body Dysmorphic Disorder

Body Image

Depression

Eating Disorders

Resilience

School Avoidance

School Failure

Sexual Development

Sexual development, also called puberty, is a normal stage of life during which adolescents experience many physical, cognitive, and emotional changes.

Not a Day at the Beach

"Mostly I'm pretty scared because I don't know if I'm normal or, you know, just strange. My body seems to be changing but not like some of my friends. I still look pretty much like a little kid and my best friend looks like he's 18 or something. I don't want to go near the gym anymore because then I'll have to take a shower. I know the other guys are going to laugh at me because I, well, you know, just don't look developed."—John, age 13.

"Now I have zits all over my face, my nose is too big and my breasts are too small. It really bothers me. I don't think guys will ever notice me, let alone like me if my body stays like this—I'm a disaster."—Dominique, age 14.

"No one had told me anything about menstruation. When I started to bleed and nobody was at home, I got so scared I called 911."—Aisha, age 12.

During adolescence the body a child has had for several years seems to become different and sometimes strange. This phase of development is referred to as puberty and involves rapid changes in the body, including sexual maturation. Bodies change, attitudes about self and others change, thinking abilities change, and interest in sexual activities changes as well. The good news is that puberty does not last forever—most people get through it by age 18.

Changing Bodies

Adolescence in Western societies spans the age range from about 8 to 20. During this period there are major physical and emotional changes associated with sexual development. This time is called puberty.

Puberty is the growth stage in which the reproductive organs mature. Girls begin puberty, on average, about two years before boys. For girls, the body changes associated with puberty usually begin between the ages of 8 and 13. For boys, the normal age range for the start of puberty is between 10 and 14. What starts puberty is unknown, but the hypothalamus, a small area located deep within the brain, plays a key role. During puberty the hypothalamus and pituitary gland, a pea-sized organ located just beneath the hypothalamus, send out chemical messages that cause the gonads, or sex glands (testes in boys, ovaries in girls), to increase production of sex hormones* (testosterone in boys and estrogen in girls). With the increase in these hormones, the body begins to

* **hormones** are bodily substances that originate in a gland or organ. The hormones most commonly referred to in regard to sex are androgens and estrogens.

319

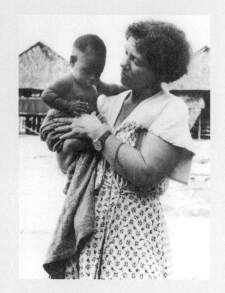

▲

Anthropologist Margaret Mead studied the sexual development of adolescents across cultures, discovering that different cultures have different rites of passage to mark the milestones in an individual's sexual development. Her landmark book *Coming of Age in Samoa: A Psychological Study of Primitive Youth for Western Civilization* was published in 1928 and still is a best seller. *AP/Associated Press*

develop secondary sex characteristics (body hair, breasts, deeper voice, etc.) as well as to undergo a growth spurt.

The organs involved in sexual reproduction also enlarge and develop. For girls this series of changes leads to menstruation and signals that the body is capable of sexual reproduction, or having babies. For boys these changes lead to the production of sperm. While boys may have experienced erections throughout childhood, ejaculation, the release of sperm in a fluid called semen, is only possible when this developmental level has been achieved.

Unfortunately, many studies continue to show that neither girls nor boys are prepared for the physical changes that make their bodies seem strange and foreign. Most girls report they knew little if anything about what usually is referred to as a "period" before their first experience. It also is typical for boys not to understand their newly acquired potential for ejaculation. Menstruation and ejaculation can be quite shocking and frightening experiences if one is unaware and unprepared.

Changing Attitudes, Changing Thoughts, Changing Emotions

Puberty is a normal developmental stage that involves rapid and dramatic changes. In addition to physical changes, adolescents also experience changes in mood, thinking, and in social interests.

Mood Changes in hormones in the adolescent body can trigger sudden and unpredictable changes in moods. One minute a boy or girl may be laughing and then, for no apparent reason, he or she can suddenly become angry or tearful. The different feelings that adolescents experience often make them feel like their emotions are on a roller coaster. The increased production of sex hormones is just one of many factors that contribute to these mood swings.

Cognition During this stage of life, adolescents develop the ability to think in more abstract and logical ways. They have a greater ability to examine their own, as well as other's, thoughts. These improved cognitive abilities often contribute to the disagreements between adults and adolescents as the adolescent is trying out new ways of thinking about issues and the world. If adults are not prepared for the changing nature of the adolescent's thought process, then the adolescent may feel as if he or she is being misunderstood or "treated like a child." Similarly, since adolescents are just beginning to develop these different cognitive abilities, there may be times when they want to think and act more like their younger selves. The adults around them need to respond to these changes and provide appropriate, challenging opportunities, but not opportunities that will overwhelm or frustrate the adolescent. The adults surrounding the adolescent are also learning about this changing, new person and are undergoing a "development" process, too!

Sensitivity Adolescents are also changing the way they think about themselves and others. Adolescents at this developmental stage are quite involved with their own thoughts and feelings. Many adolescents believe that everyone is as absorbed with himself or herself as he or she is. Additionally, adolescents at this time believe that others are looking at them or thinking about them in a critical manner. This may cause some adolescents to be very sensitive about body image, minor mistakes they make, or differences between themselves and others. Sometimes people refer to adolescents as "hyper-sensitive," which means that others feel that adolescents care too much about relatively minor things. For the adolescents, however, this hypersensitivity is part of the normal process of developing an understanding of who they are.

Uniqueness Adolescents have a new sense of personal uniqueness or "egocentrism." At this stage, adolescents believe that no one else can ever understand how they feel, not parents or even friends. Sometimes, to maintain a sense of personal uniqueness, adolescents may have ideas and beliefs that seem inaccurate or unrealistic. This is a normal reaction to the changes that the adolescent is undergoing.

Invulnerability Sometimes adolescents feel they are indestructible or invulnerable to danger. This can lead to reckless behaviors such as drug use, fast driving, "daredevil" behaviors, suicidal thoughts, or sexual promiscuity. The adolescent may be unable to comprehend accurately the potential risks and negative outcomes of these reckless acts. This is another area of potential conflict between adolescents and adults: adults are responsible for keeping adolescents safe, and adolescents perceive adult actions to be overly controlling, overly cautious, or "out of touch."

What About Sex?

Adolescent development comes with many new and different physical and emotional feelings. Some of the most confusing may be the sexual thoughts that cause sensations or reactions in the body. Both girls and boys experience sexual feelings. These feelings are pleasurable and exciting and perfectly normal. Sometimes it is difficult to understand what one is expected to do with these new sexual feelings. Adolescents are aware that adults and the society in which they live have many, often conflicting, ideas about sex. For example, even though masturbation is a normal part of human sexuality, many people feel embarrassed to talk about it or may feel it is harmful or sinful. Adults are important resources who can help adolescents learn that sexual development and the physical changes of their bodies are normal. Unfortunately many adults are reluctant to discuss these issues, and adolescents are left with the impression that there is something wrong or shameful about the natural functioning of their bodies.

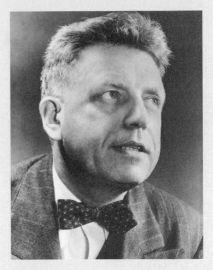

Alfred C. Kinsey and his colleagues interviewed men and women about their sexual behaviors and published two influential reports, *Sexual Behavior in the Human Male* (1948) and *Sexual Behavior in the Human Female* (1953). *Archive Photos*

Menstruation

When girls reach a particular stage of development, usually between ages 9 and 15, menstruation (MEN-stru-A-shun) begins. Often referred to as a "period," the word "menstruation" comes from the Latin word "mensis" meaning month. Each month an egg (ovum) is released from a woman's ovaries. This is called ovulation. The egg carries half of the genetic information needed to create a baby. The other half is contained in the sperm cell provided by the male. If the egg is fertilized by sperm, the embryo implants in the uterus where it will grow. If the egg is not fertilized, the soft lining of the uterus is shed and passes out of the woman's body. Every month a woman's body readies for a possible pregnancy. The time between one menstruation and the next is about a month and is called the menstrual cycle.

Information Menstruation is a normal and important fact of a woman's life. Many young women are not adequately informed about menstruation. One study found that 43 percent of women felt frightened, panicky, or ill when they started to menstruate for the first time. About one-third of women in another survey did not know about menstruation before they began menstruating. It is important for girls to be told about the various physical and emotional changes surrounding menstruation. For example, it is common for a woman's breasts to feel swollen and tender before her period begins. Other women experience temporary weight gain of a few pounds or sudden cravings for carbohydrates such as chocolate prior to their periods. Some women feel they are absent-minded or disorganized or that their emotions are out of control before their periods begin. Many women experience cramps, pains in the lower abdominal area, at the start of their periods. All of these experiences are normal and it is important that young women are aware of these potential feelings as a natural part of menstruation.

Erections and Ejaculation

When boys reach puberty they may begin to experience more frequent erections. Erections occur when blood rushes into the penis, causing it to grow and stiffen. Ejaculations occur when sperm mixes with fluids from a gland called the prostate gland, and exits through the opening of the penis. It is through ejaculation that sperm leaves the male's body to enter the female's body when they combine during sexual intercourse to begin a pregnancy. Not all erections lead to ejaculations or sexual intercourse. As boys mature they may also have erections and orgasms during sleep or pleasurable dreams. These are often called "wet dreams" or nocturnal emissions. Nocturnal emissions are usual and normal for boys. If a boy's pajamas or sheets are wet and sticky upon awakening, he has probably had a wet dream. Sometimes a full bladder may cause an erection so it is not uncommon for males to awaken with an erection. Because there are many ways to excite the penis to erection, sometimes men have erections for no apparent reason, or even at inconvenient times. Boys may have erections at times that can be embarrassing, perplexing, or even anxiety provoking. While it may seem embarrassing and troublesome, it is all quite normal. Discussing these confusing moments with someone the young man trusts and is comfortable with can help to reassure him about these experiences.

Masturbation

Masturbation is the self-stimulation of the genitals to achieve pleasurable sensations, sometimes resulting in sexual orgasm. It is one of the most common human sexual expressions. Children from about the age of 2½ may masturbate. A recent study has shown that one-third of females and two-thirds of males report masturbating before they reached adolescence. Many parents are hesitant to condone or express their approval of masturbation. Many religions feel that masturbation is improper. It is a difficult topic to discuss openly even though the majority of teenage boys and girls report having masturbated by the end of puberty.

While masturbation is a safe and available release for sexual tension, many people masturbate and many do not. It is a matter of personal choice, guided by one's beliefs and values.

Staying Safe

While most people engage in some form of mutual sexual interaction at some time in their lives, when, with whom, and why are big questions that should be carefully considered before activities begin. In addition to the emotional price of having sex before one is ready, it can also pose some potential health risks and other problems. Pregnancy and sexually transmitted diseases are two health issues that may arise from sexual intercourse.

Pregnancy Pregnancy is a natural outcome of sexual intercourse. Unless an adult couple is prepared and ready to start a family, an unexpected pregnancy can cause many problems. This is one of the reasons it is so important to consider the consequences of acting on one's sexual desires before engaging in intercourse. There are many ways to prevent pregnancy. These methods are called contraception or birth control. The most effective method of contraception, and the only one that is 100 percent effective, is to refrain from all sexual intercourse until ready for pregnancy. This is sometimes called "abstinence." Many religious groups and many parents support the idea that sexual intercourse should only occur within a marriage.

Contraception There are many methods of contraception. Using no "protection" against pregnancy by trying to time sexual contact or trying not to ejaculate during intercourse are generally not considered effective. There are other methods of contraception that allow a couple to engage in sexual intercourse with protection against unwanted pregnancy.

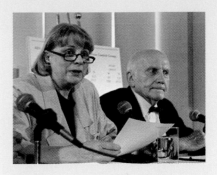

William H. Masters and Virginia E. Johnson were a married couple who studied sexual desire, arousal, and orgasm. They published their findings in the books *Human Sexual Response* (1966) and *Human Sexual Inadequacy* (1970). *AFP/Corbis*

Men may use a condom, sometimes referred to as a rubber or jimmy, during intercourse. A condom is a soft, thin latex or polyurethane cover that fits over an erect penis.

Other forms of contraceptives include birth control pills, diaphragms, intrauterine devices or IUDs, cervical caps, Norplant, or Depo Provera. These methods are all prescribed forms of contraception that can only be obtained from a doctor or health clinic. These methods are only used by women and require a thorough physical examination before they are prescribed.

It is important to understand that any decision about contraception, like any decision about sex, should be an informed decision. Discussions with parents, health professionals, counselors, and trusted adults should be part of making mature and informed decisions about sexual activity. Many states regulate the age at which a person can receive prescription birth control methods. Often people who are younger than 18 years of age must have the permission or consent of parents or guardians to obtain these birth control measures.

Sexually transmitted diseases   Although the proper use of condoms can decrease the risk, abstaining from intercourse or other risky sexual activities is the only sure way to prevent the spread of HIV/AIDS, gonorrhea, chlamydia, syphilis, herpes, and other sexually transmitted diseases.

Sexual Orientation

Sexual orientation refers to one's feelings for and sexual attraction to other people. People can be heterosexual, homosexual, or bisexual. Most people's orientation is heterosexual (attraction to the opposite sex), but homosexual (attracted to the same sex) and bisexual (attracted to both sexes) orientations are normal as well. It is estimated that as many as 10 percent of people are homosexual and there are no reliable estimates for the prevalence of bisexuals. There are many problems with obtaining reliable estimates of the numbers of gays, lesbians, and bisexuals in the population because of the ongoing discrimination they face due to their sexual orientation.

Experimentation   During adolescence one's sexual orientation is often unsettled. Some people engage in various forms of sexual experimentation during early adolescence. This experimentation is generally due to opportunities that present, curiosity, or family or peer pressure. These may not always be consistent with a person's natural sexual orientation or attraction.

What this means is that some people might have some alternative sexual feelings or activities (for example, homosexual sex) during adolescence. These people may go on to be fully heterosexual. Similarly, individuals who identify themselves as homosexual may have heterosexual experiences during adolescence. For some people, adolescence is a time of curiosity and exploration. This is considered normal and generally has nothing to do with how someone will "grow up."

How does sexual orientation develop? Sexual orientation is a natural fact of human life and central to everyone's core identity. This question is most often asked about same-sex and bisexual orientations. Do people choose to be homosexual or bisexual? Are they born that way? This has been a long-standing and controversial debate. Many scientists now believe that sexual orientation is not a matter of choice. These scientists think people are born with their sexual orientation, just like they are born with their eye or hair color. Other scientists believe that experiences during a person's childhood contribute to his or her sexual orientation. Up to this point, there is no conclusive scientific evidence that completely answers the question of what makes a person gay or straight.

Resources

Books

Bell, R. *Changing Bodies, Changing Lives: A Book for Teens on Sex and Relationships.* New York: Random House, 1988.

Harris, R. H. *It's Perfectly Normal.* Cambridge, MA: Candlewick Press, 1996.

Madaras, L., and A. Madaras. *My Body, My Self for Girls.* New York: Newmarket Press, 1993.

Madaras, L., and A. Madaras. *My Body, My Self for Boys.* New York: Newmarket Press, 1995.

Marcus, E. *What If Someone I Know Is Gay?* New York: Price Stern Sloan, 2000.

▶ *See also*
Body Image
Gender Identity

Shyness   *See* Social Anxiety

Sibling Rivalry   *See* Families

KEYWORDS
*for searching the Internet
and other reference sources*

Circadian rhythm

Melatonin

Sleep disorders

Sleep medicine

Sleep research

*metabolism (me-TAB-o-liz-um)
includes the chemical
processes in the body that
convert foods into the energy
needed for body functions.

*hallucinate (huh-LOO-sin-ate)
means to hear, see, or otherwise sense things that are not
real.

Sleep

Sleep is a state marked by a lowered level of consciousness, decreased movement of the body's muscles, and slowing of metabolism*.

Asleep for Twenty-Five Years

While it might sound like the title of a new science fiction movie, this phrase actually describes the typical experience of most people who live to the age of 75. The fact that people spend about one-third of their lives asleep (roughly eight hours out of every twenty-four-hour day) suggests that sleep is very important to how their brains and bodies function.

Why Do People Need to Sleep?

The desire for sleep is strong. People may be able to deny themselves food or water for a few days, but they cannot go without sleep. Research has shown that severely sleep-deprived people become very uncomfortable and anxious and may even start to hallucinate*. This explains why prisoners-of-war sometimes are forced by their captors to stay awake for long periods of time: the captors know that prisoners are likely to become so desperate for sleep that they will eventually break down and share important information.

Researchers have not been able to precisely explain the function that sleep serves. At one time it was thought that sleep provided a time for the brain to rest, but studies have shown that the brain's neurons, or nerve cells, are just as active during sleep as when a person is awake. Some neurons are even more active during sleep. Another theory about the function of sleep is that sleep is essential for the proper storage of long-term memories by the brain. A study by researchers at Harvard University found that performance of a newly learned task actually improves after a good night's sleep. Yet another theory is based on the observation that the brain makes proteins at a much faster rate when people are asleep than when they are awake. These proteins are necessary for maintaining the structure and function of neurons, so it may be that sleep gives the brain the chance to replenish its store of these important substances. This would explain why people report feeling "burnt out" when they are not getting enough sleep; the brain literally may be burning through its proteins faster than it can replace them.

What Are the Stages of Sleep?

While researchers are still trying to figure out why people need to sleep, they have learned a great deal about what happens during the sleep process itself.

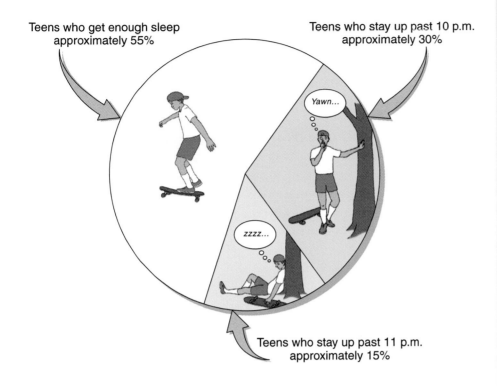

Teens who get enough sleep approximately 55%

Teens who stay up past 10 p.m. approximately 30%

Yawn...

zzzz...

Teens who stay up past 11 p.m. approximately 15%

Research shows that the brain makes proteins essential for neuron function at a faster rate during sleep than during waking hours. But close to half of all teens do not get as much sleep as they need, leading to feelings of "burn out," possibly because the brain is burning through proteins faster than it can replace them.

Measuring brain waves with electroencephalography (EEG)

Throughout the nervous system, neurons communicate with each other in a language that is both chemical and electrical. Researchers can use specialized equipment to measure the waves of electricity generated by the hundreds of thousands of brain cells. This test, which is called electroencephalography (eh-lek-tro-en-sef-uh-LAH-gruh-fee), or EEG, involves placing electrodes on the scalp and attaching them to a machine that amplifies the electrical changes that are occurring. A special recording pen then translates these changes onto paper, generating waves of various sizes. The appearance of the EEG changes according to whether a person is excited or anxious, calm or relaxed. For instance, when a person is relaxed, the brain generates what are known as alpha waves from the back of the head. People can actually learn how to generate alpha waves by thinking calm, soothing thoughts and entering a state of total relaxation.

Shallow sleep and deep sleep

Thanks to sleep studies using EEG, researchers have been able to identify four stages of sleep that are distinguished by different wave patterns recorded from the brain: stage four is the deepest, and stage one is the shallowest. Within forty-five minutes of falling asleep, most people descend very rapidly to level four, which is marked by larger, slower brain waves on the EEG. Heart rate

"Get a Good Night's Sleep" May Be Good Advice

Instead of cramming all night for the weekly math quiz, a person might be better off practicing the new concepts until bedtime and then getting a good night's sleep. A team of researchers at Harvard University found that college students who got a full night's sleep after they learned a new task were much more likely to improve their performance on the task the next day than those who did not get enough sleep. The researchers taught the students to spot visual targets on a computer screen and to press a button as soon as they were certain they had seen one. With about an hour of practice, students were able to perform the task well. When retested later that same day, the students

(continued)

showed no improvement over their best times. When tested the next day, students who had slept six hours or less showed no improvement. Other students who slept more than six hours performed better than their best times from the previous day.

Did the extra sleep really make the difference? In another study with a different group of students, the researchers allowed half of the students to sleep at the end of the day but kept the other half awake until the next night. Then both groups were allowed to sleep on the second and third nights. On the fourth day, both groups were tested. The researchers found that the students who slept the first night performed better than the students who did not, even though the others had two nights of catch-up sleep. This finding seems to provide even more evidence that sleep plays a key role in helping the brain absorb and retain new material.

and blood pressure decrease, the muscles relax, and it is very difficult to awaken the sleeper. Throughout the night, the person surfaces from level four to levels three, two, and one (progressively shallower states of sleep in which the brain waves get smaller and faster) and then back down to level four again. This cycle happens several times during the night.

Rapid Eye Movement (REM)   During the shallow sleep stages, people enter into yet another stage of sleep known as Rapid Eye Movement, or REM. This is when dreaming occurs. The eyes move rapidly behind the closed eyelids, and the person's muscles become very rigid. In addition to moving through the four non-REM sleep stages, people can experience as many as four or five periods of REM sleep per night; in general, younger people spend more time in REM sleep than do older people. Because dreams are quickly forgotten after moving out of the REM phase, most people probably dream much more than they think they do. Ordinarily, a person will only remember the dreams that he or she had during the REM phase that occurred just before waking.

Research studies have shown that all mammals, not just humans, experience REM sleep, and that the brain knows the difference between this stage and the non-REM stages. Sleep studies have been done in which people are persistently awakened before they can enter REM sleep. After this goes on for a few nights, the people are allowed to sleep normally. Measurements show that they tend to spend more time in REM sleep on successive nights than they usually would. In a sense, the brain seems to be making up for lost REM-sleep time. This holds true for the deep sleep stages (non-REM stages three and four) as well; if people are deprived of these stages, they will spend more time in them on successive nights.

The red regions of these PET scans show the difference in brain activity during normal sleep *(left)* and REM sleep *(right)*. During REM sleep dreams occur, and the brain strengthens memories by processing experiences and new information. The PET scan of the REM brain actually looks similar to a PET scan of a brain that is fully awake. *Photo Researchers, Inc.*

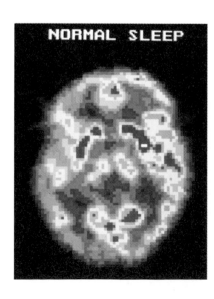

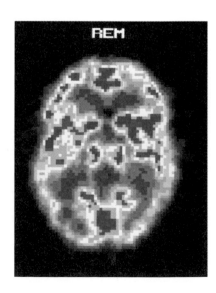

What Makes a Person Fall Asleep?

There are a variety of physical, psychological, and environmental factors involved in the sleep process.

Brain chemistry Levels of alertness in the brain are controlled by different groups of chemical neurotransmitters* in certain areas of the lower portions of the brain. Levels of these chemicals vary at different times of the day and as emotions change. The lower portions of the brain communicate with the higher portion of the brain, the cortex*, signaling it to increase its activity or to slow down. Slow-down signals come just before bedtime or at certain other times of the day; many students can relate to feeling sleepy during an early afternoon lecture. However, the cortex has some say in the matter as well. People who are nervous or under stress often have trouble falling asleep because they cannot stop thinking about what is bothering them. And the tired student can force herself to stay awake if she knows the lecture is important. In other words, the brain's cortex can override the signal to fall asleep.

Melatonin Another chemical substance, a hormone* called melatonin (mel-uh-TOE-nin), also seems to play a role in producing sleep. Melatonin is released into the bloodstream by a tiny gland located in the center of the brain. The amount of melatonin in the blood fluctuates widely over the course of a twenty-four-hour period, with levels being up to ten times greater at night than during the day.

Circadian rhythm People also have a main "biological clock" that is located within the area in the center of the brain known as the hypothalamus*. This area receives direct input from the eye, responding to the light changes of day and night and keeping the body on a twenty-four-hour cycle. This cycle, also referred to as the circadian (sir-KAY-dee-un) rhythm, involves predictable changes in body temperature, heart rate and blood pressure, sleepiness and wakefulness, and other functions. For example, body temperature drops to its lowest point between 2 A.M. and 5 P.M. and reaches its highest point in the afternoon or evening.

Light and dark The cues of light and dark help to keep a person's sleep patterns and other bodily rhythms on track. However, studies have shown that when a person is deprived of light, his or her body resets its internal clock to a twenty-five-hour schedule. People who have taken part in such studies—living in darkness for weeks at a time—tend to underestimate the amount of time they spent living without the normal cues of day and night. Clearly, then, our environments have some effect on the patterns on sleep and wakefulness that structure our lives.

* **neurotransmitters** (NUR-o-tranz-mit-erz) are brain chemicals that let brain cells communicate with each other and therefore allow the brain to function normally.

* **cortex** (KOR-teks) is the part of the brain that controls conscious thought. It is where people experience conscious, subjective feelings.

* **hormones** are chemicals that are produced by different glands in the body. A hormone is like the body's ambassador: it is created in one place but is sent through the body to have specific effects on other parts of the body.

* **hypothalamus** (hy-po-THAL-uh-mus) is a brain structure located deep within the brain that plays a part in regulating automatic body functions such as heart rate, blood pressure, temperature, respiration, and the release of hormones.

Researchers believe that the body's daily "clock," also called its circadian rhythm, is linked to the pineal gland and to the suprachiasmatic nucleus region of the hypothalamus. These structures within the brain receive information from the eye's retina about daylight and darkness, and send signals about regulating body responses to the spinal cord and elsewhere in the nervous system. ▶

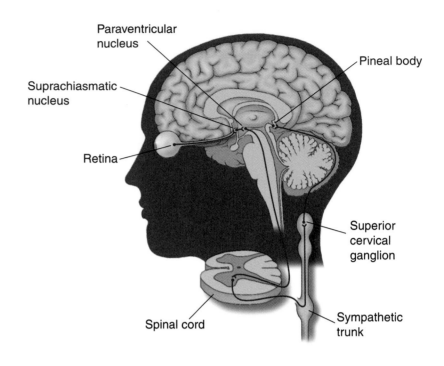

Paraventricular nucleus

Pineal body

Suprachiasmatic nucleus

Retina

Superior cervical ganglion

Spinal cord

Sympathetic trunk

* night terrors occur during deep (stage 4) sleep, usually within an hour after a person goes to bed. People experiencing night terrors may sit up in bed, scream, cry, sweat, and appear to be extremely frightened, but they are still asleep and are unaware of their environment. Night terrors most commonly affect young children, although anyone can experience them.

What Are Sleep Disorders?

There are many types of disorders that can make sleeping difficult, including:

- Insomnia (in-SOM-nee-uh) is the best-known sleep disorder. It means simply that a person has trouble falling asleep. Just about everyone experiences insomnia at some point in their lives, but for some people this is a condition that persists night after night.

- Parasomnias (par-uh-SOM-nee-uhs) are a wide range of disruptive sleep-related events, such as sleep walking, sleep talking, eating while asleep, or night terrors*. Often the person is completely unaware of what he or she is doing during these episodes.

- Periodic limb movement disorder is a condition in which people repeatedly twitch or jerk their limbs in their sleep.

- Restless leg syndrome is a condition in which people feel uncomfortable sensations in their legs prior to falling asleep. People with this condition often feel the irresistible urge to move their legs; they may also experience cramping, burning, pain, or a creeping or crawling sensation.

- Sleep apnea (AP-nee-uh) involves having trouble breathing while asleep; the sleeper might snore loudly or sound as if he or she is gasping for air.

Physicians who specialize in sleep medicine are trained to diagnose and treat these and other sleep problems. Typically, patients need to discuss their symptoms with the doctor and undergo overnight testing in a sleep lab. A combination of medications and behavioral therapy can usually help.

Resources

Organizations

American Academy of Sleep Medicine, 6301 Bandel Road NW, Suite 101, Rochester, MN 55901.
Telephone 507-287-6006
http://www.aasmnet.org

National Sleep Foundation, 1522 K Street NW, Suite 500, Washington, DC 20005
Fax: 202-347-3472
http://www.sleepfoundation.org

▶ *See also*
Bedwetting (Enuresis)
Brain Chemistry (Neurochemistry)
Consciousness
Hypnosis
Relaxation

Smoking *See* Tobacco Addiction

Social Anxiety Disorder

Social anxiety (ang-ZY-e-tee) disorder is an intense, long-lasting fear of social situations in which embarrassment might occur.

Kim was shy. She did not like to raise her hand in class, but when the English teacher asked her a question, she answered in a soft voice. Angie, on the other hand, was so afraid of being called on that she began skipping English class. Her problem went beyond ordinary shyness. She was suffering from social anxiety disorder.

What Is Social Anxiety Disorder?

Social anxiety disorder, also known as social phobia (FO-bee-a), is an intense, long-lasting fear of embarrassment in social situations. It is different from shyness or stage fright, however. Social anxiety disorder involves extreme anxiety, an unpleasant feeling of fear, worry, or nervousness. It may cause people to avoid social situations, or to feel intensely self-conscious or uncomfortable and may lead to problems at home, work, or school.

KEYWORDS
for searching the Internet and other reference sources

Anxiety

Selective mutism

Shyness

Social phobia

Some people with social anxiety disorder are afraid of one particular type of situation, such as giving a speech, talking in class, eating in a restaurant, or going to a party. Others, however, have a broad form of the disorder, in which they fear and avoid almost any interaction with other people. In its most extreme form, the disorder can greatly limit people's lives. It makes it hard for them to go to school or work. It also makes it almost impossible for them to have any friends at all. Some children who have a particular and intense form of social phobia that causes them to be too anxious to speak in certain situations may have another type of disorder, known as selective mutism.

What Causes Social Anxiety Disorder?

There are probably several causes for social anxiety disorder. People may learn their fear in part from watching how other people behave and what results from their behavior. Research also suggests that some people may inherit a tendency for anxiety. Research points to the possible role of the amygdala (a-MIG-da-la), a small structure inside the brain that is believed to be the seat of fear responses, whether learned or inherited. In addition, some studies have looked at the role of various hormones*, which have an effect on how the body responds to stress. Scientists are exploring the idea that certain hormones may influence some people to overreact to criticism shown by others.

What Are the Symptoms of Social Anxiety Disorder?

Children with social anxiety disorder may cry, throw tantrums, freeze, shy away from others, or avoid or refuse to participate or perform in certain situations without really understanding what the problem is. Teenagers and adults, on the other hand, realize the source of their fears. While they know their fears can be extreme, unreasonable, or out of proportion they feel they cannot control them. Instead, they avoid the feared situation, or they face it with great distress. People with social anxiety disorder commonly fear situations including:

- giving a speech
- performing on stage
- eating in a restaurant
- using a public restroom
- talking in class
- talking to a teacher
- going on dates
- going to parties
- meeting someone new
- talking on the phone

---

*__hormones__ are chemicals that are produced by different glands in the body. A hormone is like the body's ambassador. It is created in one place but is sent through the body to have specific effects on other parts of the body.

Speaking Up

The most common form of social anxiety disorder is fear of public speaking. Many people have a less extreme form of this fear. Toastmasters International is a group with more than 8,000 clubs and more than 170,000 members worldwide. The aim of this group is to help people become more comfortable with and skilled at speaking in public. Some of the group's tips for successful public speaking include:

- Know the material that you will present. Practice your speech, and change it if necessary.

- Imagine yourself giving the speech successfully. Imagine your voice as loud, clear, and confident.

- Realize that people do not want you to fail. They want you to be interesting and fun to listen to.

- Do not apologize for nervousness or glitches. This just calls attention to any problems you have.

- Think about what you are saying, not how you are saying it. Focus on getting your message across.

About 4 percent of adults in the United States show symptoms of social anxiety disorder in any given year. The problem typically starts in childhood or the early teen years. It occurs twice as often in women as men, but a higher percentage of men who have social anxiety disorder seek treatment for it.

How Are Teenagers Affected?

Most teenagers feel self-conscious at times, but those who are gripped by social anxiety disorder may be so overcome by self-doubt and worry that they find it hard to join in social activities. Instead, they may withdraw to the point where they have trouble making and keeping friends or participating in class. Their constant fear of being judged harshly or criticized may lead them to fret too much about their health and appearance. Some teenagers may try to escape the anxiety by drinking alcohol or using drugs. Others may try to mask fear by acting like class clowns. Still others may stop going to school or taking part in after-school activities and may avoid opportunities to socialize with friends. As a result, their grades may fall, and their self-esteem may decline.

How Is Social Anxiety Disorder Treated?

Medications Four out of five people with social anxiety disorder feel better when treated with medications, psychotherapy, or both. Several kinds of medications have been shown to help people with the disorder. Though they cannot cure social anxiety, certain medications, called selective serotonin* reuptake inhibitors, can decrease the intensity of anxiety, allowing people to learn and practice new ways to feel comfortable in social situations. These medications work to correct imbalances in neurotransmitters* (like serotonin), which play a part in mood conditions such as anxiety and depression. Other medications that are sometimes used include benzodiazepines (BEN-zo-dy-AZ-a-peenz), fast-acting agents that help people relax and decrease physical symptoms of anxiety like sweating, trembling, and a pounding heart.

Psychotherapy In psychotherapy (sy-ko-THER-a-pee), people talk about their feelings with a mental health professional, who can help them change the thoughts, behaviors, or relationships that play a part in their problems. With social anxiety, certain approaches to therapy can be especially helpful. Exposure (ex-PO-zhur) therapy is the name of a technique in which people are gradually introduced, in a relaxed and supportive environment, to situations that frighten them, until they begin to feel more and more comfortable. Anxiety management training refers to various techniques, such as deep breathing, that people can be taught to use to help control their distress. Cognitive techniques help

* **serotonin** (ser-a-TOE-nin) is a chemical in the brain that is associated with feelings of well-being.

* **neurotransmitters** (NUR-o-tranz-mit-erz) are chemical messengers that let brain cells communicate with each other and therefore allow the brain to function properly.

people learn to identify their beliefs that might not be reasonable (for example, "I will die if I have to give this talk") and replace them with more realistic ideas about the likelihood of danger in social situations (for example, "It might be uncomfortable, but I know the material, and I will be okay.").

Resources

Organizations

Anxiety Disorders Association of America, 11900 Parklawn Drive, Suite 100, Rockville, MD 20852. This group sponsors a public education program on social anxiety disorder.
Telephone 301-231-9350
http://www.adaa.org

Anxiety Disorders Education Program, U.S. National Institute of Mental Health, 6001 Executive Boulevard, Room 8184, MSC 9663, Bethesda, MD 20892-9663. This government program provides reliable information about social anxiety and other anxiety disorders.
Telephone 888-8ANXIETY
http://www.nimh.nih.gov/anxiety

► See also

Anxiety and Anxiety Disorders

Medications

Phobias

School Avoidance

Selective Mutism

Self-Esteem

Therapy

KEYWORDS
for searching the Internet and other reference sources

Encopresis

Enuresis

Soiling (Encopresis)

Soiling, also called encopresis (en-ko-PREE-sis), is having uncontrolled bowel movements in one's underwear.

Young children routinely have bowel movements in their diapers or underwear, but by about age 3 most children are able to maintain good bowel control and can be toilet-trained. When people who have established bowel control begin to have a bowel movement in their pants, the condition is called soiling, or encopresis. This soiling is often a leaking and not a full bowel movement. Most people who have a problem with soiling do not even realize that it is happening, because they do not feel as if they are having a bowel movement. In the majority of cases, encopresis is a medical problem. This medical problem can have serious psychological effects, ranging from embarrassment to family stress to teasing.

Why Does Soiling Happen?

Soiling is related to constipation (kon-sti-PAY-shun). Constipation is infrequent, hard, and painful bowel movements. When food goes through the digestive system, it is broken down into a thick, sludgelike liquid. The nutrients that the body needs, such as sugars, are absorbed from this liquid in the small intestine. The rest of the material passes into the large intestine, where water is reabsorbed. The remaining solids, called feces (FEE-seez), are then passed out of the body as a bowel movement.

When the bowels move infrequently, the large intestine reabsorbs so much water that the feces become hard and compacted. As a result, bowel movements are painful, causing many people to try to avoid having them. This only makes the problem worse. Eventually, the mass of hard solids in the large intestine causes it to stretch out of shape. As it stretches, small amounts of liquid sludge from the small intestine seep around the hard mass of feces in the large intestine and then leak out of the body. This is the material that causes soiling.

Some adults think that children soil on purpose or that soiling is evidence of a psychological problem. In reality, soiling accidents are not intentional. In fact, people often do not know that soiling is happening until feces are noticed or others smell it. At times the person with encopresis may not even smell the accident. Sometimes children who are teased or embarrassed about soiling can have emotional or behavior problems. Generally, once the soiling is treated and stops, these problems will disappear.

How Is Soiling Treated?

There are three steps to treating soiling:

- Empty the large intestine
- Establish regular bowel movements
- Maintain regular bowel movements.

An enema or a laxative medication often is used to empty the large intestine. With an enema, liquid is pushed into the large intestine to soften the hard mass of feces and create the urge to expel it. Sometimes strong laxatives are used instead, to encourage the intestine to contract and push out the feces.

Once the large intestine is unblocked, it is important to establish regular bowel movements to keep it clear. A doctor may recommend laxatives taken by mouth, such as milk of magnesia, products that contain senna, or mineral oil. These laxatives keep waste material moving quickly through the large intestine so that it remains soft. Setting aside time each day to try to have a bowel movement (usually after breakfast or dinner) also helps establish a regular schedule.

Once a person is having regular bowel movements daily, laxatives are reduced and then gradually eliminated so that a regular schedule can be maintained without artificial assistance. Eating a high-fiber diet and drinking plenty of liquids also help maintain bowel regularity. Once

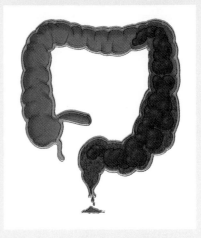

▲

Soiling results when solid body waste becomes hard and compacted in the large intestine, blocking it and causing it to stretch out of shape. If softer waste (liquid stool) seeps around the blockage, it can leak out of the anus, causing soiling.

feces move through the large intestine in a regular, painless way, the problem of soiling disappears. Unfortunately, it often takes time for soiling to be diagnosed correctly and properly treated. Sometimes consultation with a mental health professional, who works with a person's doctor, helps in developing a good behavioral treatment program that also minimizes emotional difficulties.

▶ *See also*
Bedwetting (Enuresis)

KEYWORDS
for searching the Internet and other reference sources

Conversion disorder

Hypochondria

Psychosomatic illness

Somatization disorder

Somatoform Disorders

Somatoform (so-MAT-a-form) disorders are a group of conditions in which physical symptoms suggest a disease or medical condition, but no physical cause can be found. The term "somatoform" is derived from the Greek "soma," meaning "body." A "somatoform disorder" is one in which emotional problems are transformed into body symptoms. These disorders include hypochondria (hy-po-KON-dree-a), conversion disorder, and somatization (so-ma-ti-ZA-shun) disorder. Somatoform disorders do not include malingering or Munchausen syndrome, both of which involve pretending to be physically ill or intentionally producing the symptoms of an illness.

How Can Somatoform Disorders Be Told Apart?

Somatoform disorders are alike in that they each involve physical symptoms without evidence of physical disease. The symptoms stem from an emotional cause. To understand how the disorders differ from each other, consider three young people in a doctor's waiting room who are all having trouble with their voices. Tommy, a teenager, was only hoarse, but he feared this meant that he was getting throat cancer. Nine-year-old Mary had suddenly lost her voice completely and could not speak. Lilian, who was 25, was also hoarse and coughing, but she had many other symptoms, including dizziness and a stomachache.

As it turned out, Tommy was suffering not from cancer but from hypochondria. He had been much too worried about his hoarseness, which had come from cheering for his high school football team. The doctor could find nothing wrong with Mary's larynx, or voice box. Her mother said that Mary had been punished severely for "talking back," and the doctor suspected that she had lost her voice because of conversion disorder. None of Lilian's many symptoms, which had come and gone for years, could be traced to any physical disorder. The doctor thought that she must have somatization disorder. Tommy, Mary, and Lilian were referred to mental health professionals for treatment.

More Symptoms of Somatoform Disorders

Hypochondria   People with hypochondria have the fear or belief that they have a serious illness, such as heart disease or cancer, even though medical tests show no sign of disease. People with this condition may be excessively concerned with a wide range of common, usually minor, symptoms, such as coughing, nausea, dizzy spells, and various aches and pains. When their physicians reassure them that these symptoms do not mean that they are seriously ill, they are not always convinced and may remain anxious, worried, and preoccupied with their symptoms. They may then go to one doctor after another for a "true" diagnosis of the same symptoms.

Conversion disorder   Conversion disorder, a much rarer somatoform disorder, might cause people to lose their voice, sight, or hearing or to become paralyzed in one or more of their limbs. They also may have trembling or lose feeling in various parts of their bodies. The condition is psychological, because medical examination can find no physical explanation for the symptoms. It typically begins suddenly after an extremely stressful event in a person's life. The symptom or affected body part is usually related in some way to the trauma or stress that triggered the conversion reaction. For example, a soldier who is extremely distressed after killing people during battle might develop "paralysis" in his weapon arm. Conversion disorder resulting from war experience has also been called shell shock or battle fatigue. Someone who has witnessed the murder of a loved one may develop "blindness" as a conversion symptom.

Somatization disorder   In somatization disorder, there are many different recurring symptoms in various parts of the body. They may include headache, backache, and pains in the abdomen, chest, and joints. There also may be digestive symptoms, such as nausea and abdominal bloating, or symptoms that involve the reproductive and nervous systems. As in other somatoform disorders, medical examinations and testing generally find no clear physical cause for the symptoms.

Pain disorder and body dysmorphic disorder   Two other kinds of somatoform disorders are pain disorder and body dysmorphic (dis-MOR-fik) disorder. Pain disorder is similar to somatization disorder, except that pain is the main symptom. The pain may be in one or several areas of the body, but it doesn't fit a pattern of any particular medical illness or injury, and diagnostic tests fail to show the presence of any disease. In body dysmorphic disorder, a person becomes extremely concerned about some imagined or very slight body defect. Sometimes called "imagined ugliness," body dysmorphic disorder can cause great distress and cause a person to avoid being seen in public. In some cases, a person may seek unnecessary plastic surgery.

*anxiety (ang-ZY-eh-tee) can be experienced as a troubled feeling, a sense of dread, fear of the future, or distress over a possible threat to a person's physical or mental well-being.

▶ *See also*

Anxiety and Anxiety Disorders

Body Dysmorphic Disorder

Body Image

Conversion Disorder

Hypochondria

Malingering

Munchausen Syndrome

Stress

Causes of Somatoform Disorders

The causes of somatoform disorders are not clearly understood. In hypochondria, a person may be overly sensitive to body sensations or overinterpret the meaning of normal body sensations. A distressing memory of childhood illness may also play a part. It is believed that conversion disorder, somatization disorder, and pain disorder are all caused by the conversion, or shifting, of stressful emotional events or feelings of conflict into body symptoms to relieve anxiety*. Body dysmorphic disorder involves a distorted body image, and may be influenced by cultures that emphasize the importance of physical appearance, and early experiences which may have interfered with developing self-esteem.

Diagnosis and Treatment of Somatoform Disorders

Somatoform disorders are diagnosed by performing a medical evaluation and testing to determine whether there is a physical reason for a patient's symptoms and complaints. If there is not, a somatoform disorder may be diagnosed by looking closely at the particular signs and symptoms. A correct diagnosis is important, in order to avoid unnecessary surgery and other medical procedures and to begin proper treatment for the particular disorder.

Psychotherapy Psychotherapy is the appropriate treatment for somatoform disorders. With the help of a mental health professional, a person tries to understand and resolve anxiety, trauma, or conflicts that are behind these conditions. Treatment may take varying lengths of time, depending on the severity of a disorder in a particular person.

Resources

Organizations

U.S. Surgeon General Dr. C. Everett Koop
http://www.drkoop.com

Nemours Center for Children's Health Media, A. I. duPont Hospital for Children, 1600 Rockland Road, Wilmington, DE 19803. This organization is dedicated to issues of children's health. Their website has much valuable information for children, teens, and parents. http://www.KidsHealth.org

Stealing *See* **Conduct Disorder**

Stress

Stress is the body's natural response to demands placed upon it. This response affects children, teenagers, and adults. Relaxation and stress management techniques help people deal with stress.

Good Stress and Bad Stress

Everyone experiences stress, which is the body's general response to any event, real or imagined, that requires an adaptation or extra effort. In most cases, an event or situation is not stressful by itself. Rather, it is how people view the event and what they believe about their own ability to respond to it that create stress. About 10 percent of modern stress can be linked to actual physical threats to life or safety, such as being threatened with a weapon or needing to slam on the brakes to avoid an accident. The other 90 percent of stress seems to result from our perceptions of life events, such as fights with friends or family, worries about school or work, or problems we do not know how to solve. The majority of doctor visits are believed to be stress-related.

Stressors   Stressors are the triggers for the body's stress response. These triggers are unique to each person. An event that one person finds relaxing may create tension in another. Stressors fall into several different categories:

- Physical stressors affect a person's body. These biological stressors may include exercise, illness, or disabilities.

- Environmental stressors include noise, overcrowding, poverty, natural disasters, or even technology that causes too much change in too short a period of time.

- Life situations create both good and bad stressors. These may include moving to a new home, changing schools or jobs, or experiencing changes in the family structure, such as marriage, divorce, the birth or adoption of a new sibling, or the death of a friend or family member.

- Behaviors also can be stressors. These may include smoking cigarettes, taking drugs, not sleeping enough, eating too little or too much, or exercising too little or too much.

- Certain patterns of thinking (cognitive actions) can be stressors, too. These may include fearing change or challenge, remembering hard times that have passed, interpreting minor losses as catastrophes, or having too little self-esteem.

Stress and anxiety (distress)   Most often, stress is associated with negative events or thoughts, which are difficult experiences that most

KEYWORDS
for searching the Internet and other reference sources

Anxiety

Depression

Post-traumatic stress

Relaxation

Resilience

Stress inventories

Stress management

Stressors

Coping with Stress

Tips for coping with stress:

- Be realistic.
- Don't try to be perfect.
- Don't expect others to be perfect.
- Take one thing at a time.
- Be flexible.
- Share feelings.
- Maintain a healthy lifestyle.
- Meditate.
- Ask for help when necessary.

Tips for helping others cope with stress:

- Pay attention.
- Take them seriously.
- Be patient.
- Offer help when necessary.

people find unpleasant, frightening, or anxiety-producing. Stress may result from teasing by peers, being bullied, anxiety about homework or tests, disappointment about not achieving a goal, encountering unfamiliar people or places, or efforts to cram too many activities into too little time. Job stress and caregiver stress often fall into this category. So does being a pessimist and "worrywart" who believes that whenever something can go wrong, it will go wrong. Stress is the body's natural response to the difficult demands it encounters everyday.

Stress and excitement   Take a deep breath when faced with stress, and sometimes anxiety turns into excitement. That is because some stressors are positive. An audition, a stage performance or applause (instead of stage fright), an A grade or a game point (instead of anxiety), or a date to the prom with someone brand-new are positive stressors. Stress also is the body's natural response to the exciting new challenges it encounters everyday.

Trauma and stress   Some events are so stressful that they overwhelm us, and no amount of deep breathing or positive thinking can help. Accidents, injuries, abuse, violence, war, serious threats to physical safety, or the sudden death of a loved one are examples of traumas that cause a stress response within the body.

What Is the Stress Response?

Stressors good and bad set off a series of events within the body's neuroendocrine system. Often called the "fight or flight" response, these events are triggered by the brain, which alerts the body's autonomic nervous system to prepare all systems to react to an emergency. The autonomic nervous system sends a message in a split second through nerve fibers, which signal all the other body systems.

During this alarm period, many different hormones are activated with many dramatic effects on other body systems. The heart beats faster, blood pressure is raised, and blood vessels dilate (open wider) to increase blood flow to the muscles. The pupils dilate to aid vision. The digestive system slows down so that the body's resources and energy can be used wherever else they are needed, and the production of saliva decreases. The bronchi dilate to aid breathing. The skin sweats to cool the body, and the liver releases its stores of glucose, the major fuel of the body, to increase the person's energy level. The body stays in overdrive until the brain tells it that the emergency has ended.

Events that trigger the stress response usually are emergencies that do not last for very long. This allows the body to relax and recover after the emergency has ended so that it can respond correctly the next time its emergency response system is needed.

Long-term stress (chronic stress), frequently recurring stress, or extreme stress from trauma or a life-threatening event can keep the body's

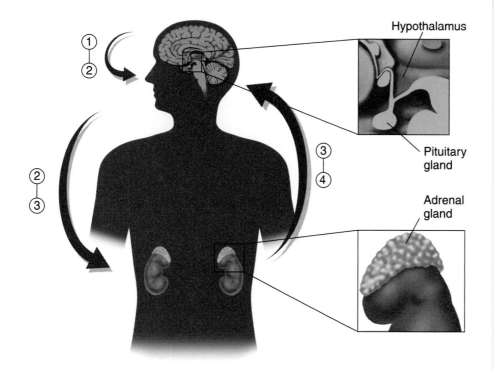

Hypothalamus

Pituitary gland

Adrenal gland

The body's stress hormone response: When the brain perceives stress, the hypothalamus releases corticotropin-releasing factor (1), which triggers the release of adrenocorticotropin (ACTH) (2) from the pituitary gland. ACTH (2) travels through the bloodstream and (along with signals from the brain sent through the autonomic nervous system) stimulates the adrenal glands to release cortisol and epinephrine into the bloodstream (3). Cortisol and epinephrine (3) help provide energy, oxygen, and stimulation to the heart, the brain, and other muscles and organs (4) to support the body's response to stress. When the brain perceives that the stress has ended, it allows hormone levels to return to their baseline values.

◀

stress response system activated at too high a level or for too long a period of time. This may interfere with the body's ability to recover from the stress response. Chronic stress or post-trauma stress also may lead to physical, emotional, or behavioral problems, post-traumatic stress disorder, or even the development of stress-related illnesses.

What Happens with Too Much Stress?

Researchers have found that chronic stress and post-trauma stress can suppress the immune system, interfering with the body's natural ability to defend itself against infection. Chronic stress also may contribute to many other problems of mind and body, including:

- headaches or stomachaches
- allergic responses, such as skin rashes or asthma
- irritability, aggression, or conduct disorders
- bruxism (grinding the teeth)
- sleep disorders
- eating disorders
- alcoholism or substance abuse
- anxiety
- phobias
- depression

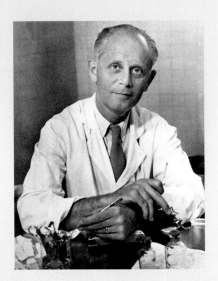

▲

Dr. Hans Selye of the University of Montreal is considered the founder of modern stress research. *Bettmann/Corbis*

HANS SELYE AND STRESS RESEARCH

Dr. Hans Selye (1907–1982) is considered the founder of modern stress research. He authored 39 books, wrote more than 1,700 scholarly papers, and was cited as a source in more than 362,000 scientific papers, not to mention countless articles in magazines and newspapers around the world. He also established the International Institute on Stress at the University of Montreal. The body's "general adaptation syndrome" often is called "Selye syndrome."

Dr. Selye defined stress as "the nonspecific response of the body to any demand," which means the body's reaction to any change in its environment. Dr. Selye linked physical illnesses not just to bacterial and viral infections, but also to hormones within the body that become activated whenever the body responds to external stressors, such as temperature extremes, pain, and threats to safety. Dr. Selye determined that many of the body's hormonal responses to stress were helpful and "adaptive," but others were "maladaptive" and placed physical demands on the body that could result in disease.

Still, Dr. Selye described stress as the spice of life, which might make one person sick while invigorating another. In one of his best-selling books, *The Stress of Life,* Dr. Selye offered this rhymed advice: "Fight for your highest attainable aim/But never put up resistance in vain." By choosing wisely where we invest effort and emotional energy, we can reduce the damaging side effects of stress, keep distress to a minimum, and increase our enjoyment of life.

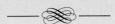

Chronic stress is believed to be a factor in many cases of abuse, violence, and suicide. Over the long term, chronic stress also may contribute to the development of cardiovascular problems, such as high blood pressure, heart disease, and stroke. People who experience chronic stress can benefit from working with a doctor or therapist to learn stress management techniques.

What Is the Antidote for Too Much Stress?

The antidote for stress is relaxation, creating a state of ease, rest, and repose within the body. Taking a deep breath almost always is the first step toward relaxation, allowing us to figure out that the emergency that triggered the body's stress response has ended.

Relaxation response   At the end of a stress response cycle, the body begins a relaxation response: Our breathing slows down, our hearts stop racing, our muscles stretch out, our minds become quieter, and levels of stress hormones in our bodies return to their baseline values. Techniques for achieving a relaxation response are many and varied. Some people listen to music or sing, go for a long walk or a run in the park, or practice meditation. Other techniques that promote a relaxation response include yoga, abdominal breathing, progressive muscle relaxation, biofeedback, guided imagery or visualization, hypnosis, prayer, support groups, or spending time with pets or loved ones. Because stress is an inevitable part of living, the long-term antidote for stress is to learn coping strategies that allow us to live with it successfully.

Resilience Resilient people who experience high levels of stress but recover quickly and show low levels of illness often are referred to as "stress-resistant personalities." According to researchers, such resilient people seem to have several common characteristics:

- They view change as a challenging and normal part of life, rather than as a threat.
- They have a sense of control over their lives, they believe that setbacks are temporary, and they believe that they will succeed if they work toward their goals.
- They have commitments to work, family, friends, support networks, and regular activities that promote relaxation, including hobbies, vacations, sports, yoga, and meditation.

Some people seem to be born with resilient personalities and good stress management skills. They know instinctively how to "get by with a little help from their friends." However, at times when a little help is not enough and only extra-strength help will do, or when a person needs some coaching to improve coping skills, it is always a good idea to turn to a doctor, counselor, or therapist.

Resources

Organizations

American Institute of Stress, 124 Park Avenue, Yonkers, NY 10703. This organization publishes the newsletter *Health and Stress* and provides informational packets about job stress, holiday stress, stress management, and other topics.
Telephone 914-963-1200
http://www.stress.org

International Stress Management Association. This organization publishes the *International Journal of Stress Management* for professionals. Its website features stress inventories, Internet links, and other resources.
http://www.stress-management-isma.org

The Relaxation Response

Dr. Herbert Benson of Harvard coined the term "relaxation response" for the body's antidote to its stress response. Triggered by a 20-minute period of meditation, the relaxation response leads to decreases in heart rate, breathing rate, blood pressure, muscle tension, metabolic rate, oxygen consumption, lactic acid production, and anxious thoughts.

To achieve the relaxation response, Dr. Benson recommended a quiet environment, a comfortable position, a focal point (a repeated word or sound, such as "Om"), and a passive attitude toward distracting thoughts that enter the mind.

▶ *See also*
Anxiety and Anxiety Disorders

Chronic Illness

Depression

Disability

Post-Traumatic Stress Disorder

Relaxation

Resilience

Stress Management Briefs. These fact sheets on children and stress, coping with change and loss, occupational stress, identifying stress factors, and other topics are provided by the University of Minnesota Extension Service.
http://www.extension.umn.edu/distribution/familydevelopment/DE7269.html

Stuttering

Stuttering is a speech disorder in which the normal flow of speech is broken by sounds that are repeated or held longer than normal, or by problems with starting a word.

People who stutter may repeat a speech sound over and over (st-st-stuttering), or they may hold a sound longer than normal (ssssstuttering). In some cases, they may have trouble starting a word, leading to abnormal stops in their speech (no sound). Yet many people who stutter learn to control the problem. The list of famous people in history who overcame stuttering includes Isaac Newton, Charles Darwin, Clara Barton, King George VI of England, Winston Churchill, and Marilyn Monroe.

What Is Stuttering?

Stuttering is a speech disorder in which the normal flow of speech is broken. Along with the effort to speak, some people who stutter also make unusual face or body movements, such as rapid eye blinking or trembling of the lips. Certain situations, such as speaking on the phone, tend to make stuttering worse. On the other hand, people usually do not stutter when they sing, whisper, or speak as part of a group, or when they do not hear their own voices. No one is sure why this is so.

Most children go through a stage of choppy speech when they are first learning to talk. In addition, teenagers and adults often add extra sounds (for example, "uh" and "um") to their speech, and they occasionally repeat sounds. This is perfectly normal. Such problems are considered a disorder only when they last past the age when most children outgrow them and get in the way of communicating clearly. Treating stuttering even in young children may help prevent a lifelong problem. Treatment may be considered for children who stutter longer than 6 months or for those who seem to struggle when they speak. Sometimes, however, no treatment is the best treatment, especially in the case of children whose stuttering worsens when attention is focused on the problem.

What Causes Stuttering?

Stuttering usually begins between the ages of 2 and 6 years. About 1 percent of children stutter, and boys are three times more likely to do so than girls. The most common form of stuttering is thought to arise when children's developing speech and language abilities are not yet able to keep up with their needs. Stuttering occurs when they search for the right word. This kind of stuttering usually is outgrown.

Another form of stuttering is caused by signal problems between the brain and the nerves or muscles involved in speech. The brain is unable to control all the different parts of the speech system. This kind of stuttering sometimes is seen in people who have had a stroke or brain injury. Yet another, less common form of the disorder is caused by severe stress or some types of mental illness. Some kinds of stuttering seem to run in families, and it is likely that stuttering is genetic* (je-NE-tik) in some cases, although no gene for stuttering has been found yet.

How Is Stuttering Linked to Fear?

Contrary to popular belief, there is no evidence that stuttering is caused by anxiety (ang-ZY-e-tee), an intense, long-lasting feeling of fear, worry, or nervousness. Yet people who stutter may become fearful of meeting new people, speaking in public, or talking on the phone. In such cases, it is the stuttering that causes the fear, not the reverse.

How Is Stuttering Diagnosed?

Stuttering usually is diagnosed by a speech-language pathologist (pa-THAH-lo-jist), a professional who is specially trained to test and treat people with speech, language, and voice disorders. The speech pathologist will ask questions about the problem, such as when it first started and when it is most and least noticeable. The speech pathologist also will test speech and language abilities. In addition, some people may be sent to other professionals for hearing tests and medical tests of the nervous system.

How Is Stuttering Treated?

There are several treatments that may improve stuttering, although none is an instant cure. With young children, the focus often is on teaching parents how to help the child at home. Parents typically are told to have a relaxed attitude and give their children plenty of chances to speak. They may be warned not to criticize their children's speech problems or even not to pay attention to them at all. Instead, they can be good role models, speaking in a slow, relaxed manner themselves and listening patiently when their children talk.

With older children, teenagers, and adults, speech therapy can help them relearn how to speak or unlearn faulty ways of speaking. Some

*__genetic__ means having to do with genes, which are chemical substances that help determine a person's characteristics such as hair or eye color, and also determine some health conditions. Genes are contained in the chromosomes, threadlike structures found in the cells of the body. A person's genes are inherited from his or her parents.

Being a Good Listener

When talking to someone who stutters, you should:

■ Be patient. Do not finish sentences or fill in words for the person. This might be taken as an insult, or you might guess the wrong words.

■ Make normal eye contact. Try not to look embarrassed or concerned.

■ Be understanding. Do not make remarks such as "slow down" or "relax." The person probably has tried this already, so your comments will not help.

■ Set a relaxed pace. Try to keep your own speech at a medium speed.

■ Be sensible. If you do not understand what someone says, politely ask the person to repeat it. This is better than risking a misunderstanding.

people who stutter have fears related to the disorder, such as a fear of speaking in public. Such problems caused by the stuttering can be helped with psychotherapy (sy-ko-THER-a-pea), in which people talk about their feelings, beliefs, and experiences with a mental health professional who can help them work out issues that play a part in their speech problems.

Resources

Books

De Geus, Eelco. *Sometimes I Just Stutter.* Mempis, TN: Stuttering Foundation of America, 1999. This book tells young people about the causes of stuttering and discusses the fears and embarrassment of people who stutter. It is available to buy or to read at the foundation's website: http://www.stuttersfa.org.

Sugarman, Michael, and Kim C. Swain. *The Adventures of Phil Carrot: The Forest of Discord.* Anaheim, CA: National Stuttering Association, 1995. This is the story of an unusual day in the life of a boy who stutters and his classmates.

Organizations

American Speech-Language-Hearing Association, 10801 Rockville Pike, Rockville, MD 20852. This professional association for speech-language pathologists offers reliable information on stuttering.
Telephone 800-638-TALK
http://www.asha.org

National Stuttering Association, 5100 East La Palma, Suite 208, Anaheim, CA 92807. This organization is the largest self-help and support group in the United States for people who stutter.
Telephone 800-364-1677
http://www.nsastutter.org

Stuttering Foundation of America, 3100 Walnut Grove Road, Suite 603, P.O. Box 11749, Memphis, TN 38111-0749. This nonprofit group works toward the prevention and improved treatment of stuttering.
Telephone 800-992-9392
http://www.stuttersfa.org

U.S. National Institute on Deafness and Other Communication Disorders, 31 Center Drive, MSC 2320, Bethesda, MD 20892-2320. This government institute is a source of facts and figures on stuttering.
Phone 301-496-7243
http://www.nih.gov/nidcd

▶ *See also*
Anxiety and Anxiety Disorders
Selective Mutism
Social Anxiety Disorder

Substance Abuse

Substance abuse is an unhealthy pattern of alcohol or drug use that usually leads to frequent, serious problems.

The statistics are startling: In 1998, 1 out of every 10 young people ages 12 through 17 in the United States said they were a current user of illegal drugs. In that same year, over 10 million Americans under age 21 reported that they drank alcohol. Of this group, 5 million were binge drinkers, meaning they drank five or more drinks at one time. This group also included 2 million who were heavy drinkers, meaning they drank five or more drinks on five or more days during the previous month.

What Is Substance Abuse?

Substance abuse is an unhealthy pattern of alcohol or drug use that usually leads to frequent, serious problems at home, school, or work. Substance abuse also can cause stress in relationships. For example, a teenager might get into frequent arguments with parents or fights with friends. Substance abuse can even lead to trouble with the law. For example, a young person might be arrested for underage drinking or disorderly conduct. People who abuse substances also may put themselves in dangerous situations, such as driving under the influence of alcohol or drugs or having unsafe sex.

Substance abuse is one step along the path from occasional drinking or drug use to outright addiction (ad-DIK-shun). When people are addicted, they develop a strong physical or psychological need for a substance. One hallmark of addiction is tolerance (TOL-er-uns). This means that over time, people start to need more and more of a substance to get drunk or feel high. Another is withdrawal, which means that people who are addicted will have physical symptoms and feel sick if they stop using the substance.

Drugs and alcohol cause intoxication (in-TOK-sih-KAY-shun), the medical term for a temporary feeling of being high or drunk that occurs just after using a drug. Intoxication leads to changes in the way people think and act. For example, people may become angry, moody, confused, or uncoordinated. These changes increase the risk that people will make poor choices, have accidents that hurt themselves or others, or behave in a way that they will later regret.

What Causes Substance Abuse?

People give many reasons for starting to drink alcohol or use drugs. Some teenagers are looking for an easy way to escape stress at home, school, or elsewhere. Others hope that alcohol or drugs will help them fit in or make them seem older. Some may be using substances to "treat"

KEYWORDS
for searching the Internet and other reference sources

Drug abuse

Marijuana

Hallucinogens

Inhalants

Narcotics

Sedatives

Stimulants

Everyone *Isn't* Doing It

Sometimes it can seem as if everybody else is drinking alcohol, smoking cigarettes, or using drugs. Monitoring the Future is a yearly survey, funded by the U.S. National Institute on Drug Abuse, that aims to find out just how common substance abuse really is among teenagers in eighth through twelfth grades. The facts are:

- 1999 was the third year in a row that drug use in this age group stayed the same or went down for most substances.

- Among eighth-graders, half had never drunk alcohol, 3 out of 5 had never smoked cigarettes, and 4 out of 5 had never used marijuana.

- Among twelfth-graders, 9 out of 10 had never tried cocaine or LSD, and 98 percent had never tried heroin.

or "self-medicate" depression or boredom. Still others are simply curious. Whatever the original reason, no one can say for sure which teenagers will go on to have a serious substance abuse problem. However, certain factors raise the risk that this will happen. Risk factors for substance abuse include:

- family history of substance abuse
- using alcohol or tobacco at a young age
- depression
- low self-esteem
- feeling like an outsider
- poverty
- child abuse or neglect
- family stress

Some of these factors can be changed or controlled by the teenagers themselves, but others cannot. However, that does not mean that those who come from stressed families or poor neighborhoods are doomed. Certain other factors raise the odds that young people will be able to cope with problems without turning to alcohol or drugs. These factors include:

- learning to do something well
- being active at school or in church
- having a caring adult to talk to

What Are Some Commonly Abused Substances?

People abuse an amazing variety of drugs, both legal and illegal. Legally available substances include alcohol, tobacco, chemicals in certain household products, drugs bought in a drugstore, and medicines prescribed by a doctor. Illegally sold substances include numerous street and "party" drugs.

Alcohol Alcohol affects virtually every organ in the body, and longtime use can lead to a number of medical problems. The immediate effects of drinking too much include slurred speech, poor coordination, unsteady walking, memory problems, poor judgement, and the inability to concentrate. Drinking too much alcohol at one time can cause alcohol poisoning and sudden death. The recklessness that comes from drinking too much also is a leading cause of traffic accidents and other injuries. In addition, alcohol drinking by pregnant women is the cause of the most common preventable birth defect, called fetal alcohol syndrome. Long-term risks of heavy drinking include liver damage, heart disease, sexual problems for men, and trouble getting pregnant for women.

Tobacco Tobacco contains nicotine (NIK-o-teen), a highly addictive chemical. Nicotine is readily absorbed from tobacco smoke in the lungs, whether the smoke comes from cigarettes, cigars, or pipes. Smoking is the number one cause of preventable death in the United States. The long-term health risks include cancer, lung disease, heart disease, and stroke. Smoking by pregnant women also has been linked to miscarriage*, still-birth*, premature* birth, low birth weight*, and infant death. Nicotine is readily absorbed from smokeless tobacco as well. Like smoking, dipping or chewing tobacco can have serious long-term effects, including cancer of the mouth, gum problems, loss of teeth, and heart disease.

Inhalants   Inhalants (in-HALE-ants) are substances that a person can sniff ("huff") or inhale to get an immediate "rush" or high. They include a varied group of chemicals that are found in household products such as aerosol sprays and cleaning fluids. Using inhalants even one time can lead to suffocation, severe mood swings, seeing or hearing things that are not really there, and numbness or tingling of the hands and feet, and even sudden death. Long-term use can lead to permanent brain damage, headache, muscle weakness, stomach pain, loss of the sense of smell, nose-bleeds, liver disease, kidney damage, lung disease, violent behavior, irregular heartbeat, dangerous chemical imbalances in the body, and loss of control over urination.

Marijuana   Marijuana (mar-ih-HWAH-nuh; nicknames: pot, herb, weed, blunts, Mary Jane) is the most widely used illegal drug. It is typically the first illegal drug tried by teenagers. It is a mixture of dried, shredded flowers and leaves from the cannabis plant. Marijuana usually is smoked in a cigarette, pipe, or water pipe, but some users also mix it with foods or use it to brew tea. Short-term effects of marijuana use include euphoria*, sleepiness, increased hunger, trouble keeping track of time, memory problems, inability to concentrate, poor coordination, increased heart rate, paranoia*, and anxiety. Long-term risks include lung disease, changes in hormone levels, lower sperm counts in men, and trouble getting pregnant in women.

Hallucinogens   Hallucinogens (huh-LOO-sih-no-jenz) are drugs that distort a person's view of reality. They include LSD (short for lysergic acid diethylamide; nickname: acid), PCP (short for phencyclidine; nicknames: angel dust, loveboat), psilocybin (SY-lo-SY-bin; nickname: magic mushrooms), mescaline (MES-kuh-len), and peyote (pay-YO-tee or pay-YO-tay). People who use these drugs may lose all sense of time, distance, and direction. They also may behave strangely or violently, which can lead to serious injuries or death. Since everyone reacts differently to hallucinogens, however, there is no way to tell in advance who will have a bad experience.

■   LSD is one of the most potent of all mind-altering drugs. It may be taken in pills. A drop may be placed on a square of paper and eaten. LSD can last a long time in the body—up to 12 hours. The physical effects of LSD use include dilated (widened)

***miscarriage** is the loss of a fetus before birth.

***stillbirth** is the birth of a dead baby or fetus.

***premature** (pre-muh-CHOOR) **birth** means born too early. In humans, it means being born after a pregnancy term of less than 37 weeks.

***low birth weight** means born weighing less than normal. In humans, it refers to a baby weighing less than 5.5 pounds.

***euphoria** is an abnormal, exaggerated feeling of well-being.

***paranoia** refers to either an unreasonable fear of harm by others (delusions of persecution) or an unrealistic sense of self-importance (delusions of grandeur).

Same Problem, Different Solution

In the United States, using and selling drugs such as marijuana and heroin is illegal, and people who break the drug laws go to jail. In the Netherlands, the government is trying a different approach that stresses treatment rather than punishment.

In the mid-1970s, the Netherlands was hit by a sharp upswing in heroin use. In response, the government launched a policy called harm reduction, which aims to lower the harmful effects of drug use for both users and society. The policy is based on the belief that "soft" drugs, such as marijuana and the related drug hashish (hah-SHESH), are less dangerous than "hard" drugs, such as heroin, cocaine, amphetamines, and MDMA. To encourage people not to try hard drugs, the government allows the sale of small amounts of marijuana and hashish in adults-only coffee shops, much the way alcohol is sold in bars. Hard drugs are still banned, but users are treated as people with an illness rather than as criminals.

There is much debate over how well this policy works. However, the number of drug addicts in the Netherlands is lower than in many countries. In addition, the average age of addicts is rising, which suggests that fewer young people are getting hooked. On the other hand, the rate of marijuana and hashish use has gone up in recent years, although it is still lower than in the United States. Another problem is the rise of Dutch crime gangs that are selling illegal drugs throughout Europe.

pupils, increased heart rate, higher blood pressure, sweating, loss of appetite, trouble sleeping, dry mouth, and shaking. The psychological effects are much more dramatic, however. Users may feel several different emotions at once, or they may swing from one emotion to another, euphoria to paranoia. They may have bizarre or terrifying thoughts, or they may see things that are not really there, like walls melting. Some users later have flashbacks, in which they relive part of what they experienced while taking the drug, even though the drug use has stopped.

- PCP can be snorted through the nose, smoked, or eaten. It has a bad reputation for causing bizarre and sometimes violent behavior. Other possible effects of PCP use include increased or shallow breathing rate, higher blood pressure, flushing, sweating, numbness, poor coordination, and confused or irrational thinking. High doses can lead to seeing or hearing things that are not really there, paranoia, seizures, coma, injuries, and suicidal behavior.

Stimulants Stimulants (STIM-yoo-lunts) are drugs that produce a temporary feeling of euphoria, alertness, power, and energy. As the high wears off, however, depression and edginess set in. Stimulants include cocaine (ko-KANE; nicknames: coke, snow, blow, nose candy), "crack" cocaine, amphetamine (am-FET-uh-mean), methamphetamine (METH-am-FET-uh-mean; nicknames: speed, meth, crank), and crystallized methamphetamine (nicknames: ice, crystal, glass).

- Cocaine is a white powder that is either snorted into the nose or injected into a vein. Crack is a form of cocaine that has been chemically changed so that it can be smoked. Both forms are very addictive. Possible physical effects of cocaine and crack use include increased heart rate, higher blood pressure, increased breathing rate, heart attack, stroke, trouble breathing, seizures, and a reduced ability to fight infection. Possible psychological effects include violent or strange behavior, paranoia, seeing or hearing things that are not really there, feeling as if bugs are crawling over the skin, anxiety, and depression. In the end, cocaine addicts often wind up losing interest in food, sex, friends, family—everything except getting high.

- Methamphetamine is taken in pills, or it can be snorted or injected. Crystallized methamphetamine is a more powerful form of the drug that is smoked. Both forms are highly addictive. Possible physical effects of methamphetamine use are similar to those of cocaine. Possible psychological effects include trouble sleeping, crankiness, confusion, anxiety, paranoia, and violent behavior. In the 1960s and 1970s there was a popular expression, "Speed kills." This saying was meant to alert users to the sad end of methamphetamine addiction.

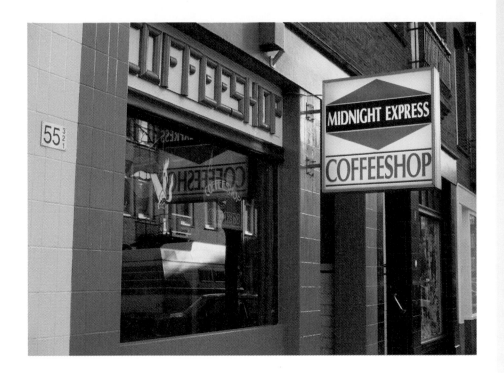

In Amsterdam, the Netherlands, marijuana use is legal. The city has coffee shops such as this one, in which people are free to purchase and use the drug. *Corbis*

Narcotics Narcotics (nahr-KOT-iks) are addictive painkillers that produce a relaxed feeling and an immediate high, followed by restlessness and an upset stomach. They can also be deadly. Drugs in this class include heroin (HAIR-oh-in; nicknames: smack, H, skag, junk), morphine (MOR-feen), opium (OH-pee-um), and codeine (KO-deen).

■ Heroin is made from morphine, a natural substance that comes from the poppy plant. It is a powder that is injected, snorted, or smoked, and it is highly addictive. Immediate effects of heroin use include a heavy feeling in the arms and legs, warm flushing of the skin, dry mouth, clouded thinking, and going back and forth between being wide awake and feeling drowsy. In addition, street heroin varies in strength, and users never know if they are getting a particularly strong dose. If they do, they can easily overdose ("OD"), resulting in coma or death. Long-term effects include collapsed veins, infection of the heart lining and valves, liver disease, and HIV/AIDS from sharing needles.

Sedatives Sedatives (SED-uh-tivz), sometimes called as tranquilizers (TRANK-will-LY-zerz) or sleeping pills, include barbiturates or "downers." They are drugs that produce a calming effect or sleepiness. Physicians prescribe them to relieve anxiety, promote sleep, and treat seizures. When they are abused or taken at high doses, however, many of these drugs can lead to loss of consciousness or even death. Combining sedatives with alcohol is particularly dangerous. Possible effects of sedative abuse include poor judgment, slurred speech, staggering, poor coordination, and slow reflexes.

351

Cocaine is a mood-altering drug that interferes with normal transport of the neurotransmitter dopamine, which carries messages from neuron to neuron. When cocaine molecules block dopamine receptors, too much dopamine remains active in the synaptic gaps between neurons, creating feelings of excitement and euphoria. ▶

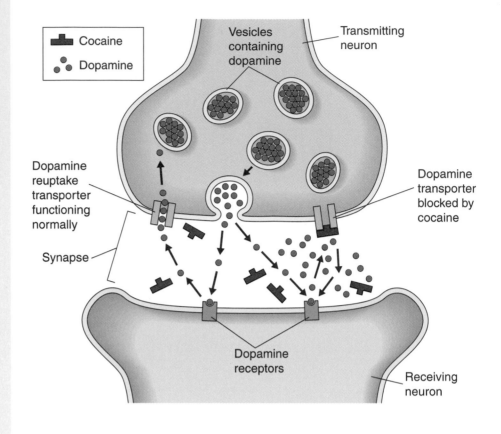

Cocaine

Dopamine

Vesicles containing dopamine

Transmitting neuron

Dopamine reuptake transporter functioning normally

Dopamine transporter blocked by cocaine

Synapse

Dopamine receptors

Receiving neuron

Club drugs   Club drugs are drugs that are mainly used by young people at parties, clubs, and bars. While users may think these are harmless fun drugs, research has shown that they can cause serious health problems and sometimes even death. When combined with alcohol, they can be particularly dangerous. Drugs in this category include MDMA (nicknames: ecstasy, Adam, XTC) GHB (nicknames: liquid ecstasy, Georgia home boy), Rohypnol (nicknames: roofies, roach), and ketamine (nickname: special K).

■ MDMA or XTC combines some of the properties of hallucinogens and stimulants. Possible effects include euphoria, confusion, paranoia, increased heart rate, higher blood pressure, blurred vision, faintness, chills, and sweating. Because this drug is increasingly abused at dances, kids may forget to drink, become dehydrated, and need to be rushed to the emergency room for immediate treatment. Possible psychological effects include confusion, depression, sleep problems, anxiety, and paranoia. Recent research also has linked MDMA to long-term damage in parts of the brain that are critical for thought, memory, and pleasure.

■ GHB, Rohypnol, and ketamine are often colorless, tasteless, and odorless, which makes it easy for someone to slip one of these drugs into another person's drink. As a result, these substances are sometimes called "date rape" drugs, because they have been used in rapes against women who were drugged unknowingly. To make matters worse, people may be unable to remember what happened to them while they were under the influence of one of these drugs.

Anabolic steroids   Anabolic steroids (AN-uh-BOL-ik STER-oidz) are drugs that are related to testosterone (tes-TOS-tuh-rone), the major male sex hormone. While these drugs have medical uses, many athletes and bodybuilders today are abusing them because they can increase muscle build-up with weight lifting or strength training. Although steroids may seem like a shortcut to improved sports performance and a more muscular body, they carry serious health risks. In boys and men, steroids can reduce sperm production, shrink the testicles, enlarge the breasts, and cause problems with sexual performance. In girls and women, they can lead to unwanted body hair, a deep voice, and irregular periods. Steroids also can damage the heart, liver, and kidneys. In teenagers, they can stunt bone growth, making the person reach a shorter final height than he or she would have otherwise. High doses of testosterone can also cause outbursts of aggressive or violent behavior ("steroid rage").

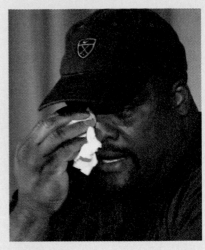

▲

C. J. Hunter, world shotput champion, breaks down during a press conference at the 2000 Summer Olympic Games. It had just been revealed that Hunter was using a steroid banned for all Olympic athletes. *AFP/Corbis*

What Are Some Other Risks of Substance Abuse?

One thing most abused drugs have in common is that they can lead to unclear thinking and unpredictable behavior. Many also cause poor coordination and slow reflexes. It is little wonder, then, that substance abuse is closely tied to accidents and injuries. Alcohol and other drugs play a role in half of all fatal car crashes, which are the leading cause of death in young people. Alcohol also is involved in nearly 60 percent of fatal falls and at least half of adult drownings.

Substance abuse is also now the single biggest factor in the spread of infection with HIV (human immunodeficiency virus), the virus that causes AIDS, in the United States. It is a direct cause, because many drugs are injected into a vein, and people can catch HIV by using or sharing unclean needles. It is also an indirect cause, because people whose thinking is clouded by alcohol or other drugs are more likely to have unsafe sex, which increases their risk of catching HIV from an infected partner.

What Are the Signs of Substance Abuse?

Substance abuse can lead to physical and psychological problems that affect people's relationships and everyday lives. Typical warning signs of substance abuse in young people include:

Violent Objections

Anyone who needs one more reason to avoid substance abuse should consider the latest statistics on alcohol, drugs, and violence.

- Alcohol is a key factor in more than 60 percent of assaults and over half of murders or attempted murders in the United States.

- Over 40 percent of convicted rapists say they were under the influence of alcohol or other drugs at the time of their crime.

- Almost two-thirds of reported child abuse and neglect cases in New York City have been linked to alcohol or drug use by the parent.

- Up to 35 percent of suicide victims have a history of alcohol abuse or were drinking shortly before they killed themselves.

- **Physical:** tiredness, unexplained health problems, red and glazed eyes, long-lasting cough
- **Psychological:** personality changes, sudden mood swings, crankiness, carelessness, low self-esteem, poor judgment, depression, loss of interest in friends and activities
- **Social:** new friends who abuse alcohol or drugs, problems with the law, changes in dress or appearance
- **Home:** starting arguments, breaking rules, withdrawing from family life
- **School:** loss of interest, bad attitude, drop in grades, frequent absences, getting into trouble

How Is Substance Abuse Diagnosed and Treated?

People who abuse alcohol or other drugs often need help to get help, since they may be tempted to deny the problem or feel as if their situation is hopeless. However, they should know that help is out there for those who seek it. The first step is to see a physician, psychologist, or counselor, or visit a health center for screening. To make a diagnosis, the health care professional will ask about present and past alcohol and drug use. If possible, the clinician also will talk to the person's family or friends. In addition, the clinician may sometimes order blood or urine tests for drugs.

Treatment for people who abuse alcohol or drugs but are not yet addicted to them usually centers around "talk" therapy. Several kinds of therapy may be used, either individually or in a group.

Cognitive therapy   Cognitive (COG-nih-tiv) therapy targets the faulty thinking patterns that lead to alcohol and drug use. One approach helps people understand and change the poor decision making that leads to a relapse (RE-laps), a slip back into their old, bad habits.

Group therapy   Individual therapy involves only the person and a therapist, while group therapy involves the person, a therapist, and other people with similar concerns. Group therapy often is used in substance abuse treatment, because it lets people get emotional support and practical tips from others who are struggling with the same kinds of problems.

Family therapy   Family therapy works on problems at home that may play a role in a person's alcohol or drug abuse. It may be especially helpful when there is severe conflict within the family or when there are other family members who are themselves depressed or abusing substances.

Self-help groups   Self-help groups can be very helpful to both people with substance abuse problems and their family members. Many are 12-step groups, patterned on the 12 steps that are the guiding principles of

Alcoholics Anonymous. Those who take part in such groups receive personal support from other people who have faced the same kinds of difficult situations.

Resources

Book

Packer, Alex J. *Highs! Over 150 Ways to Feel Really REALLY Good . . . Without Alcohol or Other Drugs.* Minneapolis: Free Spirit, 2000. For ages 13 and up.

Organizations

U.S. National Clearinghouse for Alcohol and Drug Information, P.O. Box 2345, Rockville, MD 20847-2345. This government clearinghouse is the world's largest resource for current information and materials on substance abuse and addiction.
Telephone 800-729-6686
http://www.health.org

U.S. National Institute on Alcohol Abuse and Alcoholism, 6000 Executive Boulevard, Bethesda, MD 20892-7003. This government institute provides in-depth information on alcohol abuse and addiction.
Telephone 301-443-3860
http://www.niaaa.nih.gov

U.S. National Institute on Drug Abuse, 6001 Executive Boulevard, Bethesda, MD 20892-9561. This government institute provides detailed information about drug abuse and addiction.
Telephone 301-443-1124
http://www.drugabuse.gov

Websites

ClubDrugs.org. The National Institute on Drug Abuse launched this site to provide reliable information about popular club drugs.
http://www.clubdrugs.org

Join Together Online. This site, a project of the Boston University School of Public Health, features the latest news on substance abuse.
http://www.jointogether.org

SteroidAbuse.org. The National Institute on Drug Abuse set up this site to provide facts about anabolic steroid abuse.
http://www.steroidabuse.org

▶ *See also*
Addiction
Alcoholism
Consciousness
Tobacco Addiction

Suicide

Suicide is the intentional taking of a person's own life.

KEYWORDS
for searching the Internet and other reference sources

Depression

As shocking as it may seem, in the United States every year there are more suicides than murders and twice as many suicides as deaths from acquired immunodeficiency syndrome (AIDS). Yet suicide gets far less press than murder or AIDS. Why? It may be because talking about suicide makes people very uncomfortable, because there are religious prohibitions against suicide, because suicide is thought of as a shameful act, or because many people simply cannot believe that someone they know and love could intentionally take his or her own life.

Who Commits Suicide?

Suicide is a complex act that results from many factors, not all of which are understood. It is not clear or predictable why the setbacks, losses, or difficulties that would lead one person to feel very unhappy may lead another person to be suicidal.

It is estimated that about 30,000 Americans die as the result of suicide each year, while about 20,000 people are murdered. Some experts, however, believe that the number of suicides is even higher. Many "accidents," such as self-inflicted gunshot wounds or single-car crashes, actually may be unrecognized or unreported suicides. Although no official record is kept of suicide attempts, it is estimated that there are between 8 and 25 attempts for each completed suicide. Overall, suicide is the eighth leading cause of death in the United States.

Suicides are not spread equally throughout the population. Although more women than men attempt suicide, about four times more men die, because they use more lethal means. Men of European ancestry committed 72 percent of all suicides in 1997, while women of European ancestry accounted for about 18 percent of these deaths. The rate of suicide among people of Native American ancestry, especially young men ages 15 to 24, is particularly high. The suicide rate among men of African ancestry ages 15 to 19 doubled between 1980 and 1996. Age is another factor in suicide. After age 65, the rate of suicide among men of European heritage increases steadily as they get older. Men of European heritage who are older than 85 have a suicide rate that is six times the national average. The reasons for the different rates of suicide among people of different ethnic backgrounds, gender, and ages vary. Some factors include increased rates of alcoholism, poverty, loneliness, and violence for particular groups at a particular time of life.

Young people also have higher than average rates of suicide. Suicide is the third leading cause of death among people 15 to 24 years old. A 1997 survey found that 1 in 13 high school students said that they had attempted suicide. Meanwhile, the number of children ages 10 to 14 committing suicide has increased sharply during the past decade. The most common methods of committing suicide are by intentionally taking a drug overdose (prescription or over-the-counter medicines), inhaling carbon monoxide from car exhausts, or using guns.

What Factors Make People More Likely to Commit Suicide?

About 90 percent of people who commit suicide have a diagnosed psychiatric disorder. Depression and substance abuse (either alone or in combination) are the two most common disorders that play a part in suicide. This does not mean that everyone who has depression or an alcohol or drug problem will commit suicide. The majority of people with these problems are not suicidal.

People who are more likely to kill themselves also may:

- have previously attempted suicide
- live alone and have no social support network
- have chronic (long-lasting or recurring) physical pain or a terminal (life-ending) illness
- have a family history of suicide
- be unemployed
- be impulsive
- keep a gun in the home
- have spent time in jail
- have experienced family violence, child abuse, or sexual abuse.

What Are the Signs That a Person Is Thinking of Committing Suicide?

It is a myth that people who talk about killing themselves do not do it. Four of five people who attempt suicide have given clues about their intentions before they acted on them. It is important to take seriously any talk about suicide or any indication that suicide is a possibility.

Some common warning signs that a person is thinking about suicide include:

- talking about death or making suicide threats
- making such statements as "You would be better off without me" or "I'm no good to anybody" (even if these are said jokingly)
- having any of the symptoms or signs of depression
- exhibiting major personality changes or unexplainable odd behavior
- making a will or giving away cherished possessions
- seeking isolation and becoming uncommunicative
- being fascinated with death

■ taking a sudden interest in religion if previously not religious, or rejecting religion if previously devout.

Why Do People Commit Suicide?

No one can explain why some people commit suicide and others do not. One theory is that suicide is an act of rage or anger. Another theory is that people may commit suicide because they feel they have no other choice. Hopelessness and distorted thinking may prevent a person from seeing solutions to their problems.

For a mentally healthy person, the idea that a person would have no choice except to seek death sounds absurd. But depression, substance abuse, and other mental illnesses, such as schizophrenia, alter the healthy mind. People with these problems may feel that they are in a deep, dark hole from which there is no escape and that life is so painful that there are no alternatives except death.

Researchers are finding that there may be inherited tendencies for depression, schizophrenia, alcoholism, substance abuse, and certain personality disorders. All of these problems can increase a person's vulnerability to suicidal thoughts when things go wrong. Some studies suggest that the brain chemistry of people who commit suicide is abnormal. Research is under way to examine the effects of certain medications that alter brain chemistry in a way that could decrease suicidal behavior.

If You Suspect Someone Is Suicidal

People who are thinking about committing suicide need professional help. They have usually sunk so deeply into their mental and emotional black holes that they may be unable to recognize that they are in trouble

▶

Trained adults staff a suicide hotline. These crisis lines are entirely confidential, and can be called 24 hours a day, 7 days a week. *Stock Boston*

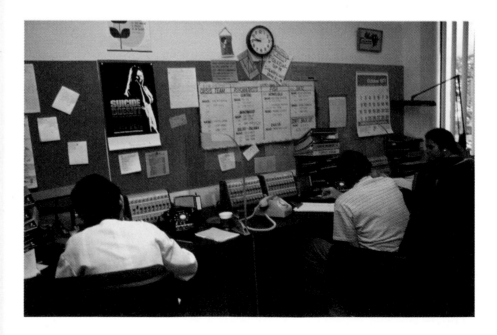

or to seek help on their own. It is important to pay attention when people talk about wanting to die and to take their words seriously. Having another person approach the subject directly is often a relief to them. It is sometimes thought that speaking to people about their possible wish to commit suicide will "put thoughts in their heads." But people who talk about suicide often are already thinking about suicide.

Professional help is available through suicide prevention and crisis intervention centers, mental health clinics, hospitals and emergency rooms, family doctors, health maintenance organizations, mental health practitioners, and members of the clergy. When a person is possibly suicidal, it is a good idea to talk to another mature, responsible person and ask that person to join in helping to deal with the crisis. Many telephone books have community service sections that list suicide and mental health crisis hotlines. Immediate help can be obtained by calling emergency services (911 in most communities).

Other ways of possibly minimizing the risk of suicide include:

- removing guns and ammunition from the house
- locking up medications and alcohol
- staying with the person, since suicide is an act most often performed alone
- talking calmly, without lecturing, being judgmental, or pointing out all the reasons a person has to continue living.

Suicide places a heavy emotional burden on the survivors. People who have been close to someone who has attempted or completed suicide might consider mental health counseling to help them deal with their own emotions.

Resources

Books

Cobain, Bev. *When Nothing Matters Anymore: A Survival Guide for Depressed Teens.* Minneapolis: Free Spirit Publishing, 1998. A guide to depression treatment and prevention. For ages 13 and up.

Crutcher, Chris. *Chinese Handcuffs.* New York: Bantam Doubleday Dell Publishing Group, 1991. A fictional account of teens dealing with suicide.

Hahn, Mary Downing. *The Wind Blows Backward.* New York: William Morrow and Co., 1994. A fictional account of teens dealing with suicide.

Organizations

American Psychiatric Association, 1400 K Street NW, Washington, DC, 20005. This professional organization provides online information on suicide (especially teen suicide) and depression at its website.

Telephone 888-357-7924
http://www.psych.org

National Center for Injury Prevention and Control, Mailstop K65, 4770 Buford Highway NE, Atlanta, GA 30341-3724. The website of this organization provides up-to-date statistics and research findings about suicide.
Telephone 770-488-1506
http://www.cdc.gov/ncipc

U.S. National Institute of Mental Health (NIMH), 6001 Executive Boulevard, Room 8148, MSC 9663, Bethesda, MD 20892-9663. This government agency conducts research on suicide and depression and provides information to the public through pamphlets and a website.
Telephone 301-443-4513
http://www.nimh.nih.gov

▶ *See also*

Bipolar Disorder

Brain Chemistry (Neurochemistry)

Death and Dying

Depression

Substance Abuse

Therapy

Testing and Evaluation

Evaluation (ee-val-yoo-AY-shun) is the process of examining a problem or condition so that it can be understood and diagnosed. Testing is one of the ways to evaluate possible behavioral and mental health problems. Tests also can be used to measure normal abilities, such as intelligence, personality, certain brain functions, learning capabilities, and school progress.

KEYWORDS
for searching the Internet and other reference sources

Intelligence testing

Standardized testing

Neuropsychological evaluation

Neil was glad that he had remembered to bring an extra pencil with him to school today. He tapped it nervously on the desk while the teacher passed out booklets for the standardized test his class was about to take. Even though he knew this test did not count for his report card, he wanted to do well. As soon as the teacher finished giving the instructions, Neil opened the test booklet and began to read the first question.

What Are Standardized Tests?

A standardized test is a test that is given under the same conditions to everyone who takes it. The questions on the test, the instructions, the time allowed for taking the test, and the rules for scoring it are the same every time the test is given and for every person who takes it. For example, students in classrooms across the country may take the same standardized test to measure school progress. At each school the same test booklets, answer sheets, and instructions are used.

Standardized tests make it possible to compare the scores of a large group of people. For example, the math scores of all sixth grade students in the country can be compared using a standardized test. It would not be possible to make such comparisons with the regular tests teachers make for their own classes, because those tests most likely would differ in ease or difficulty or might include different material. Using such tests, it would not be possible to make fair comparisons among students in different classes.

What Does a Score on a Standardized Test Mean?

The results of a standardized academic (schoolwork) test can show how well a student scored in certain subjects, such as reading comprehension (com-pree-HEN-shun) or math problem solving, compared with other students in the same grade throughout the country. Scores usually are given as percentiles in this type of test. For example, a student may score in the 86th percentile in reading comprehension. This means that the student could read and understand the readings as well as or better than 86 percent of all the students in the same grade who were tested.

What Do Standardized Tests Measure?

There are many types of standardized tests. Different tests measure different things. There are standardized tests that can measure school progress, intelligence, memory, and behavior capabilities. Some standardized tests are given to a whole group of people at once, while others are given individually. Group tests generally are given in a classroom, such as tests that measure school progress. Scores show how well a student is doing in school subjects compared with all other students in the same grade. A typical standardized test to measure academic progress consists of a test booklet with multiple-choice questions and a separate answer sheet on which the student fills in a circle to mark the correct answer.

Group standardized tests can measure academic progress at every level. Colleges and universities often use these tests to help decide whether to accept someone as a student. For example, colleges and universities often require applicants to take a standardized test called the Scholastic Aptitude Test (SAT), graduate schools may require a standardized test called the Graduate Record Exam (GRE), and medical schools usually require a standardized test called the Medical College Admission Test (MCAT). Scores from these tests help a college or university compare the abilities of students who are applying and decide which students to accept. These tests measure how much a student has learned in school and how well a student can solve problems, as well as other learned skills or natural aptitudes that may make someone a good student. Tests are just one measure of someone's capabilities, and they are generally just one of several factors used in evaluating an applicant for a college or university.

What Are Psychological Tests?

Some tests are given only by psychologists (sy-KAH-lo-jists), and they are called psychological (sy-ko-LAH-ji-kal) tests. Among the most common psychological tests are those that measure intelligence. Intelligence tests are examples of standardized psychological tests. Some other psychological tests are not standardized, but they can still provide important information about a person's personality, feelings, ideas, and concerns and can help evaluate and diagnose problems they may have. Most psychological tests are given individually and involve a face-to-face meeting with the psychologist during testing.

One commonly used psychological test to measure intelligence (IQ) in childhood is the Wechsler Intelligence Scale for Children (ages 6 to 16). There is also the Wechsler Adult Intelligence Scale, which can be given to anyone over the age of 16. Intelligence tests also can help evaluate a person for possible learning disabilities, attention problems, and mental retardation. These tests can accurately measure a person's intelligence under most circumstances, but some things may prevent a person from scoring her best, such as not feeling well or being extremely nervous about taking the test. The psychologist takes these possibilities into account and decides whether the test on that day should be considered an accurate reading of the person's true capabilities.

Placing Students in the Right Classroom

Paula was not sure what to expect when it came time for her to meet with Dr. James, the school psychologist. She knew there would be tests, but she did not know what type. As she walked from her classroom to Dr. James's office, she felt just a little nervous. But as Dr. James showed her what to do, Paula felt more at ease. Paula found that taking the tests was interesting. Some things were easy, and others were more difficult. There were vocabulary words, number problems, puzzle pieces to put together, and pictures to arrange in order. There were about a dozen tests in all. Dr. James asked Paula to work quickly but carefully, and she used a stopwatch to time how long it took Paula to do certain parts of the test, like arranging blocks to match a design. Paula was excited when, a few weeks later, she found out that she had done well enough on the tests to be placed in the gifted students class next year. The test Paula had taken was the Wechsler Intelligence Scale for Children.

Paula's best friend, Kim, took the same tests, as well as some others, with Dr. James, but for a different reason. Kim had been having trouble with her schoolwork and was finding it hard to remember what she read. In Kim's case, the tests helped Dr. James diagnose a learning disability. The tests showed that although Kim was quite intelligent, her learning disability was preventing her from doing her best work. Kim started to go to a learning support class and knew it was helping when she got a B+ on her reading test.

What Are Personality Tests?

Certain psychological tests assess personality. Some personality tests are standardized, while others are not. An example of a standardized personality test is the Myers-Briggs Type Indicator (MBTI), which can measure a person's usual personality style. Although this test is designed for adults, it can be used for teens and there are variations that are made for younger children. Another standardized personality test for older teens and adults is called the Minnesota Multiphasic Personality Inventory–Adolescent (MMPI-A), which helps identify problems with personality.

Projective tests also give information about someone's personality. Projective tests are not standardized, but psychologists follow certain guidelines for scoring and interpreting them. Projective tests usually include pictures that could have many possible meanings. People are asked to say what they see in the picture or to tell a story about it. Examples are the Thematic Apperception Test (TAT) for older teens and adults and the Children's Apperception Test (CAT) for younger children. The Rorschach Test is a projective test in which a person is shown a series of inkblot designs on cards and asked what they see in the inkblot. These tests are called projective tests because people project their own imagination, ideas, and personality onto the inkblots or pictures.

What Are Neuropsychological Tests?

A specialized group of psychological tests measure brain capacities that can affect a person's behavior. These tests can help evaluate brain damage. These neuropsychological (nur-o-sy-ko-LAW-ji-kal) tests can measure such brain functions as memory, attention, eye-hand coordination, mental processing, and reaction speed*. Neuropsychological tests may be used to evaluate the effects of a brain injury, brain infection, or stroke or to assess people who have problems with memory, balance or learning or people who might have dementia*. Examples of neuropsychological test batteries include the Halstead-Reitan and the Luria-Nebraska tests. Each battery* includes a number of tests that are analyzed to find a pattern of functions. For example, some tests might examine language functions (left brain activities), some might compare motor coordination with each hand (comparing how each side of the brain works), and some might evaluate rapid decision making and problem solving (examining frontal brain regions).

Other Tests

Adaptive behavior tests can measure people's capabilities to care for themselves and carry out other types of behavior important for daily living, such as counting money, shopping, and taking public transportation. They also can assess various job skills. Adaptive behavior tests often are used to evaluate the strengths, capabilities, and needs of someone who has mental retardation.

Vocational* tests can assess people's interests, skills, and aptitudes for particular jobs. There are also many kinds of tests that allow people to choose words or phrases that best describe them. Such "self-report" tests include checklists about behavior, feelings, or problems. These checklists can help identify important issues and start a discussion with a mental health professional who may be evaluating a person's needs and how best to help that person. For example, a self-report measure to examine possible attention deficit hyperactivity disorder might include symptoms of hyperactivity, impulsivity, and poor concentration. Scores are rated against how others self-report to give an indication of how significant the symptom pattern might be within a person's age group.

Evaluation Interviews

Tests are not the only means of finding out about a person. In fact, the most commonly used method of evaluation by psychologists and other mental health professionals is the interview. Interviewing, which consists

reaction speed is the time it takes to respond to a stimulus.

dementia (de-MEN-sha) is a condition that causes a person to lose the ability to think, remember, and act. There also may be changes in personality and behavior.

battery in this case refers to a group of related tests that are given together.

vocational (vo-KAY-shun-al) means relating to training in a particular job skill.

of questions and answers and in-depth discussion, is a very important and effective way to evaluate a person's emotional and behavioral condition. Mental health professionals are trained to use interviews to understand the many aspects of someone's situation and to begin to diagnose possible problems.

How Evaluation and Testing Can Help

Evaluation, which sometimes includes testing, is the first step toward diagnosing a person's mental health condition and possible behavioral, emotional, or learning problems. Evaluation and testing lead to a greater understanding of a problem or condition and pave the way for effective treatment. Evaluation and testing also can provide greater understanding of a person's intelligence, vocational interests, aptitudes, and learning needs, so that an educational plan can be put in place that is best suited to that person's strengths and needs.

▶ *See also*
Attention
Attention Deficit Hyperactivity Disorder
Intelligence
Learning Disabilities
Mental Retardation
School Failure

Therapy

Therapy is short for the term "psychotherapy." Psychotherapy uses talking, learning, feeling, and remembering to help people solve mental, emotional, and behavioral problems and change their lives for the better.

Many people believe that therapy is one of the most effective ways to achieve and maintain good mental and behavioral health. Therapy can help people understand, solve, and prevent problems as well as live more comfortably with problems that cannot be solved or prevented. Therapy also can support people during especially stressful times of their lives. In addition, it can teach people skills and strategies for coping with lifelong stresses, and it can make medications and other treatments work more effectively.

Therapy Is About People and Relationships

Therapy most often is provided by mental health professionals who have been trained and licensed to offer counseling. Therapists may include psychiatrists, psychologists, marriage and family therapists, social workers, ministers, and school counselors. People who work with therapists often are called patients or clients.

Therapeutic alliance Different types of therapists use different methods of therapy to work with different kinds of problems, but all therapeutic methods involve an active partnership and alliance between the therapist and client. To create a safe and trusting alliance, or relationship, therapists follow several basic principles:

KEYWORDS
for searching the Internet and other reference sources
Behavior
Cognition
Gestalt
Hypnotherapy
Psychoanalysis
Psychodrama
Psychodynamic processes
Psychology
Psychiatry

■ Therapists protect the privacy and confidentiality of the information their clients share with them during therapy sessions.

■ Therapeutic settings provide clients with safe environments and safe boundaries. Clients are not judged, disrespected, or intruded upon.

■ Therapists strive to inspire confidence, encourage emotional expression, and increase their clients' expectations for success in therapy and in the world outside therapy.

■ Therapists encourage self-knowledge and self-awareness in their clients so that clients can learn to manage their own thoughts, feelings, and actions after therapy has ended.

Clients and therapists work together to help the client learn to decrease distress, improve health, and increase quality of life.

Transference   When a patient develops trust in the relationship with a therapist, the therapy setting may become right for transference to occur. Transference represents the "transfer" of the patient's feelings onto the therapist. Complex feelings from childhood experiences and from important relationships can transfer to the therapeutic setting. These may include frustration about not getting the expected love or approval from parents and teachers, fear that parents or loved ones will abandon (leave) us, anger that authority figures (teachers, parents) want us to follow rules, and all aspects of love, hate, pride, shame, disappointment, grief, hope, and affection. Because the therapist is not the parent or loved one who was involved in the original relationship, the therapist and client are able to discuss how those earlier hurts might feel in the safe therapy setting. The client might then learn how to change his or her behaviors in current relationships outside therapy.

Individuals, families, and groups   Therapy also can involve different groups of people. In individual therapy, a client works with a therapist in a one-to-one relationship. This often is referred to as a therapeutic "dyad," from the Greek word that means "two." In group therapy, several people with similar problems work together with one or two therapists. This form of therapy can be particularly helpful for people whose problems tend to occur when they must function in groups or teams at school or work. In family therapy, a married couple or an entire family attends therapy sessions, with individuals working together as a unit to understand and resolve the problems the family is experiencing. The family therapist helps members of the family feel safe as they learn both to express their own emotions and to listen to and understand the emotions of other family members.

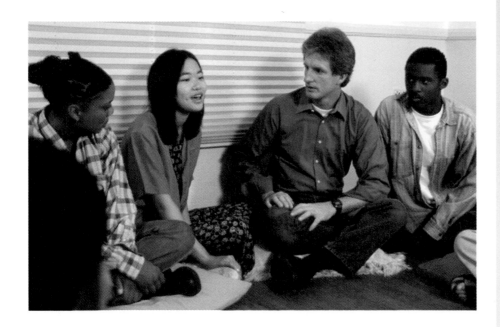

Group therapy sessions help people with similar problems learn to understand themselves, understand each other, and ask for and accept help and support from others whenever necessary. *PhotoEdit, Inc.*

Therapeutic Techniques

Therapists use many different approaches to create the trusting partnership that allows people to change their thoughts, feelings, and behaviors. No one method is better than the others, and many therapists use "eclectic" approaches that combine techniques from many different methods.

Psychoanalysis   Psychoanalysis is the original form of "talk therapy." During psychoanalysis, people talk about their dreams, desires, wishes, and fantasies from early childhood through the present day. Feelings or information of which people are unaware are called unconscious, but they still may affect their behavior. By "making the unconscious conscious," people can bring this material into awareness and understand how it may be affecting their daily lives. For example, angry feelings about a parent may be affecting a person's relationship with her boss. Insight and awareness can be used to create change and resolve conflicts. Psychoanalysis is considered a "psychodynamic" therapy because it emphasizes change, growth, and development.

Cognitive behavioral therapy (CBT)   CBT is a form of therapy that helps people learn to understand and change harmful thoughts, habits, and behaviors. It also can help people learn more effective ways to react to mental problems, emotional problems, and stressful situations. For example, people who think negatively about themselves and the world around them can learn to change these pessimistic thought patterns into thoughts that might be more adaptive. CBT often helps people with anxiety disorders, phobias, addictions, attention deficit hyperactivity disorder, and conduct disorders.

Gestalt therapy Gestalt therapy, based on the German word that means "form" or "pattern," focuses on the entire shape of a person's life: body and mind, habits and beliefs, experiences and actions, home and family, school and friends. This holistic approach to change focuses on making small shifts in body and behavior (for example, chewing food a different way or putting on clothing in a different sequence) that eventually may transform many larger aspects of a person's life. This form of therapy often is associated with the psychologists Frederick "Fritz" Perls (1893–1970) and Paul Goodman (1911–1972).

Play therapy Play therapy is used with younger children who may not be old enough to put their thoughts and feelings into words. Play therapists use dolls, toy soldiers, building blocks, games, and sand trays that allow children to express their problems in nonverbal ways. By observing the child's actions and choices during play, the therapist gradually is able to understand what the child cannot say, help the child learn to understand and put words to the problems expressed through play, and work out solutions during play that can be used in the outside world.

Art, music, dance, and pet therapy These forms of therapy work in much the same way as play therapy. They use sensory experiences, such as drawing, dancing, drumming, or petting dogs and cats, instead of talk therapy or as a supplement to it.

Hypnotherapy Hypnotherapy, also known as medical hypnosis, uses an altered state of consciousness called a trance that allows the client to relax, concentrate, listen to the therapist's suggestions, and learn new behaviors. Hypnotherapy is a recognized form of treatment and is not the same as "stage hypnosis," where the hypnotist "makes" the volunteer act "like a chicken." Researchers do not yet understand exactly how hypnosis influences the brain, but they have used it successfully to help people stop smoking, manage eating disorders, and control chronic pain.

Eye movement desensitization and reprocessing (EMDR) EMDR is a newer approach that combines talk therapy with a series of eye movements. The eye movements are believed to "reprogram" the brain's information processing systems. EMDR is used most often with people who have had a severe emotional experience (for example, witnessing a car accident) and need to "unlearn" the stress responses created by past trauma.

Psychoanalysis and Psychodynamic Therapy

Psychoanalysis and psychodynamic therapy follow a set of psychological theories that emphasize change, growth, and development. Psychoanalysts believe that change and development are achieved by understanding the internal motivations, drives, forces, and impulses that determine behavior.

Talk therapy The specific focus of psychoanalysis is unconscious mental activity—the experiences and feelings that people are unaware of but may still influence them. People in psychoanalysis are encouraged to talk about their dreams, wishes, desires, and fantasies so that the unconscious forces that shape and control their behavior can be brought into awareness and be understood. This form of therapy allows people to understand emotional conflicts, disappointments, and traumas that they experienced during childhood and to reconstruct them in the present with the therapist's guidance.

Change As with other forms of therapy, change is the goal of psychoanalysis. Change can help ease emotional pain, redirect troublesome behaviors, and improve relationships with the important people in an individual's life. The techniques that psychoanalysts use to create change include:

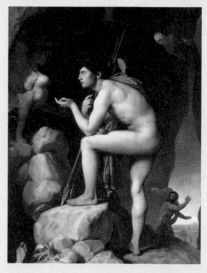

Sigmund Freud used the ancient Greek drama *Oedipus Rex*, written by Sophocles, as a metaphor for parent-child relationships. In this complex drama, Oedipus is a king who unknowingly kills his own father and marries his own mother. In Freud's "Oedipus complex," a son may be jealous of the attention and love his father gets from his mother. When he grows up, the son may even marry a woman who reminds him of his mother. *The Bridgeman Art Library International*

- **Insight:** This refers to awareness and understanding. Often it is described as "making the unconscious conscious."
- **Affective expression:** This involves expressing feelings, conflicts, and impulses. It sometimes is referred to as "catharsis."
- **Developing an observing ego:** This allows people to monitor and control their own emotions and behaviors.
- **Transference:** This allows people to "transfer" leftover feelings from other relationships to the therapist, who helps them deal more effectively with difficult feelings.
- **Conflict resolution:** This allows people to create newer and more helpful patterns for dealing with old and new stresses and problems.

Analytic psychology and psychotherapy Sigmund Freud (1856–1939) was responsible for most of the original concepts of psychoanalysis. Alfred Adler (1887–1937) shifted its focus from sexual issues to issues of power and authority, introducing the term "inferiority complex." Carl Gustav Jung (1875–1961) expanded analytic psychology to include the "collective unconscious" of entire populations as expressed in their myths, fairy tales, metaphors, and artistic creations. Freud's daughter, Anna Freud (1895–1982), and one of Freud's students, Melanie Klein (1882–1960), expanded Freud's theories and techniques to include drawing and playing, which made analysis more useful in the treatment of young children. Even though therapists disagree on how useful Freud's theories are today, most modern therapists agree that the basis of all forms of psychotherapy originated with the work of Dr. Sigmund Freud.

Cognitive Behavioral Therapy (CBT)

Rather than focusing on the unconscious conflicts that are important in psychoanalysis, CBT uses the way people think and interpret their experiences to understand why they sometimes react to stressful situations in harmful ways. CBT helps people understand their troublesome thoughts and behaviors, learn more helpful ways to behave, and practice the new behaviors until they feel comfortable substituting new thought patterns and new behaviors.

SIGMUND FREUD AND THE UNCONSCIOUS MIND

Sigmund Freud (1856–1939), a doctor of neurology, is considered to be the founder of the modern science of psychiatry. Freud developed the technique of psychoanalysis and introduced many important concepts about the human mind and human behavior.

Freud's theory described the human mind as having three parts, which he called the id, ego, and superego. Freud thought this structure provided the underlying organization for human experience, with each part of the psychic structure performing specific functions:

- The id exists from birth and controls all the basic drives that motivate people to find pleasure and seek satisfaction. Many of these drives are unconscious, meaning that they occur outside the awareness of the individual.

- The superego maintains moral standards, conscience, goals, and ideals. The superego controls feelings such as self-esteem and guilt.

- The ego is the part of the mind that balances the drives of the id and the controls of the superego. The ego represents a person's sense of self and is the part of the mind that organizes, directs, and synthesizes the personality.

According to Freud's theory, all three parts of the mind function together, with the ego acting as a brake on both the id and the superego, keeping them functioning at a healthy balance. Freud believed this balance could be achieved through a therapeutic process that he called psychoanalysis.

Freud introduced many other important concepts that are used today to understand how the mind works, including unconscious motivation, transference, and the Oedipus complex. Some of his best known concepts include:

- Defense mechanisms: These are emotional protectors that help the ego or self defend against overwhelming ideas or harmful thoughts.

- Denial: This is a defense mechanism that helps people refuse to believe thoughts or feelings that are intolerable.

- Repression: This is a defense mechanism that helps people forget events that are too painful to remember.

- Libido and psychosexual development: Freud believed that sexuality begins to develop at birth and that children go through phases he called oral, anal, and genital even before they reach puberty.

- Jokes and "Freudian slips": Freud believed that unconscious thoughts sometimes slipped into conversation as jokes or "accidental" word combinations.

Many of Freud's ideas and innovations are used in everyday language and communication today. There even is a comic strip called *The Wizard of Id*. For many people, Freud remains synonymous with the concept of psychotherapy.

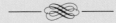

Thoughts, beliefs, and assumptions Cognitive activities keep our brains busy most of the time. We think about ourselves, our friends, our families, our everyday activities, and our futures. Cognitions include core beliefs, automatic thoughts and assumptions, self-talk, self-images, and even behavioral choices, since most of us think before we act. Sometimes, however, our beliefs, assumptions, and thoughts influence or motivate feelings that create behaviors we want to change. "I always mess up when I try something new," for example, is a thought or cognition that may lead to fear of change, fear of failure, and not taking action when needed. Working with the progression from thoughts to feelings to behaviors, CBT therapists help people learn to change their assumptions, which leads to changes both in emotional reactions and in behaviors. "Sometimes I succeed when I try something new" and "everyone makes mistakes when they try something new" are different cognitions that can lead to new behaviors.

Behaviors CBT therapists use therapeutic techniques to help people first identify the thoughts and behaviors they want to change, then identify the factors and situations within their environment that create or maintain the targeted thoughts and behaviors. Once people have done this, the next step is to learn new methods for thinking and acting whenever they encounter the situations that trigger the behaviors they want

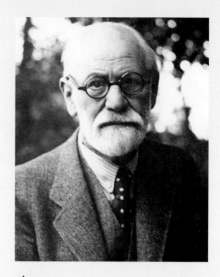

▲

Sigmund Freud is considered to be the founder of the modern science of psychiatry. *Corbis*

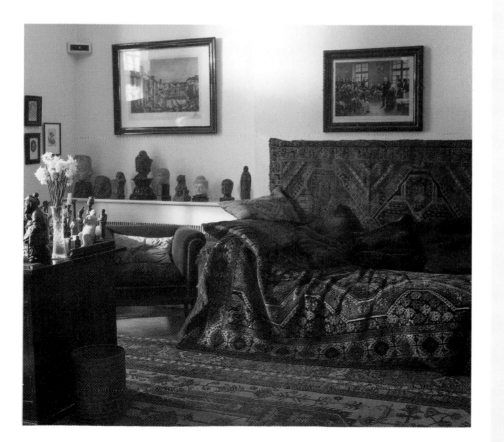

◄

This picture shows the interior of Dr. Freud's office, on display at the Freud Museum in London. Instead of using a stethoscope or scalpel, Freud treated his psychoanalytic patients by encouraging them to lie on a couch and talk about how their fantasies, dreams, wishes, and desires affected their daily activities. Today, patients sit up in chairs more often than they lie on couches, but psychoanalysis continues to be "talk therapy." *Peter Aprahamian/Corbis*

to change. For example, hearing the message "you always mess up when you try something new" from a parent, teacher, or older brother or sister might be the situation that a CBT therapist would help a client work on. Some of the specific techniques of CBT include:

- **Assertiveness training:** learning how to "stick up" for ourselves and practicing it with the therapist until we can do it on our own.
- **Desensitization training:** gradually learning how to deal with situations that trigger fear and anxiety by rehearsing similar situations and learning new response patterns in the safety and privacy of the therapist's office under the therapist's supervision.
- **Token economy:** using rewards, such as extra play time or new videos, to strengthen and reinforce new behaviors. The more difficult the new behavior, the more tokens the client is likely to receive from the therapist.

Often, a CBT therapist will choose a combination of techniques, but all of them will focus on step-by-step change in a safe and private environment with a mental health professional who inspires confidence, encourages emotional expression, and has patience while the client learns to succeed.

Marriage and Family Therapy

In marriage and family therapy, the "client" is a married couple or an entire family. The couple or the family is thought of as a complete system in which each member has influence on the system as well as on the other individual members. At the beginning of the process, one member of the family is the patient (often called the "identified patient") who "brings" the family to therapy. However, during the process of therapy, the family becomes the patient and learns how to improve all of the interactions that affect relationships among members (the system).

Some of the techniques that family therapists use include:

- using family trees (genograms) to help families understand how the family structure works
- encouraging each member of the family to share his or her thoughts and feelings without fearing the reactions of other family members
- training each member of the family to listen to the thoughts and feelings of other family members in a nondefensive manner, without blaming or feeling threatened
- role-playing with the family so that each member learns to understand the family from all other points of view
- role-playing with the family to model new patterns of behavior that involve sharing, communicating, disciplining, caregiving, and adjusting to illnesses or changes in the family structure
- assigning family homework that gives the family practice in using the new skills they have learned during their therapy sessions

PAVLOV, WATSON, AND SKINNER

Cognitive behavioral therapy was developed from the science of behaviorism, which originated with the work of the Russian physiologist Ivan Pavlov (1849–1936).

Pavlov's Dogs

Pavlov used dogs to study the digestive system, focusing on the salivary glands, pancreas, and liver. During his research, Pavlov noticed that the dogs began to salivate whenever they heard a bell. He remembered that the bell always rang before the dogs were fed, and he realized that the bell had become a stimulus for the dogs' digestive systems, because the dogs had linked the bell to food. This discovery led to the development of the science of classical conditioning (also called Pavlovian conditioning), in which "unconditioned" (natural) stimuli are deliberately linked to other events, turning them into "conditioned" stimuli. Pavlov was awarded the Nobel Prize for medicine or physiology in 1904 for his work on the digestive system in dogs.

John Watson

John Watson (1878–1958) often is referred to as the founder of behaviorism. Watson's work focused on the "response" aspect of classical conditioning. Watson knew from Pavlov's work that conditioned stimuli (such as a bell ringing before feeding) provoked conditioned responses (such as dogs salivating when they heard a bell). But Watson also observed that stimuli similar to the conditioned stimulus could lead to similar conditioned responses. For example, Watson observed that a boy afraid of rabbits might also be afraid of white furry creatures like guinea pigs. This observation was particularly important in the study of phobias. One approach to treating phobias involves slowly approaching the feared object. The further away, the less the fear. Gradually the person becomes used to being close to the object of their phobia.

B. F. Skinner

B. F. Skinner (1904–1990) is the psychologist who elaborated on Watson's theories and developed a system for behavior change called "operant conditioning." This system used rewards ("positive reinforcement") and punishments to increase or decrease specific behaviors. Skinner helped develop much of our understanding about behavior, and his theories formed the foundation of modern behavioral therapy, the forerunner of CBT. The token economy technique in CBT relies on Skinner's theories of operant conditioning.

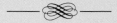

Family therapy can be especially effective for families during periods of stressful change or when families are affected by abuse, addictions, or chronic illnesses.

Choosing a Therapist

With so many different forms of therapy, how is it possible to choose the right therapist? In fact, most people rely on referrals from a family doctor, school counselor, hospital social worker, or trusted friend who has been helped by a therapist and understands the complexities of the process. Because feelings of safety, trust, privacy, and confidence in the therapist are such key aspects of healing, it is important to discuss any doubts, fears, and dislikes frankly with one's therapist. If a person feels he or she is not working well with a therapist, it is reasonable to consider changing to a different therapist. But because therapy is about improving relationships, most often, speaking up about one's doubts will help the therapist adjust his or her behaviors and techniques to make the therapeutic process even more effective.

MURRAY BOWEN AND THE FAMILY SYSTEM

In the late 1950s, a Menninger Clinic psychiatrist named Murray Bowen noticed several things in his work with people who had mental illnesses:

- Sometimes hospitalized patients with mental illnesses got worse after visits from their families.

- Sometimes symptoms of mental illness improved in one member of a family but got worse in another member of the same family at the same time.

- Sometimes parents seemed to resist change and improvement in their children with mental illnesses.

Dr. Bowen concluded that an entire family could be responsible for whether an individual family member recovered from illness or got worse. Based on his observations, Dr. Bowen developed methods of working with the entire family system in therapy. While for most therapists the individual is the patient, for family therapists the family is the patient.

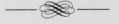

Resources

Organizations

American Academy of Child and Adolescent Psychiatry, 3615 Wisconsin Avenue Northwest, Washington, DC 20016. This professional organization has a *Facts for Families* link at its website. Its *Glossary of Symptoms* and *Mental Illnesses Affecting Teenagers* and its fact sheet *Questions and Answers About Child and Adolescent Psychiatry* explain many different aspects of psychiatric illness, evaluation, and treatment.
Telephone 800-333-7636
http://www.aacap.org

American Psychiatric Association, 1400 K Street Northwest, Washington, DC 20005. This professional association publishes a series of pamphlets and fact sheets that describe psychiatric illnesses and treatments. Its fact sheets *Psychotherapy* and *Psychiatric Medications* and its pamphlet series *Let's Talk About Facts* can help people understand the stigma sometimes attached to mental illness and psychiatric treatment.
Telephone 888-357-7924
http://www.psych.org

American Psychological Association, 750 First Street Northeast, Washington, DC 20002. This professional association publishes books, brochures, and fact sheets. It provides referrals to local psychologists, and its website includes a good search engine and a *KidsPsych* feature.
Telephone 800-374-2721
http://www.apa.org

U.S. National Institute of Mental Health, 6001 Executive Boulevard, Room 8184, MSC 9663, Bethesda, MD 20892. This division of the National Institutes of Health provides current and reliable information about psychotherapy for the public and for professionals.
Telephone 301-443-4513
http://www.nimh.nih.gov

▶ *See also*
Emotions
Families
Hypnosis
Medications
Phobias

Tic Disorders

KEYWORDS
*for searching the Internet
and other reference sources*

Tourette syndrome

*****neurological** (NUR-o-LAH-ji-kal)
relates to the nervous system.
The nervous system is made up
of the brain and spinal cord
and their connections that
regulate body functions.

Tic disorders are neurological* conditions characterized by sudden, rapid movements (for example, neck jerking) or sounds (words or other types of sounds, such as grunting or sniffing) that are repeated over and over in a consistent way many times a day.

What Are Tics?

Tics have been described as brain-activated "involuntary" movements or sounds, meaning that the person does not produce them intentionally. People with tics often can suppress them, sometimes for up to hours at a time, just as one might suppress a cough or a sneeze for a period of time. Imagine, for example, suddenly having to cough in the middle of a concert. To avoid interrupting the musicians, people might try very hard not to cough until the intermission. When they finally cough, however, they might cough several times instead of just once or twice. The experience of trying to suppress a tic is similar. After a tic is suppressed, it may erupt with even greater force or frequency.

Tics tend to get worse when people feel anxious or tired and get better when they are calm and focused on an activity. One interesting aspect of the condition is that tics usually lessen around strangers and are expressed more freely among family members and other trusted people. This does not mean that a person is producing the tics purposely around family members. It probably reflects the fact that they are working harder to suppress them in less comfortable situations, while it is natural for a person to relax their suppression when they are in more familiar surroundings. It is not uncommon for a child to be taken to a doctor to diagnose the problem, only to have the child be unable to produce tics "on command." Just as tics are experienced as uncontrollable, they cannot be voluntarily brought on. While tics may appear as early as 2 years of age, the average age at onset is about 7.

What Are the Symptoms of Tics?

Simple tics Simple tics involve a single movement, such as eye blinking or repeatedly sticking out the tongue. Tics also may be vocal, made up of a single sound, such as throat clearing or snorting, stuttering, or sniffing. The most common type of tics, and often the first to appear, are simple facial tics. Over time, more complex motor* tics may appear.

*****motor** relates to body movement.

Complex tics Complex motor tics involve several coordinated muscle movements, such as touching or smelling an object, jumping or twirling, or making deep knee bends while walking. These tics may include neck stretching, foot stamping, body twisting and bending, or mimicking the gestures of other people. Complex vocal tics can range from combining "simple" throat clearing or grunting with other vocal behaviors, to repeating a long but meaningless string of words at regular intervals.

With complex tics, the repeated phrase or gesture at first may seem meaningful, even when it is not. For example, the person with a complex motor tic may feel a need to do and then redo or undo the same action several times (for example, stretching out one arm ten times before writing or retracing the same letter or repeating the same word) before proceeding to another activity. Such forms of behavior can interfere with a person's ability to accomplish school- or work-related tasks.

Researchers have identified more than 80 tics, which are a mix of simple and complex motor and vocal tics. Some recognizable tic patterns include:

- **Echopraxia** (EK-o-PRAX-ee-a): imitating other people's movements or gestures
- **Copropraxia** (KO-pro-PRAX-ee-a): making obscene, rude, or socially unacceptable gestures
- **Palilalia** (PA-li-LAY-lee-a): repeating a person's own words
- **Echolalia** (EK-o-LAY-lee-a): repeating someone else's words
- **Coprolalia** (KO-pro-LAY-lee-a): shouting obscenities, or impolite and offensive language
- **Repetition:** repeating words or phrases out of context (for example, "Look before you leap").

What Are Tic Disorders?

Doctors usually classify tic disorders into four categories: Tourette syndrome, chronic motor or vocal tic disorder, transient (TRAN-shent) tic disorder, and tic disorder (not otherwise specified).

Tourette syndrome   Tourette syndrome is the best known of the tic disorders, and it is characterized by a frequent and long-lasting pattern of both vocal and motor tics.

Chronic motor or vocal tic disorder   In contrast to Tourette syndrome, chronic* motor or vocal tic disorder involves only one of these two basic types of tics (either motor or vocal), but not both. In other respects, chronic tic disorder has many of the same symptoms as Tourette syndrome in that:

- The tics occur many times a day, nearly every day, and the condition lasts for more than a year.
- The tics may disappear for a time, but that period never exceeds more than 3 months in a row.
- The tics first appear before the age of 18.

*__chronic__ (KRAH-nik) means lasting a long time or recurring often.

- The tics are not the result of a medication or another medical condition.
- The tics cause significant impairment at school or work.

Transient tic disorder In contrast to chronic motor or vocal tic disorder, transient tic disorder refers to a briefer problem with tics. Transient tics may be motor or vocal, or both. For a condition to be considered transient tic disorder, the tics must begin before age 18, occur several times a day, nearly every day for at least 4 weeks but for no longer than 12 months in a row. As with the other tic disorders, transient tics are not the result of another medical condition or a medication.

Tic disorder (not otherwise specified) This is a category for tic disorders when they do not fit into any of the other three groups, usually because the tics last less than 4 weeks or because they begin when a person is older than 18.

How Are Tic Disorders Diagnosed?

While there are clear differences between tic disorders, a doctor may find it difficult to make a diagnosis, because tics often change in type or frequency over time. Transient tics, for example, are short-lived tics that last for less than a year. But a child may experience a series of transient tics over several years. Neck jerking may last for several months and then be replaced by finger snapping or stamping in place. Chronic tics, on the other hand, last longer than a year and tend to remain stable and constant over time.

Transient tics that change over time are believed to affect as many as one-fourth of all school-aged children. While they last, these tics may be quite odd. They might range from sticking out the tongue again and again to repeating a word or phrase a set number of times to poking or pinching various parts of the body. These strange kinds of behavior are more common than was once believed, but often they disappear as a child matures.

Distinguishing transient tics from chronic tics often requires careful evaluation by a physician over a period of years. In addition, it is important for a doctor to gather information about other members of the family (including parents, grandparents, and siblings) who also may have tics or related conditions. It is now known that the tendency for tics to develop is passed on genetically* (inherited) from generation to generation. Because a person may inherit the genetic tendency to tics without ever experiencing tics, it is possible for the disorder to skip several generations in one family. Research is under way to identify the specific gene (or genes) for tic disorders and to understand other factors that may influence whether a person at risk actually will experience tics.

*__genetically__ means stemming from genes, the material in the body that helps determine a person's characteristics, such as hair or eye color.

Related Conditions

For most people who have tics, the real threat may not be the tics themselves but the sense of shame and social isolation that can result from this odd behavior. A child may have great difficulty dealing with these embarrassing, unwanted behaviors. It also may be hard for teachers, fellow students, and family members to understand that a person with tic disorder is not making these strange gestures and sounds intentionally, to gain attention or to avoid working. Other people can easily get that impression if the pattern of tics changes from day to day, as it often does. It can make matters even more difficult when tic disorders in children are associated with attention disorders, hyperactivity, impulsive behavior, obsessive-compulsive disorder*, irritability, or aggressiveness.

It is estimated that as many as half of the children with Tourette syndrome also have the attention and impulse-control problems that are seen in attention deficit hyperactivity disorder. Children with Tourette syndrome also have higher than average rates of learning disabilities that cause reading or language problems.

How Are Tics Treated?

There are several therapies to help children with tics cope with the frightening feelings of being out of control and with the specific types of behavior related to their condition. These include relaxation and stress-reduction techniques, and biofeedback. Often, medication is an important part of the treatment plan. Because of associated stress, anxiety, and self-esteem and relationship issues, working with a mental health professional when concerns begin to interfere with the quality of life is particularly important. A combination of treatment approaches is often required when tics and associated mental health problems are serious.

Resource

Organization

Nemours Center for Children's Health Media, Alfred I. duPont Hospital for Children, 1600 Rockland Road, Wilmington, DE 19803. This organization is dedicated to issues of children's health and produces the KidsHealth website. Its website has articales about tic disorders. http://www.KidsHealth.org.

* **obsessive-compulsive disorder** is a condition that causes people to become trapped in a pattern of repeated, unwanted thoughts, called obsessions (ob-SESH-unz), and a pattern of repetitive behaviors, called compulsions (kom-PUL-shunz).

▶ *See also*

Attention Deficit Hyperactivity Disorder

Learning Disabilities

Obsessive-Compulsive Disorder

Tourette Syndrome

KEYWORDS
*for searching the Internet
and other reference sources*

Nicotine dependence

Smoking cessation

Tobacco Addiction

Tobacco addiction (a-DIK-shun) is a strong craving for nicotine (NICK-o-teen), a chemical in tobacco that makes it hard for people to quit smoking despite the many health risks.

Cigarette smoking can be hazardous not only to your physical health but also to your social health. Contrary to popular belief, most young people do not smoke. In fact, 9 of 10 middle school students and 7 of 10 high school students reported that they were not currently smoking, according to the 1999 National Youth Tobacco Survey. Other research has found that two-thirds of teenagers say that seeing someone smoke turns them off, and more than four-fifths say they would rather date nonsmokers.

What Is Tobacco Addiction?

As encouraging as these figures are, though, they still mean that 1 of 10 middle school students and 3 of 10 high school students smoke cigarettes. Once they get started, most find it hard to stop. They quickly develop tobacco addiction, which means that they have a strong, uncontrollable craving for nicotine, a chemical in tobacco. Nicotine is an easy drug to get hooked on, as highly addictive as heroin or cocaine for some people.

One hallmark of any addiction is tolerance (TAH-le-rans), which means that over time people start to need more and more of a substance to feel its effects. Another effect is withdrawal symptoms, which means that people who are addicted to a substance have physical symptoms and feel sick if they stop using it. Tobacco addiction causes both effects. When people first start smoking, one cigarette may be enough to make them queasy and dizzy. Soon they can smoke several cigarettes without any symptoms, however, and most smokers are up to a pack or more each day by age 25. When people are forced to stop smoking even for a short time, they have unpleasant symptoms. Many rush to light up as soon as they leave a place where smoking is not allowed.

What Is Tobacco Withdrawal?

Most smokers say they do not plan to be smoking in 5 years. But, in fact, more than 70 percent of smokers continue to do so. The main reason it is so tough for them to quit is the discomfort of withdrawal. When smokers suddenly stop or sharply cut back on their tobacco use, a host of distressing symptoms quickly set in. People are tempted to start smoking again to relieve the distress. Common symptoms of tobacco withdrawal include:

- bad mood
- depression

- trouble sleeping
- irritability
- anger
- anxiety
- short attention span
- increased appetite
- weight gain

What Forms of Tobacco Are Used?

There is no such thing as a safe tobacco product. The use of any tobacco product, even ones that are labeled "low tar," "naturally grown," or "additive free," can cause addiction and health problems. Likewise, the use of tobacco in any form, including cigarettes, cigars, pipes, and smokeless tobacco (chewing tobacco or snuff), is harmful. Although cigarettes are the most popular form of tobacco, others are common too. The 1999 National Youth Tobacco Survey was the first study to look at the use of all kinds of tobacco products by young people nationwide. Of the high school students in the study, about 15 percent sometimes smoked cigars, and sizable numbers also used smokeless tobacco (chewing tobacco or snuff), kreteks (clove cigarettes), or bidis (small, flavored cigarettes from India).

What Are the Short-Term Effects of Nicotine?

Nicotine narrows the blood vessels and puts added strain on the heart. Smoking also causes shortness of breath and reduces the amount of oxygen that is available for the muscles and other body tissues to use. These changes can limit people's ability to do the things they want to do. In young people, sports performance can suffer as a result. For example, many smokers cannot run as far or as fast as nonsmokers. Tobacco use also makes people less attractive. It stains teeth and causes bad breath, yellowed fingers, and smelly clothes. In addition, even brief use of smokeless tobacco can cause cracked lips and white spots, sores, and bleeding in the mouth.

What Are the Health Risks of Tobacco Use?

Tobacco use is the primary cause of preventable death in the United States, leading to more than 400,000 deaths each year. It kills more people than AIDS, alcohol, drug abuse, car crashes, murders, suicides, and fires combined. The health risks include:

- **Cancer:** Smoking is a leading cause of cancer of the lungs, larynx*, mouth, throat, and esophagus*, and it plays a role in many other cancers. This is not surprising, since 60 of the more than 4,000 chemical compounds in tobacco and tobacco smoke are known to cause cancer, cell changes, or tumor growth.

* **larynx** (LAYR-inks) is a structure in the throat, composed of muscle and cartilage (KAR-ti-lij) and lined with a mucous (MYOO-kus) membrane, that guards the entrance to the windpipe and serves as the voice organ.

* **esophagus** (eh-SOF-a-gus) Is the tube connecting the stomach and the throat.

- **Lung disease:** Smoking is a major cause of chronic bronchitis (KRO-nik brong-KY-tis), long-lasting inflammation of the breathing tubes or passages that connect the windpipe to the lungs, and emphysema (em-fi-SEE-ma), a long-lasting disease in which the air sacs of the lungs become overly large and don't empty normally. It also worsens colds and pneumonia (noo-MO-nya), an inflammation of the lungs usually caused by infection.

- **Heart disease and stroke:** Smokers are twice as likely as nonsmokers to have a heart attack, in which the heart is damaged when the blood supply to part of the heart muscle is decreased or blocked. Smoking also raises the risk of having a stroke, in which a blood vessel to the brain is blocked or bursts, resulting in injury to brain tissue.

- **Pregnancy problems:** Smoking by pregnant women is linked to miscarriage*, stillbirth*, premature birth*, low birth weight*, and infant death. Women who smoke also are more likely to have trouble getting pregnant.

- **Dental problems:** Use of smokeless tobacco can lead to gum problems and tooth loss.

What Causes Tobacco Addiction?

Nicotine is absorbed easily from tobacco smoke in the lungs. It also is absorbed from smokeless tobacco through the inner lining of the mouth. Within seconds, it travels through the bloodstream to the brain. There it signals the brain to release chemicals that make people want to smoke more. The effect is very powerful. Some people find it especially hard to kick tobacco addiction. The younger people are when they start smoking, the harder it is to quit and the greater the risk to their health.

*__miscarriage__ (MIS-kare-ij) is the loss of a pregnancy before birth.

*__stillbirth__ is the birth of a dead infant.

*__premature__ (pre-ma-CHUR) **birth** means born too early. In humans, it means being born after a pregnancy term lasting less than 37 weeks.

*__low birth weight__ means born weighing less than normal. In humans, it refers to a full-term (pregnancy lasting 37 weeks or longer) baby weighing less than 5.5 pounds.

▶

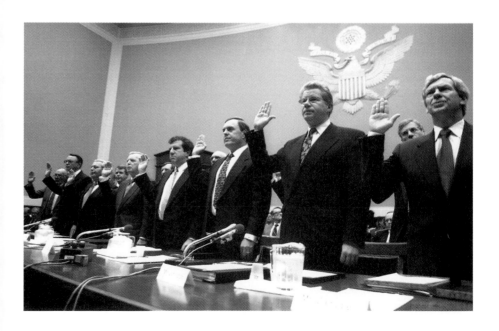

On April 14, 1994, top executives from Philip Morris, RJ Reynolds, and other major cigarette companies testified before a federal court about the addictive nature of nicotine. The tobacco industry also came under attack for targeting children and teens in their ad campaigns. In response, anti-smoking regulations have restricted cigarette sales and the ways in which cigarette companies can market their product. *AP/Associated Press*

How Is Tobacco Addiction Treated?

There are three proven ways of treating tobacco addition: using medications, getting support and encouragement, and learning new skills to resist the urge to smoke and to handle stress better.

Medications The nicotine patch and nicotine gum are sold without a prescription. The nicotine in these products passes through the skin or membranes lining the mouth and reduces the craving for tobacco. It is important to follow label directions carefully. In particular, people should not smoke while using one of these products. Young people under age 18 should check with a physician before trying the patch or gum. A nicotine inhaler* and nicotine nasal spray* are also available by prescription. Bupropion (Wellbutrin, Zyban) is another prescription drug that has been approved for use in smoking cessation. Using any of these products doubles a person's chances of success.

Counseling Counseling can give people support, and it can help them learn the skills they need to give up tobacco and handle stress without smoking. The more counseling people get, whether individually, in a group, or over the phone, the better their chances of quitting. Programs to help people quit smoking are offered at many health care centers and hospitals.

How Well Does Treatment Work?

Giving up tobacco is hard. Most people make two or more attempts before they lick the problem for good. Each time people try to quit, though, they learn more about what helps and what hurts. Half of all people who have ever smoked have been able to stop eventually.

Resources

Books

Izenberg, Neil, with Robert P. Libbon. *How to Raise Non-Smoking Kids.* New York: Byron Preiss Multimedia Company, 1997. A guide for parents that may also be useful for teen readers.

Kranz, Rachel. *Straight Talk About Smoking.* New York: Facts on File, 1999.

Organizations

American Lung Association, 1740 Broadway, New York, NY 10019. The ALA sponsors program to help people quit smoking and provides information and training about tobacco addiction and smoking cessation. Telephone 212-315-8700
http://www.lungusa.org

* **inhaler** (in-HAY-ler) is a hand-held device that produces a mist that is breathed in through the mouth.

* **nasal** (NA-zal) spray is a mist that is sprayed into the nose.

No Butts About It

Here are some quick tips for people who are trying to quit using tobacco:

- Pick a quit date. Write it down. Make a commitment to yourself and stick to your quit date.

- Tell your friends and family that you plan to quit. Ask them not to smoke around you or leave cigarettes around.

- Change your daily routine when you first stop smoking. Eat different foods, or take a different route to school.

- Plan something fun to do each day as a reward for not smoking.

- Try to distract yourself from the urge to smoke. Call a friend, go for a walk, or take up a new hobby.

- Do something other than smoking to reduce stress. Exercise, take a hot bath, or listen to soothing music.

- Drink a lot of water and other non-alcoholic fluids.

American Academy of Family Physicians (AAFP), 11400 Tomahawk Creek Parkway, Leawood, KS 66211-2672. AAFP sponsors "Tar Wars," a smoking-prevention program designed for fifth-grade students. Telephone 913-906-6000
http://www.aafp.org

Stop Teenage Addiction to Tobacco, Northeastern University, 360 Huntington Avenue, 241 Cushing Hall, Boston, MA 02115. This organization's goal is to end childhood and teenage addiction to tobacco. Telephone 617-373-7828
http://www.stat.org

Websites

Campaign for Tobacco-Free Kids. This site, run by the National Center for Tobacco-Free Kids, aims to protect children from tobacco addiction and secondhand smoke.
http://tobaccofreekids.org

Quitnet. This site, a project of the Boston University School of Public Health, offers helpful tips and tools for people who are trying to quit using tobacco.
http://www.quitnet.org

KidsHealth.org, a site run by the medical experts of the Nemours Foundation and the A. I. duPont Hospital for Children, posts information and articles on smoking, smoking prevention, and quitting for kids, teens, and parents.
http://www.KidsHealth.org

▶ *See also*
Addiction
Substance Abuse

KEYWORDS
for searching the Internet and other reference sources

Attention deficit hyperactivity disorder

Obsessive-compulsive disorder

Tics

* **genetically** means stemming from genes, the material in the body that helps determine a person's characteristics, such as hair or eye color.

Tourette Syndrome

Tourette (too-RET) syndrome (TS) is a genetically* transmitted disorder of the central nervous system* associated with several kinds of motor* tics and at least one vocal tic*.

Meet Pete

One day in the middle of a math test, Pete began to make loud sniffing noises repeatedly. Other than his periodic sniffing, his sixth grade classroom was very quiet. Mr. Carlson, Pete's math teacher, put his finger to his lips, signaling Pete to be quiet. Pete imitated Mr. Carlson's gesture, putting his own finger to his lips. He repeated the gesture several times and then stopped and began making the sniffing noises again. Pete was surprised by his own behavior. He knew that he should stop, but the more he tried to stop, the more he found that he could not.

Mr. Carlson, who always understood when Pete was late with his homework, was troubled by this new classroom behavior. Pete had had difficulty finishing homework assignments and had occasionally had trouble staying still in his seat, but he had never disrupted the class before. Mr. Carlson invited Pete out into the hallway and asked if Pete would prefer to take the math test by himself. Pete said that he would. Was Pete just trying to avoid taking the math test, Mr. Carlson wondered, or might he perhaps have TS?

What Is Tourette Syndrome?

Many people with symptoms like Pete's have TS. Their tics tend to be most noticeable when they are feeling nervous, anxious (as Pete may have been during his exam), or tired. The tics tend to ease when people are focused and concentrating on something, and they are generally not evident at all when people are sleeping.

One of the many interesting features of TS is that the tics vary from person to person, in terms of the type of tic and its severity. They also may vary in the same person over time. After several months, one tic may go away and be replaced by another. It also may disappear completely. At some point in their childhood, up to one-fourth of all school-age children have simple tics, such as eye blinking, but they do not go on to have TS. Their tics simply disappear with time. Other children may experience more complex tics as time passes. Complex motor tics involve several coordinated muscle movements, such as twirling or hopping in place while walking. Complex vocal tics include babbling, echoing sounds, and babbling meaningless strings of words.

To say that a person has TS, the tics (which usually occur several times a day) must begin before a person turns 18, and they must last for more than a year. In addition, a person must have more than one motor tic and at least one vocal tic over that period of time. The tics may occur simultaneously or at different times. In rare cases, tics may involve movements that cause the person pain or injury; for example, tics that result in biting their lips or cheeks or even banging their heads. These very severe cases are the exception and not the rule in TS. More commonly, the tics involve harmless muscle movements or vocalizations, which are mild to begin with and lessen or in some cases disappear over time. The tics also may disappear for days, weeks, or years and then recur.

TS is much more common than was once believed. It is estimated that about 100,000 Americans have TS, or 1 in every 2,000 to 2,500 people. About three times that many people have other tic disorders, such as chronic* multiple tics or transient* tics. While Tourette syndrome involves a long-lasting problem with both motor and vocal tics, chronic multiple tics involve several tics that are either motor or vocal, but not both. Transient tic disorders may look like other tic disorders but are present for less than a year.

* **central nervous system** refers to the brain and spinal cord, which coordinates the activities of the entire nervous system. The nervous system is made up of the nerve cells of the body, which communicate with each other to help regulate the functioning of the body.

* **motor** relates to body movements.

* **tics** are sudden, brain-activated "involuntary" movements (such as eye blinking or shoulder shrugging) or sounds (words or other sounds, such as sniffing, grunting, throat clearing, or even barking) that are repeated over and over in the same way.

* **chronic** means lasting for a long time or recurring often.

* **transient** (TRAN-shent) means brief or producing effects for a short period of time.

neurological (nur-o-LAH-ji-kal) relates to the nervous system.

obsessive-compulsive disorder is a condition that causes people to become trapped in a pattern of repeated, unwanted thoughts, called obsessions (ob-SESH-unz), and a pattern of repetitive behaviors, called compulsions (kom-PUL-shunz).

dopamine (DOPE-a-meen) is a brain chemical that is involved in the control of movement.

serotonin (ser-o-TOE-nin) is a chemical associated with emotions, particularly feelings of well-being.

norepinephrine (NOR-e-pi-ne-frin) is a body chemical that can increase the arousal response, heart rate, and blood pressure.

Parkinson disease is a disorder of the central nervous system that causes trembling or rigidity of muscles, uncoordinated movements, and poor balance.

What Causes Tourette Syndrome?

Until Gilles de la Tourette, a French physician, described in 1885 the group of odd and often changing tics we now associate with TS, people like Pete often were believed to be possessed by demons. Thanks to many advances in our understanding of how information is transmitted in the brain, we now know that TS is a neurological* disorder characterized by chemical changes in the brain. Although the basic cause of TS and other tic disorders is still unknown, we know that TS is an inherited condition, meaning that the likelihood of TS developing in a person is passed from parent to child.

Genetics One of the most interesting findings from studies of TS is that boys are three to four times more likely to show signs of TS than girls are. A parent with a gene for the syndrome has a one in two chance of passing it on to each child. The child who inherits the gene may show symptoms of TS or may not. In males who have the gene, there is a 99 percent chance that symptoms of the disorder will occur. In females with the gene, that likelihood is 70 percent, but girls with the gene appear to be more likely than boys with the gene to have symptoms of obsessive-compulsive disorder*, a condition that is believed to be linked genetically to TS.

Neurotransmitters New research suggests that there is an abnormality in the genes affecting the brain's handling of and levels of certain brain chemicals known as neurotransmitters. Neurotransmitters carry signals from one nerve cell to another. The transmission of these signals is involved in attention and memory, movement, and moods, such as happiness, sadness, or anxiety (ang-ZY-e-tee). The neurotransmitters that may play a part in TS include dopamine*, serotonin*, and norepinephrine*. In this regard, TS is similar to other neurological conditions, such as Parkinson disease*, which are now known to be linked to specific neurotransmitter imbalances in the brain.

How Can I Tell If Someone I Know Has Tourette Syndrome?

The short answer is that it is not always easy to spot TS. The best person to make a diagnosis of TS is a doctor who has known the person for a long time and also has gathered a detailed family medical history. Many children may have one or more simple tics, such as head turning or eye blinking, at some point in their childhood. In most cases, these tics will disappear. Besides looking for a pattern of tics that continue for a least a year, the doctor may make use of several tests, such as the Yale Global Tic Severity Scale and the Hopkins Motor/Vocal Tic Scale.

Because tics come and go, it is not unusual for a child to go to the doctor and be tic-free throughout the entire visit. Just as children may find it difficult to suppress tics at times when they may want to, they also cannot always produce tics on command. Tics tend to be more noticeable in the presence of family members and friends and less noticeable with strangers. It is important for the doctor evaluating a person for possible tics to look for related conditions and to consider the impact of the tics and related conditions on the child's ability to function in school and with friends and family.

Related Conditions

It is not uncommon for people with TS to have obsessive-compulsive disorder (OCD) as well. In this disorder, a person may have recurrent, anxiety-provoking thoughts (for example, that a person forgot to lock the door when leaving home) or behavior (for example, repeatedly checking to make sure the door is locked). In the case of both TS and OCD, the person may feel unable to resist the activity, much as a person may feel unable to resist a sneeze. An important difference is that the types of behavior (compulsions) seen in OCD are typically quite complex and are voluntary, even though they may be hard to resist (like checking the lock a number of times), while those associated with TS have a more involuntary, uncontrolled quality. Even though people with TS may be able to temporarily suppress a tic, tics occur involuntarily (like blinking, sneezing, or coughing).

There are two other conditions that are commonly associated with TS: attention deficit hyperactivity disorder (ADHD) and learning disability. ADHD is a disorder associated with physical restlessness, inattention, and poor control of impulses. People with ADHD find it very difficult to organize tasks and activities, and, as a result, they are prone to move impulsively from one unfinished task to another. Physical signs and symptoms of ADHD in school-age children include squirming in their seats, fidgeting, and shaking their feet or legs excessively. In adolescents, ADHD may take the form of getting up from the table during meals, difficulty in concentrating and finishing homework, or speaking out impulsively.

Learning disabilities, such as problems in reading, writing, or math, may interfere with a person's success in school despite good intelligence. These disabilities are diagnosed when there is a difference between children's levels of achievement on academic tests and their general levels of intelligence.

How Is Tourette Syndrome Treated?

While there is no known cure for TS at this time, there are treatments that can help ease the embarrassment and discomfort associated with the condition as well as medications that can reduce the frequency and severity of the tics. Perhaps most important of all is understanding, self-understanding as well as understanding on the part of teachers, family

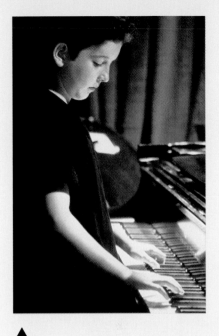

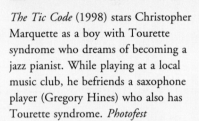

The Tic Code (1998) stars Christopher Marquette as a boy with Tourette syndrome who dreams of becoming a jazz pianist. While playing at a local music club, he befriends a saxophone player (Gregory Hines) who also has Tourette syndrome. *Photofest*

*epilepsy is a condition of the central nervous system characterized by recurrent seizures, or violent spasms, that can affect a person's movements and awareness of the environment.

*cerebral palsy (se-RE-bral PAL-zee) is a group of conditions, all of which affect a person's ability to move. They are usually caused by injury to the brain before or soon after birth.

members, and friends. It is important and helpful for all those who are involved with a person who has TS to accept that TS is a medical condition like epilepsy* or cerebral palsy* or any other neurological condition that causes involuntary responses or movements. The types of behavior associated with TS cannot be controlled, much as they might at times look or seem intentional. These types of behavior do not reflect a person's intelligence, academic ability, or potential to lead an otherwise happy and productive life.

In addition to counseling to come to terms with a diagnosis of TS, there are other measures that may help:

- **Educational alternatives:** Tutoring, smaller classrooms, private study areas, and alternative forms of testing (for example, oral exams for students who have difficulty writing) may help the child or teen with TS and related learning or attention disorders. In configuring the proper school environment, it is key to recognize that most children with TS have normal intelligence, but they may need special arrangements to achieve their full potential without disrupting other students.

- **Relaxation and biofeedback techniques:** Relaxation and biofeedback can help people with TS better manage stress that can increase the severity of the tics. With relaxation techniques, people learn to make various muscles in their bodies less tense and rigid and possibly decrease the frequency of tics. Biofeedback teaches a person to pay more attention to involuntary movements of the body, with the aim of bringing these movements under more conscious control. It is possible that relaxation and biofeedback help reduce the urge to have tics by learning to tolerate and control some of the inner tension that precedes tic behavior.

- **Behavior modification:** Behavior modification or habit reversal procedures also can be used to help "extinguish" or lessen disruptive behavior. Just as people with a fear of snakes can learn, with repeated exposures to snakes, to overcome their fear, people with TS can use exposure techniques to help desensitize themselves to the situations that are likely to bring about the tension that may produce tics.

Medications for Tourette Syndrome

Many people with TS may benefit from medications, particularly people with very severe and disruptive tics. Medications act on the neurotransmitters in the brain to help lessen the symptoms. Just as the tics themselves vary from person to person, the most effective medication for different people will vary, depending on other conditions they may have and how well they can tolerate the effects of a particular medication.

The medicine that has been used the longest to help minimize tics is haloperidol (sold under the brand name Haldol), a dopamine-blocking agent. The downside of halperidol and other similar dopamine-blocking agents is a possibly serious side effect called "tardive dyskinesia" (TAR-div dis-ki-NEE-zhah). Tardive dyskinesia is a neurological condition in which there are slow, uncontrollable mouth movements and drooling. Overall mental "dulling" is also common. There are other medications now available that may have fewer and less serious side effects. For example, clonidine (sold under the brand name Catapres) has proven to be effective in limiting tics and also in improving some of the attention problems of people with TS.

In addition to medications for the tics themselves, there are medications that have been used to treat related conditions, such as OCD and ADHD. As with any medications, those for TS are prescribed only after the diagnosis is confirmed. A doctor monitors a patient carefully for side effects. There may sometimes be problems with medications given to people who have more than one condition. For example, some medications that are used to treat children with ADHD can increase the severity of the tics seen in TS.

Living with Tourette Syndrome

TS is not a degenerative* condition that causes more damage over time. With a supportive environment and self-acceptance, the child with TS can go on to live a normal, productive life that includes not only school and work successes but also healthy friendships and relationships. In all walks of life, from sports to the arts, there are people with TS who have excelled at the activities they love. Jim Eisenreich, once a star hitter and outfielder for the Philadelphia Phillies, helped his team reach the 1993 World Series. For Eisenreich, who at one time walked off the field after twitching publicly in front of thousands of fans, the journey from shame to diagnosis, treatment, and self-acceptance paid off.

*** degenerative** means progressively worsening or becoming more impaired.

Resources

Book

Rubio, Gwyn Hyman. *Icy Sparks.* New York: Viking, 2001. A novel about a 10-year-old girl who tries to conceal her tics and the unhappiness they cause her.

Organizations

Nemours Center for Children's Health Media, Alfred I. duPont Hospital for Children, Wilmington, DE. Its website has articles about Tourette syndrome.
http://www.KidsHealth.org

National Institute of Neurological Disorders and Stoke, NIH Neurological Institute, P.O. Box 5801, Bethesda, MD 20824. This organization is a leading center for biomedical research and information.
Telephone 800–352–9424
http://www.ninds.nih.gov

Tourette Syndrome Association, Inc., 42-40 Bell Boulevard, Bayside, NY 11361-2820. This nonprofit organization for people with TS, family and friends, and health professionals funds research, provides services to patients and their families, and offers various publications and fact sheets.
Telephone 718-224-0717 or 800-4-TOURET
http://www.tsa-usa.org

Trance   *See* Hypnosis

▶ See also
Attention Deficit Hyperactivity Disorder
Learning Disabilities
Obsessive-Compulsive Disorder
Tic Disorders

Trichotillomania

Trichotillomania (trik-o-til-o-MAY-nee-a) is a condition that involves compulsive (kom-PUL-siv) hair pulling, usually the hair on the scalp or the eyebrows or eyelashes.

Penny's Story

Penny put on her favorite baseball cap and headed out the door for school. The cap hid the bald spot on the side of her head pretty well. She envied the girls who could wear barrettes and ponytails to school, and she remembered the days when she had worn them too. Over the past 2 years, Penny had started to pull out her hair and her eyebrows. It began gradually at first, but pretty soon her eyebrows were gone, and she had bald patches on her head. She did not want to pull the hair, but she felt a powerful urge to do it. She just could not stop. No one understood why she was doing it, not even Penny. The boys in her class teased her. She pretended not to listen to them, but their unkind comments made her cry when she was alone. Even the nice kids asked her why she did not have any eyebrows. Until lately, Penny did not really know what to say. Then Penny began to see a therapist, who helped her understand that she had trichotillomania.

What Is Trichotillomania?

Trichotillomania is a condition that involves strong urges to pull hair. People with this condition pluck or pull the hair on their heads, their eyelashes, their eyebrows, or hair on other body parts. For people with trichotillomania, the hair pulling is more than a habit. It is a compulsive behavior, which the person finds very hard to stop. A person with trichotillomania feels a strong urge to pull hair, an impulse that is so powerful that it seems impossible to resist.

Pulling the hair often provides a brief feeling of relief, like the feeling of finally scratching an itch but much more intense. But after the feeling of relief, which lasts only a moment, the person usually feels distressed and unhappy about having pulled the hair. Soon the urge to pull hair returns. People with trichotillomania wish they could stop, and may feel ashamed or embarrassed. Many people who have this condition try to keep it secret.

What Causes Trichotillomania?

The condition trichotillomania was first described in 1889 by the French physician François Hallopeau. The term "trichotillomania" comes from the Greek words "thrix," meaning "hair," and "tillein," meaning "to pull." "Mania," the Greek word for "madness" or "frenzy," was used in those days for any condition that affected human behavior. Dr. Hallopeau wrote that his patients with hair-pulling compulsions were, in fact, quite emotionally healthy.

Although the exact cause of trichotillomania is unknown, there is growing evidence that it is a biological disorder of neurotransmitter*

* **neurotransmitters** (NUR-o-tranz-mit-ters) are brain chemicals that enable brain cells to communicate with one another and therefore allow the brain to function normally.

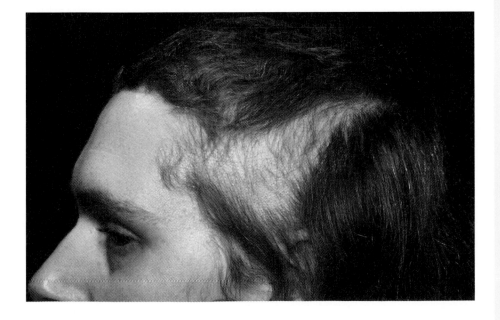

◄

About 75 percent of people with trichotillomania pull hair from the scalp. In many cases trichotillomania is a response to stress at home or school, while in others it results from a hair-pulling habit developed during childhood. *Custom Medical Stock Photos*

* **obsessions** (ob-SESH-unz) are repeated disturbing thoughts or urges that a person cannot ignore and that will not go away.

* **ringworm** is a fungal infection of the skin or scalp that appears as a round, red rash.

* **alopecia areata** (al-o-PEA-shah a-ree-AH-ta) is a condition that leads to sudden hair loss, often in small, round patches on the scalp. The cause is not known.

* **behavior therapy** is a type of counseling that works to help people change their actions.

function in the brain. Trichotillomania has some similarities to obsessive-compulsive disorder (OCD), but in trichotillomania there are no obsessions*, and hair pulling is the only compulsion. Both trichotillomania and OCD fall into the larger category of anxiety disorders. Some people with trichotillomania have other forms of anxiety as well. Trichotillomania can affect children, adolescents, and adults. Both males and females can have trichotillomania, but it seems to be more common among females.

How Is Trichotillomania Diagnosed?

When individuals lose their hair or eyebrows, doctors may first check for other conditions that might cause a person's hair to fall out, like ringworm,* alopecia areata,* or other skin diseases. But if the person tells the doctor about the hair pulling, it is probably trichotillomania. Penny's doctor sent her to see a therapist, a mental health specialist who listens to people talk about their experiences and feelings and who can help people work out ways to deal with behavior problems. The therapist explained Penny's condition to her and told her about the urges, habits, and anxiety that are part of it. She helped Penny understand that the hair pulling was not her fault. Penny felt relieved to know that she was not the only person with this problem and that there were things she could do about it.

How Is Trichotillomania Treated?

One common treatment for trichotillomania is a behavior therapy* technique called habit reversal. In habit reversal, the person first learns to notice the urge before the compulsion to pull hair becomes too strong to resist. Then the person learns to do something else instead of hair pulling until the urge grows weaker and passes. This can be more difficult than it sounds, because the person may feel increasing, uncomfortable tension and anxiety while trying to resist the urge to pull hair. With time and practice, the brain can begin to react differently to the urges, and the person can start to control the compulsive behavior. Some people also may take medication that helps with the compulsions and decreases the strength of the urges, making them easier to resist. After a few weeks of practice, coaching from her therapist, and support from her parents, Penny began to get better at resisting the urges she felt. Penny has started to see results. Her hair has begun to grow back in.

What Is It Like to Live with Trichotillomania?

Now that Penny's hair and eyelashes are growing in, she feels better about herself and more hopeful about coping with trichotillomania. Now and then, Penny may continue to feel urges to pull her hair and eyebrows, but she knows what to do to resist them. She knows that these impulses can be stronger in times of stress, but they also can arise on their own during times when Penny is bored or just relaxed. Her therapist is helping Penny learn and practice ways to cope with normal stresses, to stop the urges before they get too strong, and to control her compulsive pulling.

Resources

Book

Golomb, Ruth Goldfinger, and Sherrie Mansfield Vavrichek. *The Hair Pulling "Habit" and You: How to Solve the Trichotillomania Puzzle.* Silver Spring, MD: Writers' Cooperative of Greater Washington, 2000. A workbook and guide for kids and teens, parents and therapists that presents useful strategies and tools for conquering trichotillomania.

Organization

Trichotillomania Learning Center, 1215 Mission Street, Suite 2, Santa Cruz, CA 95060. The purpose of this organization is to advance the understanding of trichotillomania.
Telephone 831-457-1004
http://www.trich.org

▶ *See also*
Brain and Nervous System (Introduction)
Anxiety and Anxiety Disorders
Habits and Habit Disorders
Obsessive-Compulsive Disorder

Truancy *See* **School Avoidance**

V

Violence

Violence is the use of physical force to injure people or property. Violence may cause physical pain to those who experience it directly, as well as emotional distress to those who either experience or witness it. Individuals, families, schools, workplaces, communities, society, and the environment all are harmed by violence.

What Is Violence?

Violence is a social and health problem for all who experience and witness it. Violence takes many forms, including:

- Family violence, often referred to as domestic abuse, child abuse, child maltreatment, spouse abuse, and wife battering
- Peer group violence, which includes workplace violence, school violence, gang violence, and bullying*
- Sexual violence, which includes rape*, date rape, marital rape, intimate partner abuse, and child sexual abuse
- Abuse of power, which includes mistreatment of children, students, elders, people with disabilities, and others who are smaller or less powerful than the abuser
- Community violence, which includes assaults, fights, shootings, homicides, and most forms of peer violence
- Hate crimes and hate speech, which target victims based on gender, age, race, ethnicity, religious belief, or sexual orientation
- Media violence, shown on television, in film, and in video games.

Why Do People Behave Violently?

Research indicates that violent behavior may have many different causes, some of which are inborn but most of which are learned from experiencing or witnessing violent behavior by others, particularly those who are role models.

Genetics Chromosomes carry genetic messages from parents to offspring, and there is some research that suggests that, in some cases, aggressiveness may be inherited.

KEYWORDS
for searching the Internet and other reference sources

Abuse

Hate crimes

Hatred

Prevention

Self-regulation

Social modeling

* **bullying** is when a person repeatedly intimidates or acts aggressively toward those with less power or ability to defend themselves.

* **rape** is when a person forces another person to have sexual intercourse. or engage In other unwanted sexual activities.

What Is Wrong with Media Violence?

Research shows that media violence can lead to real violence in multiple ways. The U.S. Surgeon General and the U.S. National Institute of Mental Health both have reported that watching television violence is an important predictor of aggressive behavior. Children's cartoons and music videos in particular often portray violence. American children see about 16,000 simulated murders and 200,000 acts of violence on television by age 18. In nearly 75 percent of those cases, punishment is not shown to be a consequence of violent behavior.

Perhaps potentially even more serious is the link between violence and some interactive video games. During violent video games, the player identifies with the point of view of the aggressor and practices violent thoughts, feelings, and actions. For some people, with enough reinforcement, violent behaviors can become accessible or even automatic if and when the player later encounters conflict in real life.

Brain injury   Injury to the front parts of the brain may remove some personal control over anger and aggression.

Antisocial personality disorder   People with antisocial personality disorder often behave violently even as children. They may disregard their own safety and the safety of others. People with this disorder do not seem to understand that violence harms other people, and they do not seem to have a conscience that tells them right from wrong. The terms sociopath and psychopath sometimes are used to describe people with antisocial personality disorder.

Alcohol and substance abuse   Drinking and drugs often play a role in violence. For some, these substaneces interfere with otherwise good judgement or behavior. Some people try to use alcohol or drugs to treat their feelings of anger or depression, but instead feel worse. Violence toward others—or towards themselves—can result.

Desensitization   Constantly viewing violence at home, in communities, or on television can lead people to believe that violence is a normal part of life. People who are surrounded by violence may reach a point where they no longer notice violent events or remember that peaceful behavior is a possibility.

Learned helplessness   People who resign themselves to the belief that violence is an inevitable part of their lives may give up trying to avoid or escape that violence. They may become passive and unable to create safety for themselves or their families. Battered wives who remain at home with battering husbands, for example, may believe that trying to escape violence is hopeless.

Social modeling   Children learn by observation and by imitation. Children who observe their home, school, or media role models behaving in violent ways may come to believe that turning angry feelings into angry actions is acceptable behavior, or even the most effective way to solve problems. Such children may never learn peaceful behaviors or cooperative ways to solve problems.

Parents who model abusive behavior at home can create a cycle of violence, teaching children to grow up to be abusive adults. The importance of positive role models and the dangers of negative role models should not be underestimated.

Learning the boundaries between anger (emotion) and violence (physical force) is an important developmental task for all people and all cultures. It is possible to have angry feelings without turning those feelings into angry actions or violent behaviors. Expressing anger in a nonviolent way can be healthy. However, parents, adult mentors, media, and community leaders first must model nonviolent conflict-resolution skills for young people to learn them.

SOCIAL MODELING AND SELF-REGULATION

S ocial psychologist Albert Bandura has been studying social modeling, observational learning, aggression, and self-regulation since the 1970s. Bandura's theories indicate that role models (social modeling) can influence people toward creativity or toward violence. If children observe violent behavior at home, in school, or on television, they may come to believe that turning angry feelings into angry actions is acceptable behavior. When these children become angry themselves, they will display the behaviors they have observed, and they even may create new angry behaviors that go beyond what they have learned from their models.

Another important aspect of Bandura's research focuses on self-direction and self-efficacy, or people's beliefs about their own abilities to influence and affect the world around them. If children observe adults failing to control their own angry feelings or violent behaviors, or if they observe violent behavior going unpunished, they may come to believe that peaceful behaviors cannot succeed or are not worthwhile activities. They may lose their motivation to learn cooperative problem-solving skills, or they may quit before they achieve success in using these skills.

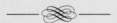

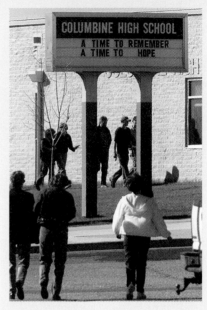

Students and faculty gather for a memorial on the one-year anniversary of the shooting at Columbine High School in Littleton, Colorado. On April 20, 1999, two students killed 12 classmates and one teacher before taking their own lives. *Reuters Newmedia Inc./Corbis*

How Is Violence Treated and Prevented?

People who experience or witness violence should react immediately. Police and violence hotlines should be called in an emergency. People who have been injured should be taken to a clinic or hospital emergency room for treatment. When an immediate crisis has ended, a family doctor or school counselor or member of the clergy should be contacted for counseling and referrals. Shelters and child protection agencies can help battered women and children. Counseling can help batterers and their families to learn better behaviors for managing stress, conflict, and anger. Therapists can help people with post-traumatic stress disorder* achieve emotional recovery from the aftermath of violence.

Those who commit violent acts or have violent or angry feelings need to receive treatment. Emotional problems, drug and alcohol abuse, and other conditions which make a person more violence-prone need to be dealt with. The social forces that prevent violence—family, friends, and the community—need to take positive steps to make violence less likely and to increase safety.

***post-traumatic stress disorder** is a mental disorder in which people who have survived a terrifying event relive their terror in nightmares, memories, and feelings of fear. It is severe enough to interfere with everyday living and can occur after a natural disaster, military combat, rape, mugging, or other violence.

Physical violence is never an acceptable form of behavior. Everyone has choices. Becoming aware of the problems, deciding not to follow violent patterns, and making a commitment to learn new ways of relating are the keys to change. It is never too late to change the pattern of violence in families, communities, or society.

Resources

Organizations

Nemours Center for Children's Health Media, Alfred I. duPont Hospital for Children, 1600 Rockland Road, Wilmington, DE 19803. This organization is dedicated to issues of children's health and produces the KidsHealth website. Its website has articles about violence. http://www.KidsHealth.org

U.S. Centers for Disease Control and Prevention. This government agency posts fact sheets at its website covering youth violence, domestic violence, intimate partner violence, and violence in the workplace. http://www.cdc.gov

▶ *See also*

Abuse

Antisocial Personality Disorder

Bullying

Conduct Disorder

Emotions

Oppositional Defiant Disorder

Personality

Personality Disorders

Post-Traumatic Stress Disorder

Rape

Bibliography

Adams, Russell L., Oscar A. Parson, and Jan L. Culbertson, eds. *Neuropsychology for Clinical Practice: Etiology, Assessment, and Treatment.* Washington, DC: American Psychological Association, 1996.

Allman, John Morgan. *Evolving Brains.* New York: Scientific American Library, 2000.

American Psychiatric Association. Diagnostic and Statistical Manual of Mental Disorders (DSM-IV), 4th ed. Washington, DC: American Psychiatric Association, 1994.

Ayd, Frank J., Jr. *Lexicon of Psychiatry, Neurology, and the Neurosciences.* Philadelphia: Lippincott Williams and Wilkins, 1995.

Barnett, Ola W., Cindy L. Miller-Perrin, and Robin D. Perrin. *Family Violence Across the Lifespan: An Introduction.* Thousand Oaks, CA: Sage Publications, 1997.

Beall, Anne E., and Robert J. Sternberg. *The Psychology of Gender.* New York: Guilford Press, 1993.

Bednar, Richard L., and Scott R. Peterson. *Self-Esteem: Paradoxes and Innovations in Clinical Theory and Practice,* 2d ed. Washington, DC: American Psychological Association, 1995.

Beidel, Deborah C., and Samuel M. Turner. *Shy Children, Phobic Adults: Nature and Treatment of Social Phobia.* Washington, DC: American Psychological Association, 1998.

Bohart, Arthur C., and Deborah J. Stipek, eds. *Constructive and Destructive Behavior: Implications for Family, School, and Society.* Washington, DC: American Psychological Association, 2001.

Brown, Ronald T., and Michael G. Sawyer. *Medications for School-Age Children: Effects on Learning and Behavior.* New York: Guilford Press, 1998.

Campbell, Anne. *Men, Women, and Aggression.* New York: Basic Books, 1993.

Carson, Ronald A., and Mark A. Rothstein, eds. *Behavioral Genetics: The Clash of Culture and Biology.* Baltimore, MD: Johns Hopkins University Press, 1999.

Carter, Rita. *Mapping the Mind.* Berkeley: University of California Press, 1999.

Cohen, Jonathan, and Bertram J. Cohler, eds. *The Psychoanalytic Study of Lives over Time: Clinical and Research Perspectives on Children Who Return to Treatment in Adulthood.* San Diego: Academic Press, 1999.

Crooks, Robert L., and Karla Baur. *Our Sexuality,* 7th ed. Pacific Grove, CA: Brooks/Cole, 1999.

DeGangi, Georgia A. *Pediatric Disorders of Regulation in Affect and Behavior: A Therapist's Guide to Assessment and Treatment.* San Diego: Academic Press, 2000.

Denham, Susanne A. *Emotional Development in Young Children.* New York: Guilford Press, 1998.

Dodgen, Charles E., and W. Michael Shea. *Substance Use Disorders: Assessment and Treatment.* San Diego: Academic Press, 2000.

Dowling, John E. *Creating Mind: How the Brain Works.* New York: W. W. Norton, 1998.

Duberstein, Paul Raphael, and Joseph M. Masling. *Psychodynamic Perspectives on Sickness and Health.* Washington, DC: American Psychological Association, 2000.

Feinstein, Robert E., and Anne A. Brewer, eds. *Primary Care Psychiatry and Behavioral Medicine: Brief Office Treatment and Management Pathways.* New York: Springer Publishing Company, 1999.

Bibliography

Gleitman, Henry. *Psychology,* 4th ed. New York: W. W. Norton, 1995.

Greenfield, Susan. *The Human Brain: A Guided Tour.* New York: Perseus Books, 1997.

Gullotta, Thomas P., Gerald Adams, and Carol Markstrom. *The Adolescent Experience,* 4th ed. San Diego: Academic Press, 1999.

Gullotta, Thomas P., and Sandra J. McElhaney, eds. *Violence in Homes and Communities.* Thousand Oaks, CA: Sage Publications, 1999.

Harrington, Anne, ed. *The Placebo Effect: An Interdisciplinary Exploration.* Cambridge, MA: Harvard University Press, 1997.

Herman, Judith Lewis. *Trauma and Recovery: The Aftermath of Violence—From Domestic Abuse to Political Terror.* New York: Basic Books, 1992.

Hibbs, Euthymia D., and Peters S. Jensen, eds. *Psychosocial Treatment for Child and Adolescent Disorders: Empirically Based Strategies for Clinical Practice.* Washington, DC: American Psychological Association, 1996.

Higgins, Gina O'Connell. *Resilient Adults: Overcoming a Cruel Past.* San Francisco: Jossey-Bass, 1994.

Imber-Black, Evan, ed. *Secrets in Families and Family Therapy.* New York: W. W. Norton, 1993.

Kendall, Philip C. *Child and Adolescent Therapy: Cognitive Behavioral Procedures,* 2d ed. New York: Guilford Press, 2000.

Kimura, Doreen. *Sex and Cognition.* Cambridge, MA: MIT Press, 1999.

Kowalski, Robin M., and Mark R. Leary. *The Social Psychology of Emotional and Behavioral Problems: Interfaces of Social and Clinical Psychology.* Washington, DC: American Psychological Association, 2000.

March, John S., editor. *Anxiety Disorders in Children and Adolescents.* New York: Guilford Press, 1995.

Micucci, Joseph A. *The Adolescent in Family Therapy: Breaking the Cycle of Conflict and Control.* New York: Guilford Press, 2000.

Mikesell, Richard H., Don-David Lusterman, and Susan H. McDaniel, eds. *Integrating Family Therapy: Handbook of Family Psychology and Systems Theory.* Washington, D.C.: American Psychological Association, 1995.

Nicholi, Armand M., Jr., ed. *The Harvard Guide to Psychiatry,* 3d ed. Cambridge, MA: The Belknap Press of Harvard University Press, 1999.

O'Connor, Kevin John, and Sue Ammen. *Play Therapy: Treatment Planning and Interventions.* San Diego: Academic Press, 1997.

Pearce, John W., and Terry D. Pezzot-Pearce. *Psychotherapy of Abused and Neglected Children.* New York: Guilford Press, 1997.

Phillips, Maggie, and Claire Frederick: *Healing the Divided Self: Clinical and Ericksonian Hypnotherapy for Post-Traumatic and Dissociative Conditions.* New York: Norton, 1995.

Plutchik, Robert. *Emotions in the Practice of Psychotherapy: Clinical Implications of Affect Theories.* Washington, DC: American Psychological Association, 2000.

Resnick, Robert J., and Ronald H. Rozensky. *Health Psychology Through the Life Span: Practice and Research Opportunities.* Washington, DC: American Psychological Association, 1996.

Roberts, Michael C., *Handbook of Pediatric Psychology,* 2d ed. New York: Guilford Press, 1998.

Rossi, Ernest Lawrence. *The Psychobiology of Mind-Body Healing: New Concepts of Therapeutic Hypnosis,* rev. ed. New York: W. W. Norton, 1993.

Sattler, Jerome M. *Assessment of Children,* 3d ed. San Diego: Jerome M. Sattler, 1992.

Savin-Williams, Ritch C. *Mom, Dad. I'm Gay. How Families Negotiate Coming Out.* Washington, DC: American Psychological Association, 2001.

Sousa, David A. *How the Brain Learns,* 2d ed. Thousand Oaks, CA: Corwin Press, 2001.

Sternberg, Esther M. *The Balance Within: The Science Connecting Health and Emotions.* New York: W. H. Freeman, 2000.

Stroebe, Margaret S., Robert O. Hansson, Wolfgang Stroebe, and Henk Schut, eds. *Handbook of Bereavement Research: Consequences, Coping, and Care.* Washington, DC: American Psychological Association, 2001.

Tangney, June Price, and Kurt W. Fischer, eds. *Self-Conscious Emotions: The Psychology of Shame, Guilt, Embarrassment, and Pride.* New York: Guilford Press, 1995.

Thompson, J. Kevin, and Linda Smolak, eds. *Body Image, Eating Disorders, and Obesity in Youth: Assessment, Prevention, and Treatment.* Washington, DC: American Psychological Association, 2001.

Walker, Lenore, with Marge Lurie. *The Abused Woman: A Survivor Therapy Approach* (video). New York: Newbridge Professional Programs, 1994.

Whittaker, Leighton C., and Jeffrey W. Pollard, eds. *Campus Violence: Kinds, Causes, and Cures.* Binghamton, NY: The Haworth Press, 1993.

Wilkes, T. C. R., Gayle Belsher, A. John Rush, Ellen Frank, and associates. *Cognitive Therapy for Depressed Adolescents.* New York: Guilford Press, 1994.

Yeates, Keith Owen, M. Douglas Ris, and H. Gerry Taylor, eds. *Pediatric Neuropsychology: Research, Theory, and Practice.* New York: Guilford Press, 1999.

Zucker, Kenneth J., and Susan J. Bradley. *Gender Identity Disorder and Psychosexual Problems in Children and Adolescents.* New York: Guilford Press, 1995.

Index

Volumes **1**, **2**, and **3** refer to the *Human Diseases and Conditions* base set; **Supp. 1** refers to the first supplement to the base set, *Behavioral Health*.

Page numbers referring to illustrations are in *italic* type.
Volume numbers are shown in **bold.**

Index

. . . .